Review and Application of Clinical Pharmacology

SUSAN E. RALSTON, R.N., B.S.N., M.Ed.

Assistant Professor, Department of Nursing

Georgia State University

MARION F. HALE, R.N., B.S., M.N.

Assistant Professor, Department of Nursing

Georgia State University

J. B. LIPPINCOTT COMPANY

PHILADELPHIA

NEW YORK   SAN JOSE   TORONTO

Dedicated with Love to Our Parents:

Stanley and Ethel Stanwyck

and

Grafton and Lillian Hale

Distributed in Great Britain by
Blackwell Scientific Publications
London · Oxford · Edinburgh

ISBN 0-397-54176-7

Library of Congress Catalog Card Number 75-42122

2 3 4 5 6 7 8 9

Manufactured in the United States of America

Library of Congress Cataloging in Publication Data

Ralston, Susan E
    Review and application of clinical pharmacology.

    Includes bibliographies and index.
    1. Pharmacology. 2. Chemotherapy. I. Hale, Marion F., joint author. II. Title. [DNLM:
1. Pharmacology—Nursing texts. 2. Drug therapy—Nursing texts. 3. Nursing care. QV4 R164r]
RM300.R34   615'.1   75-42122
ISBN 0-397-54176-7

Another pharmacology book! True. But *this* pharmacology book has been written because others fail to meet some specific student needs. *Review and Application of Clinical Pharmacology* is not a textbook, but rather a supplementary book. It can be used to supplement a pharmacology textbook or a lecture course in pharmacology; as an aid to review before state board examinations; for review before returning to clinical nursing, if you have not been practicing for a while; or for an overview of pharmacology if you have not been involved with drug therapy or have not been involved with a broad spectrum of pharmacological preparations. If the book is used for review, we suggest that you keep a medical dictionary and a medical-surgical textbook close at hand. Do not overlook any term or condition you do not fully understand.

This book is intended especially for use by students pursuing a nursing curriculum that integrates pharmacology throughout all the nursing courses. This approach allows students to learn about drugs in a more practical manner; however, many students in such curricula have told us that they are not sure how much they have actually learned. Because of this, we have divided each chapter into a review section and an application section. The various objective questions that make up the latter portion of every chapter are designed to help the student achieve a feeling of personal adequacy in knowledge of pharmacology. After answering the questions, the student can immediately check the answers at the back of the book. Answering these questions immediately after reading the review section or a pharmacology textbook will provide for active learning and immediate reinforcement.

In addition to objective questions, many chapters offer some discussion questions. These depict patient situations in which the nurse is required to answer or act upon common statements made by patients. Answers are not included with these situations, since the approach to a particular patient may depend on

more information than what is given as well as on the nurse's personality and general approach to patients. These questions may be used for discussion by a group of students, for classroom discussion, or for individual reflection about how you would react in a particular situation.

The review portion of the chapters does not by any means include all that a nurse must know about pharmacology to be a safe practitioner. Each review is just what it is claimed to be—a review. The authors feel that, insofar as is possible, the action, use, side effects, and cautions of classes of drugs are explained in a succinct, logical, and interrelated manner. Brief explanations of certain disease processes have been included wherever necessary to clarify the action of a class of drugs. Physiology and pathophysiology have been included in some areas also. As a rule, however, the reader should consult related textbooks for information about a disease or required nursing care that is not related to pharmacology. The references included at the end of each chapter direct the reader to current information available on each topic.

The only major areas of pharmacology that are not specifically covered in this book are vaccines and nutritional supplements. These two areas are so well covered in medical-surgical textbooks, pediatric textbooks, and nutrition textbooks that including them here would seem redundant.

The pages in this book are all perforated for easy removal. This will enable the student to tear out a certain section or drug chart easily and carry it as a ready reference.

The drug charts include only examples of the drugs discussed in the chapter; they list the generic and trade names, how each drug is supplied, how it is administered, the usual dose, and additional information the nurse should know when administering the drug. Knowing how the drug is supplied can enable the student to compose hypothetical dosage calculation problems and be ready to calculate a dose for an assigned patient, if necessary. Some calculation problems have been included in the application sections to help in this area.

Composing this book has been challenging, inter-esting, and enjoyable. We sincerely hope that the reader will share some of this enjoyment—and perhaps even a smile when application questions bring a former patient or situation to mind.

Acknowledgments

If we had space to acknowledge only three people in this book, they would be John Ralston, Katherine Pope, and Lars Egede-Nissen. John and Katherine deserve special thanks for their continuous support, encouragement, and good humor, and also for helping with all those daily tasks we left undone in order to complete the book. Lars is our editor, who patiently answered our endless questions and cheerfully gave us encouragement while trying to make authors out of us.

Our efforts would never have become a manuscript without our typists, Sally Hall and Linda Barker. They are both nurses, so they provided us with some professional critique as well. Linda receives our special thanks for her expertise in the operating room and in the care of burns. We also wish to thank Pam Schultheiss for her efforts in the tedious job of typing the drug charts.

We acknowledge Warren Shultz, Ph.D., who reviewed the entire manuscript and made valuable suggestions.

We fully acknowledge our indebtedness to Morton J. Rodman, Ph.D., and Dorothy W. Smith, Ed.D., for their permission to base this book on their textbook *Clinical Pharmacology in Nursing*. They have allowed us to structure our work in alignment with theirs, to draw upon their phraseology where appropriate, and to condense important concepts.

Other people we wish to acknowledge include Dave Miller, managing editor of Lippincott's nursing department, who provided us with additional guidance and confidence. Evangaline Lane and John Payne initiated the situation which made this book possible. We also wish to thank Susan Caldwell for her help in the chapters dealing with coronary care. Members of all our families—the Ralstons, Hales, Stanwycks, Popes, Thompsons, and Halls—gave us all the encouragement and enthusiasm we needed, and probably more than we deserved.

Last, but certainly not least, we wish to thank those who worked on the production of the book. Under the guidance of Rick Chafian, the designer and production coordinator, and through the efforts of Pat Foley, the copy editor, our typed manuscript became a published book.

A Note of Caution

The authors and editors of this book have expended considerable time and effort to insure that the facts and opinions offered in the text and tables of this book are in accordance with official standards and with the consensus of foremost authorities at the time of publication.

However, drug therapy is a very dynamic branch of medicine, marked by the continual marketing of new drugs and the discontinuation and withdrawal (often without notice) of older drug products. In addition, the Food and Drug Administration constantly orders changes in the labeling of even well-established drug products, on the basis of ongoing studies of their safety and efficacy. For this reason, no claims are made that statements made here concerning the current status of these drugs will continue to reflect the stated view or that the data presented in tabular form are, or will remain, complete and correct in every detail.

The most important aspect of this problem lies in the area of dosage recommendations. Every effort has been made to check that statements made in the tables are, within the limits of space, precisely correct. However, dosage schedules are frequently ordered changed in accordance with accumulating clinical experiences.

For this reason, we urge that *before administering any drug, you check the manufacturer's latest dosage recommendations* as presented in the package insert which accompanies each unit of every drug product.

Contents

Preface   iii

SECTION ONE: GENERAL PRINCIPLES
OF PHARMACOLOGY

1. **Overview of Pharmacology**   2

   Evaluation of Drugs   2
   The Nurse's Role in Drug Evaluations   2
   Government Regulations and Standards
   for Drugs   2
   References   3
   Application Questions   3

2. **Administration and Metabolism of Drugs**   5

   Administration of Drugs   5
   Drug Metabolism   6
   Nurse's Responsibility for Administration
   of Drugs   6
   References   12
   Application Questions   12

3. **Toxic Effects of Drugs and Chemicals**   16

   Drug Idiosyncracy and Allergy   16
   References   17
   Application Questions   17

4. **Drug Abuse, Dependence, and Addiction**   20

   Terminology   20
   Types of Drug Abuse   20
   References   23
   Application Questions   23

5. **Alcohol**   25

   The Action of Alcohol on the Central Nervous
   System   25
   Metabolism of Alcohol   25
   Medical Management of the Intoxicated
   Patient   25

Management of the Chronic Alcoholic
Patient   26
Ingestion of Methyl Alcohol   27
Therapeutic Effects of Ethyl Alcohol   27
References   28
Application Questions   28

SECTION TWO: DRUGS THAT AFFECT
MENTAL AND EMOTIONAL FUNCTION
AND BEHAVIOR

6. **Sedative-Hypnotics and Other
   Antianxiety Drugs**   31

   Barbiturates and Nonbarbiturate Sedative-
   Hypnotics   31
   The Minor Tranquilizers   32
   Side Effects and Cautions of the Sedative-
   Hypnotic and Antianxiety Agents   32
   References   32
   Application Questions   32

7. **Drugs Used in the Management of
   Mental Illness**   36

   The Major Tranquilizers   36
   The Antidepressant Drugs   38
   Use of Lithium Salts   39
   References   39
   Application Questions   41

8. **Psychomotor and Other Central
   Stimulants**   43

   Psychomotor Stimulants   43
   Analeptics   44
   Convulsant Drugs   46
   References   46
   Application Questions   46

viii   CONTENTS

SECTION THREE: DRUGS USED IN
NEUROLOGICAL AND MUSCULOSKELETAL
DISORDERS

9. **Neurospasmolytic Agents**   49

    Musculoskeletal Disorders   49
    Neurological Disorders   49
    Adverse Effects   50
    References   51
    Application Questions   51

10. **Antiparkinsonism Drugs**   52

    Treatment with Levodopa   52
    Other Types of Treatment   52
    References   54
    Application Questions   54

11. **Anticonvulsants**   56

    Types of Seizures   56
    Status Epilepticus   57
    The Nurse's Responsibility   57
    References   59
    Application Questions   59

SECTION FOUR: DRUGS USED FOR THE
RELIEF AND PREVENTION OF PAIN

12. **Analgesics**   62

    Drugs that Relieve Moderate to Severe Pain
    (Potent Analgesics)   62
    Drugs that Relieve Mild to Moderate Pain   65
    Management of Chronic Pain   66
    Treatment of Headache   66
    References   68
    Application Questions   68

13. **Anesthetics**   72

    General Anesthesia   72
    Local Anesthetics   73
    Care of Patients After Anesthesia   75
    References   78
    Application Questions   78

SECTION FIVE: DRUGS ACTING ON
AUTONOMIC NEUROEFFECTORS

14. **The Autonomic Nervous System**   82

    Basic Physiology of the ANS   82

    Overview of the Autonomic Nervous
    System   82
    Physiology of the Sympathetic System   83
    Physiology of the Parasympathetic System   84
    Classification of Pharmacologic Action   84
    Understanding the Terminology   84
    Application Questions   85

15. **Parasympathomimetic and
Sympatholytic Drugs**   89

    Side Effects of Parasympathomimetic and
    Sympatholytic Drugs   89
    Sympatholytic Drugs (Adrenergic Blocking
    Agents)   90
    Parasympathomimetic (Cholinergic) Drugs   90
    References   93
    Application Questions   93

16. **Sympathomimetic and
Parasympatholytic Drugs**   95

    Comparison of the Sympathomimetic and
    Parasympatholytic drugs   95
    Sympathomimetic (Adrenergic) Drugs   97
    Parasympatholytic (Anticholinergic) Drugs   97
    References   99
    Application Questions   99

SECTION SIX: DRUGS ACTING ON THE HEART
AND CIRCULATION

17. **Digitalis**   103

    Action and Use of Digitalis   103
    Side Effects of Digitalis   103
    Administration of Digitalis   104
    Digitalis Preparations   104
    References   104
    Application Questions   104

18. **Antiarrhythmic Drugs**   107

    Antiarrhythmic Therapy   107
    Antiarrhythmic Drugs   107
    Nursing Responsibilities with Antiarrhythmic
    Drugs   109
    References   109
    Application Questions   109

19. **Diuretics**   111

    Nursing Responsibilities   111
    Classification of Diuretics   111

References   114
Application Questions   114

20. **Antihypertensive Agents**   116

Primary and Secondary Hypertension   116
Diuretics   116
Sympatholytic Agents   116
Miscellaneous Antihypertensive Agents   118
References   119
Application Questions   119

21. **Vasodilators**   121

Drugs Used for Coronary Ischemia   121
Drugs Used to Treat Peripheral Vascular
Disease   122
Cerebral Vasodilating Drugs   124
References   124
Application Questions   124

22. **Antilipemic Drugs**   126

Treatment of Hyperlipoproteinemia   126
References   128
Application Questions   128

23. **Drugs That Affect Blood Coagulation**   129

Need for Anticoagulants   129
Nursing Responsibilities When a Patient is
on Anticoagulant Therapy   131
Thrombolytic Agents   131
Hemostatic Agents   131
References   133
Application Questions   133

24. **Acute Myocardial Infarction**   136

Treatment of Complications   136
General Drug Therapy   137
References   137
Application Questions   137

25. **Antianemic Drugs**   139

Types of Anemia   139
References   141
Application Questions   141

SECTION SEVEN: DRUGS FOR TREATING
ENDOCRINE DISORDERS

26. **Introduction to Endocrine Disorders and
Pituitary Hormones**   144

Posterior Pituitary   144
Anterior Pituitary   144
Parathyroid   146
References   146
Application Questions   146

27. **Hormones Influencing or Secreted by the
Gonads**   148

Pituitary and Gonad Feedback
Mechanisms   148
Male Sex Hormones   148
Female Sex Hormones   150
References   154
Application Questions   154

28. **Drug Treatment of Thyroid Disorders**   157

Hypothyroidism   157
Hyperthyroidism   158
References   160
Application Questions   160

29. **Diabetes Mellitus**   162

Insulin   162
Oral Hypoglycemics   163
Diabetic Extremes   164
References   165
Application Questions   165

SECTION EIGHT: DRUGS USED FOR
INFLAMMATION, ALLERGY,
AND RELATED DISORDERS

30. **Adrenocorticosteroid Drugs and
Corticotropin (ACTH)**   169

Adrenal Insufficiency   169
Inflammation   170
Types of Adrenocorticosteroid Drugs   170
Dosage Schedules   170
Adverse Effects of Adrenocorticosteroid
Drugs   171
Adrenocorticotropic Hormone (ACTH)   172
References   173
Application Questions   173

31. **Rheumatoid Disorders**   175

Treatment of Rheumatic Disorders   175
Treatment of Gout   176
References   178
Application Questions   178

32. **Antihistamine Drugs**   180

   Treatment of Allergy   180
   Use of Antihistamine Drugs   181
   Types of Antihistamines   181
   Side Effects and Cautions When Using
   Antihistamines   182
   References   183
   Application Questions   183

33. **Topical Drugs Used in Dermatology**   186

   Drugs Used to Decrease Inflammation, Irritation,
   and Itching   186
   Drugs Used for Their Irritating Effects   187
   Drugs Used for Thermal, Solar, and
   Pigmentation Conditions   188
   Drugs Used in the Prevention and Treatment
   of Infection   189
   References   191
   Application Questions   191

34. **Bronchodilators, Expectorants, and
   Mucolytic Agents**   193

   Bronchial Asthma   193
   References   194
   Application Questions   195

SECTION NINE: DRUGS USED
FOR TREATING INFECTIONS

35. **Antibiotics**   197

   Action and Spectrum of Antibiotics   197
   The Penicillins   198
   Alternatives to Penicillin   199
   The Tetracyclines   199
   Other Antibiotics   200
   References   202
   Application Questions   202

36. **Synthetic Anti-infectives**   205

   The Sulfonamides   205
   Other Drugs for Treating Urinary Tract
   Infections   206
   Treatment of Tuberculosis   206
   Drugs Used in the Treatment of Leprosy   207

   Antiviral Chemotherapy   207
   Antimalarial Drugs   208
   Antiamebic Drugs   208
   Anthelmintics   209
   References   209
   Application Questions   211

SECTION TEN: MISCELLANEOUS
THERAPEUTIC AND DIAGNOSTIC
AGENTS

37. **Drugs Affecting Gastrointestinal Function** 215

   The Use of Cathartics or Laxatives   215
   Drugs Used for the Relief of Diarrhea   217
   Antiemetic Drugs   217
   Drugs Used for Controlling Indigestion   218
   References   219
   Application Questions   221

38. **Drugs Used in Labor and Delivery**   223

   Oxytocic Drugs   223
   Prostaglandins   225
   Uterine Relaxants   225
   References   226
   Application Questions   226

39. **Drugs Used in Cancer Chemotherapy**   228

   Uses and Trends of Cancer Chemotherapy   228
   Anticancer Drugs Available Today   228
   Toxicity   229
   Classification of Anticancer Drugs   229
   References   232
   Application Questions   232

40. **Drugs Used in Diagnosis**   234

   Radiographic Diagnosis   234
   Diagnostic Tests of Body Function   234
   References   236
   Application Questions   236

   Answers   239

   Index   249

General Principles
of Pharmacology

SECTION ONE

Overview of Pharmacology

Pharmacology is the study of drugs. It includes study of the preparation, use, and action of every chemical having any effect on biological functioning. Although pharmacology did not really become a science until the nineteenth century, there is evidence that medicinal preparations were used even in primitive times.

EVALUATION OF DRUGS

At one time, drugs were used in accordance with folklore or the advice of a traveling medicine man. Today, extensive research and evaluation must be done before a new drug can be marketed. New drugs are subjected first to animal testing, and then to controlled clinical testing. Animal testing is done to establish a margin of safety, to study the drug's metabolism, and to study both the desired effects and the side effects. Clinical studies of a drug are done in three phases. In phase I, a qualified researcher uses the drug with only one or very few volunteers. In phase II, several physicians, specialists in the condition for which the drug is designed, administer the drug to selected patients and gather data about its efficacy and safety. In phase III, many practicing physicians use the drug on large numbers of patients and continue to submit data. Only after all three phases have been completed can the drug be considered for marketing in the United States.

THE NURSE'S ROLE IN DRUG EVALUATIONS

If a nurse is involved in the clinical study of a drug, she must familiarize herself with any available information about the drug. This is her legal responsibility. A clinical investigator's brochure or drug package insert may be obtained from the physician using the drug. The physician assisting with the clinical trials may be able to refer the nurse to journal articles or other sources of information concerning the new drug. Careful charting is of utmost importance in gathering data concerning effectiveness and side effects of the new drug. A patient taking an experimental drug may be part of a double-blind study. In this situation, some patients receive the experimental drug, and others receive *placebos,* or "dummy" medications. Placebos are made to look just like the investigational drugs but are composed of harmless substances such as sugar. In a double-blind study, no one involved with the administration of the drug knows which patients are actually receiving the drug.

GOVERNMENT REGULATIONS AND STANDARDS FOR DRUGS

Legislation

Since the early years of the twentieth century, the federal government has enacted several pieces of legislation to regulate the quality of drugs and to protect the public from dangerous and harmful substances.

The earliest federal drug legislation was the *Pure Food and Drug Act of 1906.* This law was passed to eliminate false and misleading claims on the labels of medicines. The *Federal Food, Drug, and Cosmetic Act of 1938* made it mandatory that all new drugs be tested in animals before being marketed for human use. This law did *not,* however, provide for controlled clinical trials in humans prior to widespread marketing. The *Drug Amendments of 1962* (the *Kefauver-Harris Act*) established procedures for testing new drugs in humans before marketing.

Legislation has also been enacted to decrease drug abuse. Such legislation began with the *Harrison Narcotic Act of 1914.* The *Durham-Humphrey Amendment of 1951* was passed to control marijuana traffic and to insure that habit-forming hypnotics could be obtained only on prescription. The *Comprehensive Drug Abuse Prevention and Control Act of 1970* superseded several older laws categorizing drugs according to their potential for abuse and their medicinal usefulness. Schedule I, for example, contains drugs such as heroin, marijuana, and LSD. Drugs in this category are under the strictest control because of their high potential for abuse and their very limited medical usefulness.

Government Agencies

The Food and Drug Administration (FDA) was established as an agency of the Department of Health, Education, and Welfare after the passage of the *Kefauver-Harris Act*. This administration regulates the marketing and testing of new chemicals for human use. Narcotics and other dangerous drugs are controlled in the United States by the Drug Enforcement Agency (DEA) of the Department of Justice. The Division of Biological Standards of the National Institutes of Health regulates the requirements for immunological agents. The advertising of nonprescription drugs is controlled by the Federal Trade Commission.

Official Drug Standards

There are two compendia recognized by the government as the official standards of quality and purity for drugs. They are the *United States Pharmacopoeia* (*U.S.P.*), and the *National Formulary* (*N.F.*). These compendia include information of importance to pharmacists and researchers. Of importance to the nurse, they contain the official names of drugs and information about dosage and administration. Every drug has only one official, nonproprietary, or generic name. When a pharmaceutical company markets a drug, however, the company can assign it a proprietary or trade name. The same drug, then, may have several trade names if it is manufactured by several different companies.

REFERENCES

del Baeno, Dorothy J. "Verifying the Nurse's Knowledge of Pharmacology." *Nursing Outlook* 20:462, July 1972.

Hayes, Marsden H. "Pharmacists Need Nurses—Nurses Need Pharmacists—Patients Need Both." *American Journal of Nursing* 72:723, April 1972.

Levine, Myra E. "Breaking Through the Medications Mystique." *American Journal of Nursing* 70:799, April 1970.

APPLICATION QUESTIONS

I. *True-False*

For each statement below, write **a** if the statement is true or **b** if it is false.

_____ 1. When administering an investigational drug in a double-blind study, the nurse does not have a legal responsibility to be knowledgeable of the drug's proposed action.

_____ 2. A drug may have many nonproprietary names but only one proprietary name.

II. *Multiple Choice*

For each of the following questions, indicate the letter providing the *best* answer.

_____ 1. Who assigns the proprietary name of a drug? (a) the pharmaceutical company which manufactures it (b) the Food and Drug Administration (c) the United States Adopted Name Council (d) United States Pharmacopoeia

_____ 2. Which of the following are the two *official* compendia of standards for quality and purity of drugs and authoritative information on dosage and administration? (a) *Physicians' Desk Reference* and *The United States Dispensatory and Physicians' Pharmacology* (b) *United States Pharmacopoeia* and *The American Hospital Formulary Service* (c) *National Formulary* and *The United States Dispensatory and Physicians' Pharmacology* (d) *United States Pharmacopoeia* and *National Formulary* (e) *Physicians' Desk Reference* and *The American Hospital Formulary Service*

_____ 3. The nurse is concerned mainly with which of the following subdivisions of pharmacology? (a) pharmacognosy (b) pharmacodynamics (c) pharmacotherapeutics

_____ 4. Pharmacology became a science early in what century? (a) seventeenth (b) eighteenth (c) nineteenth (d) twentieth

_____ 5. Which of the following activities is *not* included in the preclinical testing of a new drug? (a) animal testing (b) toxicity testing for margin of safety (c) study of drug metabolism in the body (d) study by one clinical investigator with one patient

III. *Matching A*

Match each agency to its controlling department.

_____ 1. Food and Drug Administration
_____ 2. Drug Enforcement Agency
_____ 3. Division of Biological Standards

(a) Department of Justice
(b) Department of Health, Education, and Welfare
(c) National Institutes of Health
(d) Department of the Treasury

IV. *Matching B*

Match each law with its resulting control.

_____ 1. *Durham-Humphrey Amendment of 1951*

_____ 2. *Comprehensive Drug Abuse Prevention and Control Act of 1970*

_____ 3. *Drug Amendments of 1962 (Kefauver-Harris Act)*

_____ 4. *Federal Food, Drug, and Cosmetic Act of 1938*

_____ 5. *Pure Food and Drug Act of 1906*

(a) Eliminates false or misleading claims in labeling

(b) Requires that habit-forming hypnotics may be obtained only on prescription

(c) Requires toxicity testing in animals before drugs are marketed for humans

(d) Requires clinical testing of new drugs in humans before marketing

(e) Categorizes drugs in accordance with their potential for abuse and their medical usefulness

V. *Matching C*

Match each agency with its appointed activity for drug control.

_____ 1. *Federal Trade Commission*

_____ 2. *Division of Biological Standards*

_____ 3. *Food and Drug Administration*

_____ 4. *Drug Enforcement Agency*

(a) Approves new drugs for marketing

(b) Enforces regulatory and control measures for habit-forming drugs

(c) Regulates advertising of nonprescription drugs

(d) Regulates requirements for vaccines, antitoxins, and other immunological agents

Answers to the Application Questions are at the back of this book.

Administration and Metabolism of Drugs

The administration and metabolism of drugs refers to how and where drugs enter the body and what happens to them in the body.

ADMINISTRATION OF DRUGS

There are many routes by which drugs can be administered. The principal routes are: oral; intramuscular (injected into the muscle); subcutaneous (injected under the skin); buccal (dissolved in the cheek); sublingual (dissolved under the tongue); intrathecal (injected into spinal canal); intra-articular (injected into a joint); inhalation; rectal; urethral; vaginal; and topical. The techniques of administering drugs are discussed thoroughly in basic nursing textbooks and in self-instructional materials.

Oral Medications

The simplest, safest, and least expensive way to administer a drug is by mouth. Medications to be given by mouth can be in the form of powders, tablets, capsules, or liquids. The nurse may occasionally crush, dissolve, or mix oral medications with food or juices to make them more palatable or easier for a patient to swallow. It is important, however, that prolonged action or sustained release tablets and capsules should never be tampered with in any manner. These preparations contain enough of a drug to last over a long period of time and are covered with a variety of coatings to delay absorption as needed. Crushing the drug or mixing it with food could destroy the coatings and cause all of the drug to be absorbed at the same time. This could lead to an overdose and toxic reaction.

Topical Medications

Medications applied topically to the skin do not usually cause systemic effects, as they are absorbed very slowly, if at all. Medications applied to mucous membranes, such as those administered by the buccal, sublingual, or rectal routes, may be given for systemic effects. Mucous membranes are so vascular that absorption occurs quickly. For absorption to occur, the medication must remain in contact with the mucous membrane. After receiving rectal medication, then, the patient should remain lying in bed to avoid expelling the medication. Patients receiving buccal or sublingual medications should be instructed not to swallow until the medication has dissolved.

Parenteral Medications

Literally, the word *parenteral* refers to anything outside the digestive tract. Generally, however, the term is used for subcutaneous, intramuscular, intravenous, and other injectable routes of drug administration. Parenteral medications are usually absorbed into the blood faster than oral drugs, and their rate of absorption can be better controlled. However, parenteral medications may be painful; they may predispose the patient to infection because they involve a break in the skin; and they often require the expense and service of a health worker to administer the drug.

The rate at which a parenteral medication is absorbed depends on the blood supply of the depository site. Intravenous medications are the most rapidly absorbed, as they are deposited directly into the blood. Since muscle has more blood supply than subcutaneous tissue, intramuscular medications are absorbed more rapidly, as a rule, than subcutaneous medications. The nurse must be aware of factors that may affect the circulation and thereby alter the absorption of an injected drug. When a patient is in shock, tissue perfusion is poor and absorption is not reliable. Medications needed for shock are usually given intravenously for this reason. If a patient has a paralyzed extremity, the circulation to that part will be more sluggish than to nonparalyzed areas. It is best to avoid injections into paralyzed or denervated muscle areas.

The subcutaneous tissue has more pain receptors than the muscle tissue, and subcutaneous injections may be quite painful if more than 2 cc. of fluid are deposited at the same site.

DRUG METABOLISM

The fate of a drug which enters the body may be discussed in terms of its absorption, distribution, biotransformation, and excretion.

Absorption

This term describes the process by which a drug enters the systemic circulation. Most orally administered medications are absorbed from the small intestine. Some medications come in enteric coated tablets which prevent dissolution until they reach the lower gastrointestinal tract thereby preventing irritation of the stomach and small intestine. Most oral drugs are absorbed more rapidly when there is no food in the stomach. Absorption is more reliable between meals, because some foods may bind with drug molecules and prevent their absorption. Other drugs may be destroyed by the gastric juices present during digestion. Some drugs are very irritating to the gastrointestinal mucosa, though, and must be taken with food in order to be tolerated.

Distribution

This term refers to transportation of drugs in the body. After a drug is absorbed, it must be transported to the fluid surrounding the reactive tissues and deposited in a concentration high enough to stimulate or depress the affected cells. Drug molecules usually become attached to plasma proteins for transportation in the blood stream. However, the drug must be free of the protein to pass through the capillary membrane into the tissue cells. Thus, at any given time, some drug molecules are free and some are attached to protein. A toxic reaction may occur when two drugs that compete for the same protein-binding sites are administered simultaneously. When this occurs, one drug displaces the other one, causing unusually high amounts of free drug molecules and a faster rate of diffusion into the tissues.

Biotransformation and Excretion

The process of converting a drug into a harmless substance for excretion is called biotransformation. Enzymes capable of detoxifying drugs are found in all body tissues; however, the liver is the most important organ in the detoxification of drugs. After a drug is detoxified, its metabolites are excreted from the body. The kidney is the major organ of excretion, but drugs may be excreted by the lungs or through the salivary, sweat, or mammary glands. Although most drugs undergo the process of biotransformation and then excretion, some anesthetics and other drugs may be excreted unchanged from the body.

Differences in Individual Response

Patients may react very differently to the same dose of the same drug. In evaluating dosage, it is important to consider the patient's body weight, age, sex, physiological state, pathological state, genetic factors, immunological factors, and psychological and emotional factors. Any of these may affect the action of a drug in the body, as may environmental factors such as climate.

Drug Interactions

Two drugs given at the same time may interact; such an interaction may affect the action of one or both of the drugs. Drug interactions may occur during absorption, distribution, biotransformation, or excretion. As a result of interaction, one drug may prolong or potentiate the action of the other to such a degree that a toxic reaction may occur with an otherwise normal dose. In some cases, antagonism may occur, in which two drugs interact and the effect of one or both of the drugs is greatly reduced. The tables in this chapter discuss some common drug interactions.

NURSE'S RESPONSIBILITY FOR ADMINISTRATION OF DRUGS

The actual procedure of administering a drug to a patient is but a very small part of the nurse's responsibility in drug therapy. Nurses need to know the intended results of the therapy and to observe for these results. They should know the action of the drug and relate this to possible side effects and contraindications. Nurses should familiarize themselves with drug interactions (see table 2–2). The nurse needs to be able to interpret standard abbreviations used for writing drug orders. Table 2–1 lists some of the common abbreviations. Calculating dosage is a responsibility of the nurse, who should be familiar with dose equivalents and remember *always* to have someone else check the dosage calculations. The nurse should never hesitate to question a medication order if the handwriting is not legible; if the dosage is not within the appropriate range for the individual patient; if there is reason to believe the drug is contraindicated for this patient; or if the patient is taking another drug that may interact with the drug just ordered.

When a medication is given, its action may be enhanced if the patient is told about the purpose of the drug. When giving a sedative, for example, say to the patient, "This drug will help you get some sleep." If a patient asks specifically for the name of the medication he is receiving, there is not usually a valid reason for withholding the information.

Table 2–1. Abbreviations.

aa	each	q.h.	every hour
a.c.	before meals	q.i.d.	four times a day
b.i.d.	twice a day	q.o.d.	every other day
c̄	with	q.4h.	every four hours
cc.	cubic centimeter	Rx	take
cap., caps.	capsule	s̄	without
dr., ℥	dram	Sc	subcutaneously
elix.	elixir	ss.	half
ext.	extract	stat.	immediately
Gm., gm.	gram	tab.	tablet
gr.	grain	T., Tbsp.	tablespoon
gtt.	drop	t., tsp.	teaspoon
h.	hour	t.i.d.	three times a day
h.s.	at bedtime	tr., tinct.	tincture
hypo, h	hypodermically	U.	unit
I.M.	intramuscularly		
I.V.	intravenously		
L.	liter		
m., min.	minim		
mEq.	milliequivalent		
mg., mgm.	milligram		
ml.	milliliter		
mm.	millimeter		
μg.	microgram		
N.P.O.	nothing by mouth		
O.D.	right eye		
oint.	ointment		
O.S.	left eye		
O.U.	each eye		
oz., ℥	ounce		
per.	by		
P.O.	by mouth		
p.r.n.	as needed		
pt.	pint		
q	every		
q.d.	every day		

Table 2–2. Drug interactions

---

1. *acetazolamide (Diamox)*
    amphetamine
        action: Alakline urine increases the reabsorption of amphetamines. Acetazolamide increases
            the alkalinity of urine.
        nursing implication: Recognize that patients receiving both drugs will have a prolonged effect
            of the amphetamines.

    methenamine (Urotropin) and related compounds
        action: The methenamine compound's pharmacological action depends on urine with a pH of 5.5 or less.
            Acetazolamide (Diamox) increases the alkalinity of urine.
        nursing implication: Recognize that these drugs should not be used in concurrent therapy as they
            are antagonistic in action.

---

2. *alcohol, ethyl (ethanol)*

    antidiabetic drugs
        action: Alcohol ingestion in patients receiving antidiabetic drugs may produce symptoms such as vomiting,
            headache and flushing. Interference with the effect of the drugs may also be a possibility.
        nursing implication: Patient teaching including information about possible outcomes if larger or
            even moderate amounts of alcohol are consumed.
    disulfiram (Antabuse)
        action: Nausea, vomiting, sweating and more severe systemic reactions occur when even small amount of
            alcohol is ingested during treatment with disulfiram.
        nursing implication: Teach the consequences of combining these substances. Non-prescription
            preparations often include alcohol and patients must be instructed to read labels.

---

3. *allopurinol (Zyloprim)*

    azathioprine (Imuran)
        action: These drugs used concurrently inhibit the chemical action necessary for the inactivation
            of azathioprine. Therefore they potentiate the toxic effect on body tissues.
        nursing implication: Call attention to this interaction calling for azathioprine (Imuran) dosage adjustment.
    mercaptopurine (6-mp)
        action and nursing implications same as above.

---

4. *cephalosporins* i.e. cephaloridine (Loridine)
    furosemide (Lasix)
        action: Furosemide (Lasix) when combined with the cephalosporins appears to increase
            the kidney tissue toxicity effect of the cephalosporins.
        nursing implication: Renal function test results should be observed closely.

---

5. *digitalis*

    chlorthalidone (Hygroton), ethacrynic acid (Edecrin), furosemide (Lasix),
    metolazone (Zaroxolyn)
        action: Diuretics such as chlorthalidone (Hygroton) produce potassium and probably magnesium
            deficiencies which create an environment conducive to digitalis intoxication.
        nursing implication: Observe the potassium and magnesium levels. Record and report promptly so
            replacement therapy can be ordered.
    amphotericin B (Fungizone)
    digitalis glycosides
        action: Digitalis toxicity is more likely to occur when potassium levels are lowered. Systemic
            treatment with amphotericin B (Fungizone) may result in hypokalemia.
        nursing implication: Observe laboratory data indicating potassium levels so that hypokalemia
            can be avoided by the proper treatment.

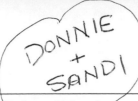

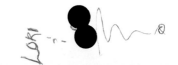

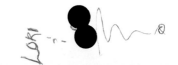

6. *diphenylhydantoin (Dilantin)*

    disulfiram (Antabuse)

        action: The metabolism of diphenylhydantoin is inhibited by the use of disulfiram (Antabuse) concomitantly.

        nursing implication: Observe and record signs of diphenylhydantoin toxicity. Reduction in diphenyldantoin dosage may be indicated.

    isoniazid (INH)

        action: Isoniazid (INH) apparently inhibits the excretion of diphenylhydantoin.

        nursing implication: Patients receiving both isoniazid (INH) and diphenylhydantoin (Dilantin) should be observed closely for diphenylhydantoin intoxication. A reduction of the diphenylhydantoin may be indicated.

7. *disulfiram (Antabuse)*

    alcohol (ethanol)

        action: Consumption of even very small amounts of alcohol can bring about symptoms such as vomiting, headache, and flushing.

        nursing implication: Patient teaching should include information about alcohol content in preparations which might bring about accidental poisoning and consequences of alcohol intake.

8. *echothiophate iodide (Phospholine iodide)*

    succinylcholine (Anectine, Quelicin)

        action: Continued use of echothiophate iodide eyedrops brings about a systemic response which depresses the body's ability to metabolize succinylcholine.

        nursing implication: Know the tests to measure the body's response to succinylcholine. Know the signs and symptoms of toxicity and report.

9. *epinephrine (Adrenalin)*

    tricyclic antidepressants

        action: The mechanism of action is unknown but patients receiving tricyclic antidepressants do have an exaggerated response to epinephrine with resulting systemic responses ranging from hypertension to cardiac dysrhythmias.

        nursing implication: Monitor vital signs. Record and report irregularities immediately.

10. *ethacrynic acid (Edecrin)*

    aminoglycosides

        action: The possibility of an untoward reaction of ototoxicity to the aminoglycosides such as kanamycin, neomycin, gentamicin and streptomycin is enhanced by the administration of ethacrynic acid (Edecrin).

        nursing implication: Observe for toxic reactions, record and report. Recommend that these drugs not be used concurrently.

11. *guanethidine (Ismelin)*

    tricyclic antidepressants

        action: Tricyclic antidepressants interfere with the adrenergic blocking mechanism of guanethidine, thereby rendering it ineffective as an antihypertensive agent.

        nursing implication: Recommend the use of another antihypertensive agent. Monitor vital signs carefully, or possibly get tricyclic changed.

12. *kaolin-pectin (Kaopectate)*

    lincomycin (Lincocin)

        action: Lincomycin absorption is restricted when given in conjunction with kaolin-pectin mixtures.

        nursing implication: Administer the kaolin-pectin (Kaopectate) at least two hours before lincomycin.

13. *levarterenol (norepinephrine)*

    tricyclic antidepressants

        action: The pressor response expected from levarterenol is exaggerated markedly when given to patients receiving tricyclic antidepressants.

        nursing implication: Recommend that the combination of these drugs be avoided. Monitor vital signs.

14. *levodopa (L-dopa)*

    pyridoxine (vitamin B$_6$)

        action: The combination of these drugs enhances the metabolism of the levodopa.

        nursing implication: Patient teaching should include instructions regarding vitamin preparations. Do not give vitamin preparation containing B$_6$ to L-dopa patient.

15. *methotrexate (Amethopterin, MTX)*

    salicylates (aspirin)

        action: The salicylates tend to free the methotrexate and prevent its secretion by the renal tubules, thereby increasing the possibility of toxic reaction.

        nursing implication: Teach patients, including information on excluding salicylates, reading non-prescription labels and self-medication.

    smallpox vaccination

        action: Methotrexate impairs the body's ability to respond normally to the vaccines.

        nursing implication: Plan patient immunological care so that vaccines are not given during the time patients are receiving methotrexate.

16. *monamine oxidase inhibitors*

    amphetamines

        action: The monoamine oxidase inhibitors increase the amount of norepinephrine present in the body. Amphetamines increase catecholamine release. This combination can bring about symptoms ranging from hypertension to death.

        nursing implication: Recommend that this combination not be given.

    antidiabetic drugs

        action: It is possible that MAOI interferes with the body response to hypoglycemia, extending the effect of antidiabetic drugs.

        nursing implication: Observe closely for signs of hypoglycemia. Teach patients signs and symptoms of hypoglycemia and how to carry out ordered regimen.

    ephedrine

        action: MAOI brings about an increase in norepinephrine. When ephedrine is administered concurrently with MAOI, the drugs exert a combined effect bringing about the release of large amounts of norepinephrine and severe systemic reactions.

        nursing implication: Know the body reaction to excessive amounts of norepinephrine. Monitor vital signs carefully.

    metaraminol (Aramine)

        action: The similar action in the body of these drugs, metaraminol and MAOI, that of increasing norepinephrine, brings about an increase or potentiating relationship.

        nursing implication: Recommend that these drugs not be given concurrently.

    phenylephrine (Neo-Synephrine)

        action: The monoamine oxidase inhibitor drugs metabolize phenylephrine (Neo-Synephrine) in the intestine and liver, thereby increasing the pressor effect of the phenylephrine (Neo-Synephrine).

        nursing implication: Recommend parenteral doses of phenylephrine if the drugs are to be combined in therapy. Teach patients to read labels on non-prescription medications to avoid accidental ingestion of phenylephrine (Neo-Synephrine).

    phenylpropanolamine (Propadrine)

        action: These drugs (like ephedrine and MAOI) exert a combined effect bringing about the release of large amounts of norepinephrine resulting in systemic reactions of nausea, headache and hypertension.

        nursing implication: Recommend that this drug combination be avoided.

17. *para-aminobenzoic acid (PABA)*

    sulfonamides

        action: This drug combination produces reaction counteracting the antibacterial effect of sulfonamides.

        nursing implication: Recommend that this combination not be given.

18. *phenylbutazone (Butazolidin)*

    antidiabetic drugs

        action: Phenylbutazone (Butazolidin) appears to prolong the hypoglycemic effect of some antidiabetic drugs particularly the sulfonylureas.

        nursing implication: Observe for signs of hypoglycemia and record and report promptly. Teach signs and symptoms of hypoglycemia to the patient and his family.

19. *polymyxin B*

    skeletal muscle relaxants

        action: The action of drugs used surgically as skeletal muscle relaxants is potentiated by polymyxin B.

        nursing implication: Recommend that this drug combination be avoided. Secure respirator as standby equipment in case of respiratory arrest.

20. *potassium chloride*

    spironolactone (Aldactone)

        action: A primary function of spironolactone (Aldactone) is to preserve potassium. Additional potassium chloride may result in hyperkalemia.

        nursing implication: Observe for signs and symptoms of hyperkalemia. Watch lab studies.

    triamterene (Dyrenium)

        action: As seen in spironolactone, triamterene (Dyrenium) preserves potassium in the body. Additional potassium salts may result in hyperkalemia.

        nursing implication: Recommend that this drug combination be avoided or careful monitoring of potassium levels be carried out.

21. *probenecid (Benemid)*

    aminosalicylic acid (PAS)

        action: It is probable that probenecid interferes with the excretion of PAS.

        nursing implication: Recommend possible reduction of PAS dosage to compensate for the reduced excretion rate.

    salicylates

        action: Probenecid enhances the excretion of uric acid. Salicylates are thought to inhibit this action.

        nursing implication: Instruct patients receiving probenecid to avoid taking aspirin and to read labels of non-prescription drugs carefully.

22. *propranolol (Inderal)*

    antidiabetic agents

        action: The mechanism by which propranolol (Inderal) reduces glycogenolysis is not clearly understood; however, blood glucose rebound is retarded and symptoms of hypoglycemia masked in patients receiving both these drugs.

        nursing implication: Observe closely for clinical indications of hypoglycemia.

23. *quinidine*

    surgical muscle relaxants

        action: The action of quinidine is one of muscle action depression. When this drug is given immediately postoperatively during which surgical muscle relaxants were given, muscle paralysis may occur.

        nursing implication: Recommend this drug combination not be used. Have respirator as standby equipment in case of respiratory failure.

24. *tetracycline*

    antacids

        action: Most antacids interfere with the absorption of the tetracyclines.

        nursing implication: Administer tetracycline at least two hours before or after antacids. Avoid the use of milk products within an hour of tetracycline administration.

    methoxyflurane (Penthrane)

        action: The toxic reaction of this combination of drugs is evidenced by kidney damage although the process is not understood.

        nursing implication: Recommend that these drugs not be given concurrently.

25. *thyroid*

    cholestyramine (Cuemid, Questran)
        action: Absorption of thyroid is impaired when given concurrently with cholestyramine.
        nursing implication: Schedule the administration of these drugs four to five hours apart.

26. *warfarin and related compounds*

    anabolic steroids
        action: Steroids have many qualities that potentiate anticoagulant therapy.
        nursing implication: Observe closely for signs or symptoms of hemorrhage.

    antidiabetic drugs
        action: The metabolism of the oral hypoglycemics is retarded when these two drugs are initially combined; however, continued use brings a reverse reaction.
        nursing implication: Observe for signs of hypoglycemia such as weakness or fatigue.

    barbiturates
        action: Barbiturates appear to increase the metabolism and decrease the absorption of warfarin.
        nursing implication: Recommend that these drugs not be used concurrently.

    chloramphenicol (Chloromycetin)
        action: Chloramphenicol acts as a potentiator when combined with warfarin.
        nursing implication: Observe closely for signs of excessive bleeding.

    clofibrate (Atromid-S)
        action: The action of clofibrate on warfarin is unknown; however, the anticoagulant effect is prolonged and control of the therapy may be lost.
        nursing implication: Recommend starting doses of warfarin be lower than average. Observe closely for bleeding.

    diphenylhydantoin (Dilantin)
        action: The interaction of these two drugs is a complex one and not clearly understood.
        nursing implication: If warfarin is given to patients maintained on diphenylhydantoin, observe closely for signs of diphenylhydantoin intoxication. If diphenyldydantoin is added to a patient on a controlled warfarin regimen, observe closely for bleeding as though control had not been established.

    disulfiram (Antabuse)
        action: The effect of disulfiram on anticoagulant therapy is not known, but it is thought that disulfiram inhibits the metabolism of the anticoagulants.
        nursing implication: Monitor laboratory test results and report results promptly.

    phenylbutazone (Butazolidin)
        action: The metabolism of warfarin is increased and the action enhanced by concomitant use with phenylbutazone.
        nursing implication: Recommend that the use of these drugs together be avoided.

    thyroid preparations
        action: Resistance to warfarin is apparent in some patients receiving thyroid hormones. Larger doses of anticoagulants may be required.
        nursing implication: Monitor laboratory data and report.

REFERENCES

DiPalma, Joseph R. "The Why and How of Drug Interactions." *RN* 33:63, March 1970.

Donn, Richard. "Intravenous Admixture Incompatibility." *American Journal of Nursing* 71:325, February 1971.

Hays, Doris. "Do It Yourself—the Z-track Way." *American Journal of Nursing* 74:1070, June 1974.

Hussar, Daniel. "Drug Interactions by the Hundreds." *Nursing 72* 2:4, January 1972.

Lambert, Martin. "Drug and Diet Interactions." *American Journal of Nursing* 75:402, March 1975.

Leary, Jean A., et al. "Self-administered Medications." *American Journal of Nursing* 71:1193, June 1971.

Lowenthal, W. "Factors Affecting Drug Absorption—A Programmed Unit." *American Journal of Nursing* 73:1391, August 1973.

Odom, Jeffrey V. "Going Metric." *American Journal of Nursing* 74:1078, June 1974.

APPLICATION QUESTIONS

I. *True-False*

For each statement below, write **a** if the statement is true or **b** if it is false.

  _b_ 1. Drugs can never be excreted from the body intact, without being detoxified or broken down into metabolites.

_a_ 2. Subcutaneous injection of a medication provides for slower absorption than intramuscular injection of the same medication.

____ 3. All drugs are excreted through either the kidneys or the lungs.

____ 4. The liver is the only organ with enzymes that have the ability to detoxify drugs.

____ 5. The term _absorption_ includes the time from the entry of a drug into the body until it is in critical concentration in the fluid surrounding the reacting cells.

____ 6. _Biotransformation_ refers to the reaction that takes place when the drug molecules interact with the cells at the site of drug action.

____ 7. The term _parenteral_ is used generally to indicate any injection route for medication.

____ 8. There are more sensory nerve endings in muscles than in subcutaneous tissues; as a result, intramuscular injections are usually more painful than subcutaneous injections.

____ 9. It is easier to inject medication accidentally into a vein when using the intramuscular route than when using the subcutaneous route.

____ 10. Sublingual medication is given for localized effect and does not have a systemic effect.

____ 11. Medication applied to the rectal or nasal mucosa can be absorbed quickly into the systemic circulation because of the high vascularity of these areas.

____ 12. Topically applied medications are usually poorly absorbed through the skin into the systemic circulation.

____ 13. The nurse must never tell the patient the name of the drug he is receiving.

II. _Multiple Choice_

For each of the following questions, indicate the letter providing the _best_ answer.

____ 1. What organ or system is mainly responsible for detoxification of drugs? (a) liver (b) kidney (c) lymph (d) intestine (e) spleen

____ 2. What organ or system is mainly responsible for excretion of drugs or metabolites? (a) liver (b) kidney (c) intestine (d) lung (e) blood

____ 3. Where does most absorption of orally administered drugs usually take place? (a) mouth (b) stomach (c) small intestine (d) large intestine

____ 4. Rank the following routes of drug administration according to the usual rate of absorption, from the most rapid to the slowest. (1) intramuscular (2) intravenous (3) subcutaneous
(a) 1–2–3 (b) 2–3–1 (c) 3–2–1 (d) 2–1–3 (e) 1–3–2

____ 5. After rectal administration of a drug, which of the following activities would best aid in absorption of the drug? (a) moving and walking about (b) lying in bed (c) sitting in a chair (d) drinking warm liquids

____ 6. As you are preparing to give him an injection of morphine, a patient asks what drug you are administering to him. Which of the following would be the best initial response? (a) "Your doctor ordered this to make you feel better." (b) "This is morphine." (c) "This medication will relieve your pain." (d) "It is the same drug you received earlier this morning." (e) "You'll have to ask your doctor about that; I cannot discuss that with you."

____ 7. What is the usual maximum amount of medication deposited at one time in any subcutaneous injection site? (a) 0.5 cc. (b) 1 cc. (c) 2 cc. (d) 3 cc. (e) 5 cc.

____ 8. When would it be best to give an oral drug that is irritating to the gastrointestinal tract? (a) between meals (b) before a meal (c) after a meal

____ 9. Why are some tablets or capsules enteric coated? (a) to prevent irritation in the mouth (b) to permit dissolving only in the stomach (c) to prevent irritation of the esophagus (d) to permit dissolving only in the upper intestinal tract (e) to permit dissolving only in the lower intestinal tract

____ 10. What is the danger of opening a prolonged-action capsule and mixing its contents with food to facilitate a patient taking the medication? (a) This practice could result in an overdose of the drug. (b) The contents would not dissolve, resulting in an underdose. (c) The drug would most likely be irritating to the stomach lining. (d) There is no danger—this is a good practice.

III. _Matching A_

Match each abbreviation to its definition.

____ 1. q.i.d.   (a) Every hour

____ 2. q.h.   (b) At once

____ 3. t.i.d.   (c) Twice a day

____ 4. stat.   (d) Three times a day

____ 5. b.i.d.   (e) Four times a day

IV. _Matching B_

Match each abbreviation to its definition.

____ 1. h.s.   (a) Before meals

____ 2. a.c.   (b) After meals

_____ 3. p.c.   (c) At bedtime

_____ 4. O.D.   (d) Right eye

_____ 5. O.S.   (e) Left eye

V. *Matching C*

Match each form of drug administration to its definition.

_e_ 1. Buccal   (a) just below surface
                                skin
_____ 2. Sublingual
                            (b) Into the subarach-
_____ 3. Intra-articular   noid space of the
                                spinal column
_____ 4. Intradermal
                            (c) Under the tongue
_____ 5. Intrathecal
                            (d) Within a joint

                            (e) In the cheek of the
                                mouth

VI. *Drug Interactions*

In each of the following situations, determine whether the pharmacologic effect of Drug X would be changed. Write **a** if its effect would be increased; **b** if it would be decreased; or **c** if it would be unchanged.

_____ 1. Two pain relievers, Drugs X + Y, given together provide relief from pain for six hours, rather than the four hours either drug would provide if given alone.

_____ 2. An antacid (Drug Y) inhibits the absorption of an antibiotic (Drug X).

_____ 3. Two drugs are given for different purposes, but Drug Y inhibits the enzyme necessary for the detoxification of Drug X.

_____ 4. Two drugs are given for different purposes, but Drug Y increases the synthesis of the enzyme necessary for metabolizing Drug X.

_____ 5. An anticoagulant (Drug X) is given with an anti-inflammatory drug (Drug Y), and the patient begins spontaneous bleeding.

_____ 6. Two pain relievers, Drugs X and Y, provide the same effect whether 5 mg of each drug is given simultaneously or if 10 mg of either drug is given alone.

_____ 7. Two drugs are given for different purposes, but Drug Y frees many more molecules of Drug X from their plasma binding sites.

_____ 8. Two drugs are given for different purposes, but Drug Y interferes with the renal excretion of Drug X.

VII. *Nursing Action*

Of the activities listed below, indicate by **a** those which are considered independent nursing functions and by **b** those which are not.

_____ 1. Establishing whether a medication to be given once a day will be given in the morning or at night.

_____ 2. Withholding a medication if there is reason for doing so based on nursing knowledge.

_____ 3. Changing a dosage of a drug if the patient is experiencing side effect.

_____ 4. Changing the route of administration of a drug if the patient is not tolerating the present route.

_____ 5. Withholding a p.r.n. medication if there is a reason for doing so based on nursing knowledge, even if the patient asks for it.

_____ 6. Giving a p.r.n. medication even if the patient does not ask for it.

_____ 7. Mixing an oral medication with food or juice to disguise its taste.

_____ 8. Refusing to give a drug after checking with the physician if the dose is excessively above the normal range.

_____ 9. Insisting that a physician write and sign a medication order before administering a drug.

VIII. *Discussion*

For each patient statement given below, write **a** if teaching is needed or **b** if no teaching is needed. If teaching is needed, outline the content you would include.

_____ 1. "I always take my heart medicine with one little cracker or else I get so very sick to my stomach."

_____ 2. "When I'm on a reducing diet I take mineral oil every night to keep me 'straight' and one multiple vitamin pill at night, too."

_____ 3. "I don't like taking that big antibiotic capsule, but it seems to go down lots easier with a big glass of milk."

_____ 4. "I know the doctor put me on a stool softener, but I take a little mineral oil too, just to be sure I don't have any problems."

_____ 5. "I remember to take my antibiotic pills by putting the bottle right on the table and taking them with each meal."

_____ 6. "Sometimes I retain a lot of water so I take one of the diuretics I have at home; but you know, even with the diuretic and the gout medicine, I seem to have more attacks of gout during that time."

_____ 7. "Aspirin doesn't seem to work for me at all; sometimes when I have a bad attack of gout, I take some aspirin with my gout medicine and it actually seems to make it worse instead of better."

_____ 8. "The doctor told me to take one or two of these pills as needed to keep me calmed down. You know, I only need one at night to help me sleep, but I usually need two during the day."

Toxic Effects of Drugs and Chemicals

Drugs and chemicals can have two kinds of adverse effects. The first is a reaction *not* related to the pharmacological effect of the drug; it is referred to as an allergic reaction or idiosyncrasy. These reactions cannot be predicted on the basis of widespread toxicity testing, since they result from the reactivity of an individual's tissues with the drug. Allergy-prone patients can be skin tested with many drugs prior to drug therapy to determine individual allergic response.

The second type of adverse reaction results from the known pharmacological effect of a drug. An example would be *excessive* depression of the central nervous system following administration of a drug whose pharmacological action is central nervous system depression. Any patient may experience this type of adverse reaction or poisoning if a massive overdose is taken. Such a reaction may also follow the normal dosage of a drug if a patient is hypersusceptible for reasons such as abnormal pathology or drug interactions; this would be considered a "relative" overdose.

Teratogenicity is an additional type of drug reaction that does not literally fit into either of the above two categories. This type of reaction occurs when the drug crosses the placenta and causes developmental deformities in the fetus.

Every drug is capable of causing adverse effects. Overdosage, whether absolute or relative, is the most common cause of adverse drug reactions.

DRUG IDIOSYNCRASY AND ALLERGY

An idiosyncratic reaction may occur the first time a patient is exposed to a drug; a drug allergy, on the other hand, does not occur if a drug is used only once. In a drug allergy, antibodies are manufactured in response to a first exposure, and allergic symptoms occur following subsequent exposures. Symptoms of allergy may be as mild as a skin rash or as severe and sudden as anaphylactic shock. The allergic response is reviewed in Chapter 32. To detect possible allergic or idiosyncratic reactions, the nurse must observe results of laboratory tests such as blood, liver and kidney studies. She must also observe for changes in the patient's skin and eyes.

POISONING

Poisoning—whether from an overdose of a drug or from ingestion of a harmful chemical—is an emergency situation. Stress to patients the importance of keeping drugs and chemicals in their original containers and keeping the labels intact so the ingredients can be known. Many household chemicals also have their antidote printed on the label. Encourage the patient to have the physician or pharmacist identify drugs by name on prescription bottles. This can save a great deal of valuable time if an accidental overdose occurs. This practice is required by law in some states; check the laws in your area.

Treatment of Poisoning

If poisoning occurs, it is important to try to identify the poisonous substance and the quantity involved. After the drug or chemical has been identified, emergency measures should be instituted in the following manner: (1) remove the poison, if this is possible and not contraindicated; (2) administer the chemical antidote; and (3) apply supportive measures to maintain vital signs and treat complications.

Vomiting and gastric lavage are the most effective means of removing poison from the gastrointestinal tract. In the following cases, however, vomiting should *not* be induced: (1) if the ingested substance is corrosive or caustic; (2) if only a small amount of a light, volatile petroleum distillate—such as a kerosene product—has been ingested; or, (3) if the patient is nonresponsive or very stuporous or shows signs of impending convulsive seizures. If vomiting is contraindicated, gastric lavage is also considered to be contraindicated. If vomiting is not contraindicated, it may be induced by touching the back of the throat or by giving an emetic drug.

Emetic Drugs.   The two most commonly employed emetic drugs are syrup of ipecac and apomorphine. One-half ounce of syrup of ipecac with a glass or two of water, repeated in fifteen minutes if vomiting does not occur, is the usual treatment. It is possible to buy a one-ounce bottle of this drug without a prescription. No more than one ounce, total dose, should ever be taken, as the emetic itself could cause toxic effects. Never confuse syrup of ipecac with the fluidextract of ipecac. The fluidextract is a much more concentrated form of the drug; a single teaspoon could cause severe poisoning. The nurse will probably not encounter this form of the drug except in the hospital pharmacy, but it is good to remember that any fluidextract is more concentrated and potent than a syrup.

Another emetic is the very fast acting apomorphine. When 5mg are injected subcutaneously, vomiting usually occurs within 5 minutes. Because apomorphine is an opium derivative, it is a central nervous system depressant and should not be used if a patient is already stuporous. A narcotic antagonist drug should be on hand to counteract any adverse reactions from the apomorphine.

Chemical Antidotes.   Antidotes are given to neutralize ingested chemicals and prevent their absorption. The most effective material for inactivating most poisons while still in the gastrointestinal tract is activated charcoal, readily available for emergency household use by scraping charcoal from burned toast. This antidote also can be purchased as a powder; it must first be mixed with a small amount of water to form a paste and then with more water to make a glass of liquid. Activated charcoal has no taste or odor. Diluted weak acids such as citrus juice or vinegar may be given to neutralize ingested bases; and weak basic solutions of substances such as baking soda may neutralize ingested acids.

Specific drug antidotes are rare, but in some cases a drug can be given to produce physiologic functions opposite to those of the poison. These agents do not neutralize the poison, but they do counteract the symptoms.

Chelating agents are given to counteract the effects of ingested heavy metals such as arsenic, mercury, gold, lead, and iron. The commonly used chelating agents are dimercaprol (BAL); calcium disodium edetate, which is specific for lead poisoning; and deferoxamine (Desferal), specific for iron toxicity.

Support of Vital Signs.   After emergency measures have been instituted, supportive measures may be needed to treat the symptoms and complications of poisoning. This usually involves assistance with respiration, circulation, and kidney function.

Information you may wish to know:
1. Where is the nearest poison control center?
2. What is the telephone number of the poison control center?

REFERENCES

Craven, Ruth, and Lester, JoAnn. "Anaphylactic Shock." *American Journal of Nursing* 72:718, April 1972.

Croft, Harriet, and Frenkel, Sallie. "Children and Lead Poisoning." *American Journal of Nursing* 75:102, January 1975.

Forrest, J. A. H. "Acute Poisoning." *Nursing Times* 70:590, April 1974.

Reed, A. Jane. "Lead Poisoning—Silent Epidemic and Social Crime." *American Journal of Nursing* 72:218, December 1972.

Rodman, Morton J. "Poisonings and Their Treatment." *RN* 35:57, November 1972.

APPLICATION QUESTIONS

I. *True-False*

For each statement below, write **a** if the statement is true or **b** if it is false.

_____ 1. An idiosyncrasy is an adverse effect of a drug which is not related to its expected pharmacological effect.

_____ 2. An allergic reaction to a drug usually occurs the first time it is given, even if the dose is small.

_____ 3. An anaphylactoid reaction is an allergic reaction occurring immediately after a drug is given.

_____ 4. Teratogenicity refers to drug reactions in children from birth to one year.

_____ 5. Following ingestion of a corrosive substance, the patient should be induced to vomit in order to stop the corrosive action on the stomach lining.

_____ 6. Fluidextract of ipecac is a more concentrated drug than syrup of ipecac.

_____ 7. Gastric lavage is usually contraindicated in treating poison ingestion whenever vomiting is contraindicated.

II. *Multiple Choice*

For each of the following questions, indicate the letter providing the *best* answer.

_____ 1. What is the best antidote to use following the ingestion of a heavy metal? (a) an absorption agent (b) a chelating agent (c) a weak acid (d) syrup of ipecac

_____ 2. What is the best and most accessible household source of activated charcoal? (a) burned toast (b) charcoal briquettes (c) wood ashes (d) burned meat

_____ 3. When a patient is receiving apomorphine, the nurse should be certain that which of the following drugs is on hand? (a) syrup of ipecac (b) BAL (c) Lorfan (d) calcium disodium edetate

_____ 4. What is the most effective antidote for treating any poisonous chemical ingestion? (a) activated charcoal (b) milk (c) lemon juice (d) syrup of ipecac

_____ 5. What is the *major* danger in giving an emetic drug to a semicomatose patient? (a) the patient might be uncooperative in swallowing it (b) the patient might aspirate the vomitus into his lungs (c) the drug will cause a deeper coma (d) the vomiting reflex is depressed and the patient will be unable to vomit

III. *Situation A*

Assuming all are available to you, indicate by letter which of the following would be your *best first* action in each situation:
- **a** Give ipecac to induce vomiting.
- **b** Give a glass of lemon juice and water.
- **c** Give a glass of milk of magnesia and water.
- **d** Give a glass of milk.
- **e** Call the poison control center.

_____ 1. A small child swallows some toilet bowl cleaner containing hydrochloric acid.

_____ 2. A child eats an insecticide containing arsenic.

_____ 3. A child drinks a small amount of chlorine bleach.

_____ 4. A child eats some drain cleaner containing lye.

_____ 5. An adult ingests a bottle of prescription capsules. The name of the drug is written on the label, but you are totally unfamiliar with the drug.

_____ 6. A child swallows some oven cleaner containing lye.

_____ 7. A child drinks carbon tetrachloride spot removing fluid.

IV. *Situation B*

Assume that you make each of the following observations during a visit to a patient's home. Write **a** if the observation suggests that teaching is needed or **b** if it does not suggest any necessary teaching. If teaching is necessary, outline the content you would include.

_____ 1. You see a woman flush the remaining pills of an old prescription down a toilet.

_____ 2. You enter the bathroom to wash your hands and notice that the light bulb is burned out.

_____ 3. You notice that the labels on the children's bottles of liquid medicines are covered with the colorful, sticky medication.

_____ 4. You overhear a mother sternly correct a child who refers to his medication as "candy."

_____ 5. While you are talking to a mother, she asks her six-year-old to bring her two aspirin from the bathroom because "Mommy has a headache."

____ 6. A young mother returns from grocery shopping and divides a new bottle of strong disinfectant evenly into two peanut butter jars. She tightens the lids securely and places one under each of the two bathroom sinks.

V. *Calculations*

____ 1. A 90-pound child is to receive calcium disodium edetate. The drug is given on the basis of 1 gram/30 pounds of body weight per day, divided into two equal doses. What amount of the drug would *one* dose contain?

____ 2. A 90-pound child is to receive BAL. The dosage reads, 2.5 mg./kg. body weight. What is the dosage for this child?

Drug Abuse, Dependence, and Addiction

Drug abuse is a very widespread social problem in the United States. Terminology associated with drug abuse has become quite confusing. The term "addiction," for example, has been used in so many ways that it does not really have a specific meaning. In this chapter we will use four terms: *misuse, abuse, habituation,* and *dependence.*

TERMINOLOGY

Misuse refers to the use of nonprescription drugs and chemicals when there is not a definite need for them. Misused drugs include laxatives, antacids, analgesics, sleeping medications, and many others. The chemical most widely misused is alcohol.

The second term, *drug abuse,* refers to use of drugs in a way that most people in a given society consider improper. It may refer to the taking of a drug or chemical in excessive quantities, either periodically or continually, or to taking a drug in the wrong situation. A person intoxicated with alcohol at a cocktail party may not be considered abusive; on the job, the same level of intoxication would be considered abusive.

The next term, *habituation,* denotes a mild form of psychological dependence. A person feels better when he has taken the chemical; although he can function competently without it, he may experience some emotional discomfort. Caffeine and nicotine are examples of habituating chemicals.

Dependence on a drug can be psychological, physical, or both. Psychological dependence involves the craving for the feeling the drug produces. This craving is such that all other goals are discarded in order to achieve the pleasurable drug-induced state. Physical dependence, which develops from continual use of drugs, involves biochemical changes, particularly in tissues of the nervous system.

A person who misuses or is habituated to a drug or chemical can usually end his consumption with individual effort; he may perhaps need some help from other individuals. Physical dependence on a drug or chemical can be relieved in a matter of days or weeks, depending on the drug involved and the amount taken. Withdrawal is not without danger, but it can be accomplished under medical supervision, without the extreme, terrifying discomforts of abrupt, "cold turkey" cessation.

Psychological dependence on a drug is most difficult to relieve. A person may be detoxified or physically withdrawn from a drug but still have a psychological dependence that will cause him to continue taking drugs. Treatment of psychological dependence requires a long period of time and the assistance of health personnel and medications specific for the situation.

TYPES OF DRUG ABUSE

There are six classifications of abused drugs: (1) the potent narcotic analgesics, such as heroin and morphine; (2) the general depressants, such as the barbiturates, tranquilizers, and alcohol; (3) the inhaled volatile solvents; (4) the psychomotor stimulants, such as amphetamines; (5) the hallucinogens, such as LSD and mescaline; and (6) the cannabis derivatives, such as marihuana and hashish. In general, chemicals in the first three categories—the narcotics, depressants, and volatile solvents—are capable of causing definite physical and psychological dependence. Psychomotor stimulants can definitely cause psychological dependence; it is uncertain whether they cause physical dependence. Substances in the last two categories —the hallucinogens and the cannabis derivatives —can produce psychological dependence, but there is no evidence that they produce physical dependence. Drugs in all categories have physical effects, some of which may be very severe. However, the ability to produce severe physical effects should not be confused with the ability to cause physical dependence. All the drugs classified above are capable of producing psychological dependence, but psychological dependence is more likely to occur in persons already disturbed emotionally or those who seem to be dependence prone. Alcoholics and previously drug-dependent persons should never be given dependence-producing drugs, even on prescription, because of the possibility of creating some degree of dependence.

Potent Narcotics

Taking opiate drugs, or the potent narcotic analgesics, makes a person indifferent to stress. He is pleasurably relaxed and experiences euphoria and freedom from anxiety and conflict. The person dependent on opiates may appear to be in a drowsy, dreamlike state. He may be nauseated and vomit; his skin will be warm and moist; his face will be flushed and his pupils pinpoint size. Overdose can cause coma or pulmonary edema and may lead to cardiovascular collapse or respiratory failure. Frequent injection of opiates over a long period of time can lead to skin problems, such as scars and abscesses from the multiple needle punctures, and to medical problems such as hepatitis and thrombophlebitis.

Physical Withdrawal. Physical withdrawal symptoms from the potent narcotics may be mild to severe. Without medical intervention, they might include any of the following: runny nose, sweating, anorexia, muscle contractions, dilated pupils, insomnia, restlessness, alternating shivering and hot flashes, vomiting, rapid respirations, heart palpitations, and high blood pressure. Severe reactions do not usually occur, because of medical intervention to decrease the discomfort. Methadone hydrochloride (Dolophine) is a drug sometimes used for detoxification. It is an opiate itself, but if used for brief periods of time, then gradually discontinued, it can decrease the discomforts of withdrawal.

During withdrawal, the patient is especially sensitive to the attitudes of others. It is important that he be listened to and that he be told what to expect during the process. The nurse should attend to comfort measures as they are needed, such as back rubs to relax aching muscles, warm blankets to counteract chills, and small, frequent meals when the patient is not nauseated.

Psychological Withdrawal As stated above, physical withdrawal can be accomplished with a minimum of

danger and discomfort; psychological dependence, however, may lead the former drug user back to the drug. Experimental programs have been instituted to help the former drug user reduce his craving for the drug and to aid him in resocialization and establishment in a job and the community. Methadone maintenance is one such program. The use of methadone over a long period of time is criticized by some because it is still an opiate drug. A daily dose of methadone, however, permits normal functioning without the interfering effects that occur when other opiates are taken. It does not provide a "high" feeling, and, while on methadone, a person is unable to experience a "high" from heroin.

The narcotic antagonists, such as nalorphine (Nalline), levallorphan tartrate (Lorfan), naloxone (Narcan) and cylclazocine are being used for withdrawal. Like methadone, the narcotic antagonists block the "high" effect if heroin is taken; but unlike methadone, they do not block the craving for heroin. Because of the short action of these drugs, it would be possible for a patient to return to opiates after missing only one dose. However, the narcotic antagonists are preferable to methadone in that they are not dependence producing. They are used for detoxification and perhaps someday will be used for maintenance programs.

General Depressants

The central nervous system depressants cause sedation, drowsiness, lethargy, sleep, deepening stupor, and coma. They are also capable of causing a period of excitement, confusion, and unpredictable boisterous behavior just before sleep occurs. This stage is often seen in persons intoxicated with alcohol. A person dependent on a central depressant may have difficulty in speaking and in walking; he may be untidy or unkempt, irritable, and confused with impaired judgment; he may appear excited or may be delirious, stuporous, in a deep sleep, or in a coma, with depressed respiration and very low blood pressure. Death from overdose of a central nervous system depressant occurs from respiratory and circulatory failure. The depressant abuser may take an overdose accidentally because of his confusion, or because of mixing two depressant drugs, such as alcohol and barbiturates.

Withdrawal. Physical withdrawal from central nervous system depressants is potentially more dangerous than from opiates. Withdrawal symptoms may include restlessness, anxiety, insomnia, muscle twitching, abdominal cramps, and vomiting. Hallucinations, delirium, and confusion can lead to grand mal seizures, or even status epilepticus, with high fever and cardiovascular collapse. Withdrawal may take weeks if gradual reduction of barbiturate dosage is necessary to avoid convulsions.

Inhaled Volatile Solvents

Inhaling the vapors of volatile solvents such as those in model airplane glues, plastic cements, and spot removers affects the central nervous system in the same way as other depressants. The person often appears as if he were intoxicated with alcohol. Death may occur from respiratory failure or cardiac arrest. The danger of these chemicals, commonly used by younger children, is the irreversible toxic damage they can cause to liver, kidneys, and bone marrow.

Psychomotor Stimulants

The amphetamines and other psychomotor stimulants have two main effects: (1) they cause an increase in wakefulness and alertness; and (2) they increase feelings of self-confidence. They also cause palpitations, headache, hypertension, dry mouth, dilated pupils, nervousness, irritability, insomnia, talkativeness, and anorexia with resultant weight loss. Continued use of amphetamines can lead to confusion, perceptual changes, hallucinations, and paranoid feelings. Amphetamines may be abused occasionally, continually, or in sprees. The truck driver making a long haul and the student or executive trying to meet a deadline would be considered occasional abusers. The continual user may be one who begins taking amphetamines by prescription for a weight problem or for lethargy. The feeling of well-being is so enjoyable that the person continues using the drug even when not available on the original prescription. This person may eventually begin taking a depressant drug to combat the unpleasant feelings of the amphetamines and become dependent on both a stimulant and a depressant.

The use of amphetamines by the spree user is the most dangerous. His use involves intravenous injections of the drug. The person may have a run of several days of being very active, talkative, and always awake. Each injection of amphetamines gives an immediate "jolt" of intense pleasure and the feeling of extreme mental and physical power. The run continues until the person "crashes" into a deep sleep. When he finally awakens, he is lethargic and deeply depressed. Continuous alternating runs and crashes result in definite mental and emotional changes. Para-

noid psychosis eventually occurs, requiring hospitalization and symptomatic treatment with phenothiazines. An overdose of intravenous amphetamine can cause severe vasoconstriction; it may result in temporary paralysis and aphasia from cerebral ischemia, or in severe chest pains from coronary ischemia. The common physical effects of long-term amphetamine abuse stem from infection and malnutrition.

Hallucinogens

The word "hallucinogen" actually refers to a drug capable of producing changes in perception. LSD and mescaline can change perception, thought, mood, and behavior, but there is no one word to describe all of these effects. The mental effects of LSD are highly unpredictable. A person may have a "good trip" or a "bad trip"—an acute panic reaction which may require hospitalization and treatment with chlorpromazine. Physical effects of the hallucinogens are mainly sympathomimetic. It has been suggested that long-term use before or during pregnancy causes breaks in chromosomes, leading to leukemia or birth defects in the infant.

Mescaline mainly causes visual hallucinations, spatial distortions, and intensified color patterns. An overdose can cause discomforting sympathomimetic effects.

Dimethoxymethylamphetamine (DOM, "STP") is a potent hallucinogen derived from amphetamine, with the effects of LSD and atropine (see chapter 16). It often causes prolonged acute panic reactions which necessitate treatment with sedatives such as pentobarbital sodium, chlordiazepoxide, or chloral hydrate. Chlorpromazine hydrochloride should *not* be used, because the psychological effects and sympathetic physical disturbances are made *worse* by the administration of this drug.

Cannabis Derivatives

Marihuana and related drugs affect people in different ways. When taken in small doses, they are mild intoxicants with effects similar to alcohol. These effects—ranging from euphoria to anxiety and depression—depend in part on the expectations of the individual and on the environment in which the drug is taken. The first effect of floating and drowsiness may be pleasurable or unpleasant. Large doses may bring about perceptual changes, hallucinations, confusion, anxiety, and panic. The nonsmoker may experience the unpleasantries of inhaling smoke, such as dry throat, coughing, and nausea.

REFERENCES

B., ELAINE, et al. "Helping the Nurse Who Misuses Drugs." *American Journal of Nursing* 74:1665, September 1974.

FINK, MAX, et al. "Narcotic Antagonists: Another Approach to Addiction Therapy." *American Journal of Nursing* 71:1359, July 1971.

FINNEGAN, LORETTA P., and MACNEW, BONNIE A. "Care of the Addicted Infant." *American Journal of Nursing* 74:685, April 1974.

FORT, JOEL. "Comparison Chart of Major Substances Used for Mind Alteration." *American Journal of Nursing* 71:1740, September 1971.

LEVINE, DAVID, et al. "A Special Program for Nurse Addicts." *American Journal of Nursing* 74:1672, September 1974.

NELSON, KARIN. "The Nurse in a Methadone Maintenance Program." *American Journal of Nursing* 73: 870, May 1973.

APPLICATION QUESTIONS

I. *True-False*

For each statement below, write **a** if the statement if true or **b** if it is false.

_____ 1. Physical dependence on a drug is characterized by a craving for the feeling that the drug produces.

_____ 2. Habituation involves a mild degree of psychological dependence and does not involve physical dependence.

_____ 3. An addict may overcome his physical dependence on a drug yet still maintain his psychological dependence.

_____ 4. Self-medication leads to psychological dependence only in individuals with a previously manifested personality disturbance or emotional disorder.

_____ 5. During withdrawal or detoxification, the heroin addict is indifferent to the attitudes of others.

_____ 6. The heroin addict will be more comfortable during withdrawal if his environment is kept cool and frequent cool sponging is done to relieve his excessive perspiration and feeling of warmth.

_____ 7. The withdrawal syndrome from the opiate drugs is potentially more dangerous than from the barbiturate drugs.

_____ 8. A patient on methadone maintenance cannot experience the euphoric effects of heroin.

_____ 9. The drug methadone is a synthetic narcotic and can cause dependence.

_____ 10. A patient maintained on daily doses of a narcotic antagonist such as Nalline or Lorfan cannot experience the euphoric effects of heroin.

_____ 11. Abusers of barbiturates achieve a state of sedation and never experience excitement similar to that induced by opiates.

_____ 12. A patient intoxicated from barbiturate or tranquilizer abuse is similar in appearance and action to a person intoxicated from alcohol.

_____ 13. One of the main differences between barbiturate abuse and alcohol abuse is that the barbiturate abuser is less likely to suffer from malnutrition.

_____ 14. Abruptly discontinuing the abused drug from a barbiturate addict may result in convulsions.

_____ 15. The "glue sniffer" may experience changes in consciousness but is in no danger of causing pathological damage to body organs.

_____ 16. Amphetamine drugs relieve fatigue and do away with the body's need for rest.

_____ 17. A spree user is a person who injects amphetamines intravenously.

_____ 18. The amphetamine abuser often suffers from skin infections and malnutrition.

_____ 19. Physical dependence does not occur with LSD.

_____ 20. An acute panic reaction caused by the hallucinogen agent LSD or "STP" is best treated with the tranquilizer chlorpromazine hydrochloride (Thorazine).

_____ 21. Marihuana is a narcotic and can cause an opiate-type dependence.

_____ 22. Marihuana does not seem to bring about damage to vital body organs.

II. *Multiple Choice*

For each of the following questions, indicate the letter providing the *best* answer.

_____ 1. What type of intoxication would you suspect if a patient appeared drowsy, with flushed warm skin, vomiting, and with constricted pupils? (a) opiates (b) amphetamines (c) hallucinogens

_____ 2. What type of intoxication would you suspect if a patient appeared thin, talkative, restless, confused, and with dilated pupils? (a) opiates (b) amphetamines (c) hallucinogens (d) barbiturates

_____ 3. What type of intoxication would you suspect if a patient appeared unkempt, staggering, drowsy, and confused, with difficulty speaking and a low blood pressure? (a) opiates (b) amphetamines (c) hallucinogens (d) barbiturates

III. *Matching*

Match each statement to the type of dependence it suggests.

_____ 1. "I finally got my
           prescription filled,
           so tonight I'll sleep
           with my pills."

_____ 2. "I'm so cold—
           give me some
           methadone quick."

_____ 3. "I don't care about
           my job; I just
           want the feeling
           that joint gives me."

(a) habituation

(b) psychological
    dependence

(c) physical dependence

5

Alcohol

Alcoholism is one of the most serious public health problems in the United States. Prolonged intake of alcohol can result in many physical and behavioral complications. In addition, many deaths and injuries have resulted from drunken drivers. This chapter deals with the actions and metabolism of alcohol in the body, the treatment of acute alcohol intoxication, and rehabilitation of alcoholic patients. The therapeutic effects of alcohol are also considered.

THE ACTION OF ALCOHOL ON THE CENTRAL NERVOUS SYSTEM

Alcohol is *not* a stimulant. It has a *depressant* effect on the central nervous system (CNS), similar to the barbiturates and some general anesthetics. The excited behavior that can result from intake of alcohol is actually caused by depression of brain areas that normally have an inhibitory effect on behavior.

The effects of alcohol on the CNS are directly related to the level of alcohol in the brain. A small amount of alcohol may exert a tranquilizing or sedative effect and reduce nervous tension. As the blood alcohol level rises toward 100 mg.%, the individual is usually mildly intoxicated and dangerously unfit to drive an automobile. He also suffers a decreased ability to evaluate reality, make judgments, and restrain his impulses. An individual with a blood alcohol level of 150 mg.% to 200 mg.% is considered moderately intoxicated; when the blood level reaches 300 mg.%, the person is markedly intoxicated. Such a person may be in a stage of acute excitement and may need to be kept from harming himself and others. This stage of intoxication may require hospitalization and the administration of medications to calm him down. When the blood alcohol level reaches 400 to 500 mg.%, the individual usually goes into a stupor or even a coma. Respirations may become very slow and shallow, and emergency measures may be required to maintain the vital functions.

METABOLISM OF ALCOHOL

Alcohol is rapidly absorbed from an empty stomach. Central nervous system effects may be delayed when the stomach contains a moderate amount of food. Foods which contain fats will especially slow the passage of alcohol into the small intestine, the main site of alcohol absorption.

When alcohol enters the blood stream, it is rapidly carried to the central nervous system because of the rich blood supply to the brain. Alcohol passes the blood-brain barrier and builds up in concentrations that depress various nerve centers. The drug is later redistributed to other tissues of the body and detoxified.

Most absorbed alcohol is eventually broken down into carbon dioxide and water, with the production of considerable energy. Some alcohol leaves the body unchanged through the breath and urine. An average person oxidizes about 7 Gms. (10 cc.) of alcohol in an hour. This means that it would take three hours to metabolize the ounce of alcohol in the average mixed drink; the body would need almost a day to rid itself of a pint of whiskey. Heavy drinkers may metabolize alcohol more rapidly; this does not, however, mean that blood levels high enough to cause intoxication will not be reached.

MEDICAL MANAGEMENT OF THE INTOXICATED PATIENT

Alcoholic Stupor and Coma

Most intoxicated patients who are found in a stupor but have normal vital signs require no special treatment. If respirations are slow and shallow, however, the respiratory rate may be increased by parenteral administration of an analeptic such as caffeine sodium benzoate. Or, respirations may be deepened by having the patient inhale 5 percent carbon dioxide periodically.

The patient who is comatose requires more vigorous treatment to prevent respiratory failure and other complications such as hypostatic pneumonia.

Attempts may be made to lower the level of alcohol in the patient's blood. Gastric lavage may be beneficial if the stomach still contains a large amount of unabsorbed alcohol. Substances such as thyroid hormone and insulin with glucose solutions and B-complex vitamins are of questionable value for lowering blood alcohol levels. Because the markedly intoxicated patient may be hypoglycemic, administration of insulin without additional glucose could compound the situation of the comatose patient.

Alcoholic Excitement

A patient in the noisy, combative stage of alcoholic intoxication needs to be calmed and kept from injuring himself and others. The use of sedatives such as barbiturates and paraldehyde may intensify the depressant effects of the alcohol and cause the patient to lapse into coma. The preferred medications, then, would be the tranquilizers, such as chlordiazepoxide (Librium) and diazepam (Valium), or the phenothiazines, such as chlorpromazine hydrochloride (Thorazine) and promazine (Sparine). The antiemetic effect of the phenothiazines may help relieve the patient's nausea, but these drugs might also bring about a severe fall in blood pressure. Intoxicated patients who receive phenothiazines should therefore be kept lying down.

Alcohol Withdrawal Syndromes

Individuals who have maintained a consistently high intake of alcohol may develop various mental and physical symptoms when alcohol is withdrawn. The severity of symptoms depends on the amount of alcohol taken and the length of time the person has been drinking. The mildest symptoms consist of the discomforts of a hangover; the most severe occur with the potentially fatal condition of delirium tremens ("D. T.s").

The agitation and tremulousness of moderate withdrawal may be treated with general depressant drugs or with tranquilizers such as chlordiazepoxide or diazepam. In such treatment, the general depressants substitute for the alcohol, whereas the tranquilizers are used solely for treating symptoms of withdrawal. If auditory or visual hallucinations occur, a phenothiazine-type tranquilizer may be added to the treatment regimen.

The condition of delirium tremens may result in quite rapid death as a result of circulatory collapse. The severe agitation may be controlled by administering one of the phenothiazine drugs with a sedative such as paraldehyde, chloral hydrate, or a barbiturate. An anticonvulsant drug such as diphenylhydantoin (Dilantin) may be given to prevent and control seizures. Cerebral edema may also occur; if it does, the patient may also receive an osmotic diuretic such as urea or mannitol. Intravenous fluids containing vitamins and electrolytes will be administered to counteract the dehydration that can result from diaphoresis and vomiting, and also to correct the avitaminosis which often occurs in chronic alcoholics. Such a patient should not be left unattended and should not be restrained, as this will only serve to increase his agitation.

MANAGEMENT OF THE CHRONIC ALCOHOLIC PATIENT

Continued heavy drinking leads almost inevitably to organic damage. This may occur either by the damaging effects of alcohol or through malnutrition; the chronic alcoholic may fail to eat. The heavy drinker can satisfy a large part of his daily energy requirement with alcohol, because of its high caloric value when metabolized in the tissues. Oxidation of one gram of alcohol produces seven calories—more energy than that obtained from an equal amount of carbohydrate or protein, and almost as much as that obtained from an equal amount of fat. Because alcohol has no nutritional value other than calories, the chronic alcoholic often shows symptoms of vitamin and protein deficiencies.

Heart muscle damage may result from a deficiency of vitamin B_1. This myocardopathy may result in congestive heart failure. Prolonged excessive drinking of alcohol may also have a direct toxic effect on the myocardium, resulting in cardiac arrhythmias during bouts of acute intoxication.

Deficiency of the B-complex vitamins may result in various central nervous system complications including Wernicke's encephalopathy, Korsakoff's psychosis, and alcoholic polyneuropathy. Wernicke's disease is characterized by ocular muscle paralysis, ataxia, and mental confusion. These symptoms may be reversed with massive doses of thiamine. The intellectual impairment of Korsakoff's psychosis is characterized by disturbance in memory and an inability to learn new material. These symptoms are *not* reversible with large doses of vitamins, and because of the nature of this disorder, many patients with Korsakoff's psychosis must be institutionalized. Chronic alcoholics may also demonstrate signs of damage to the peripheral motor and sensory nerves. Symptoms of alcoholic polyneuropathy may include muscle weakness, numbness and tingling of the skin, burning pain in the feet and hands, and aching of the legs. Analgesics may help relieve some of these discomforts; the patient is placed on a high calorie, high protein diet with massive daily doses of vitamins.

Alcohol is directly irritating to the mucous membranes lining the stomach. Heavy drinkers of "straight" alcohol are especially likely to develop acute and chronic gastritis. Acute gastritis is relieved when the alcoholic stops drinking and begins eating again. Antacids, antispasmodics, and antiemetics may bring symptomatic relief of this condition. Alcohol has not been proven to *cause* peptic ulcer, but gastric bleeding is common in alcoholic patients who already have ulcers.

Liver disease is also common among chronic alcoholics. Acute alcoholic hepatitis is characterized by anorexia, nausea, vomiting, abdominal pain, jaundice, and an enlarged liver. The incidence of cirrhosis and fatty liver is much higher among chronic alcoholics than in the general population. Because of the remarkable regenerative properties of the liver, much of the liver damage may be reversed if the alcoholic can be helped to stop drinking soon enough. The patient with liver pathology is also treated with a high protein and high vitamin diet.

Rehabilitation

Rehabilitation of the alcoholic patient requires long-term treatment. There are many forms of rehabilitation therapy; they are all based on the premise that the alcoholic *cannot* drink in moderation. It is absolutely essential, then, that the alcoholic totally abstain from alcohol.

Because alcoholics often abuse other depressant drugs and may become addicted to them, long-term use of tranquilizers and sedatives is not desirable. The major tranquilizers and antidepressant drugs are claimed to be less likely to cause dependence; they may, therefore, be used during periods of anxiety and depression that might cause the alcoholic to start drinking again. Other drugs may be used in two types of rehabilitation therapy—deterrent therapy and aversion therapy. It must be remembered, though, that during rehabilitation, drug therapy is less important than psychotherapy and the personal acceptance and support of other people. Organizations such as Alcoholics Anonymous may assist in meeting those personal needs.

Deterrent Therapy. If the alcoholic really wants to stop drinking, his desire may be reinforced by a daily dose of a deterrent drug such as disulfiram (Antabuse), citrated calcium carbimide (Temposil), or me-

tronidazole (Flagyl). If a patient drinks alcohol after taking a dose of disulfiram, his skin turns bright red and warm; he experiences a pounding headache; his blood pressure drops; he feels faint, dizzy, and weak; and he becomes nauseated. Ingesting such a drug and realizing what consequences will occur if he drinks alcohol may relieve the patient of having to make decisions about whether to drink alcohol. However, the patient's sincerity about wanting to stop drinking must be ascertained before these drugs are given, for fatal complications *have* resulted when a patient continues to drink while taking such drugs. Disulfiram must be used with caution in combination with drugs such as diphenylhydantoin and anticoagulants; Disulfiram may potentiate the action of these drugs and necessitate a reduction in dosage. Other drugs to be avoided are paraldehyde and metronidazole.

Aversion Therapy. Aversion therapy is an attempt to create a distaste for alcohol. The patient receives an injection of the potent emetic drug apomorphine after drinking alcohol; the drug causes violent vomiting. The patient may thus begin to associate drinking with the unpleasant vomiting reaction.

INGESTION OF METHYL ALCOHOL

Methyl alcohol (methanol or wood alcohol) has less of a depressant effect on the CNS than ethyl alcohol. However, it can cause serious poisoning, since it is metabolized into formic acid and formaldehyde in the body. Ingestion of wood alcohol has caused blindness and acidosis, and can prove fatal. Treatment includes correction of acidosis by intravenous infusions of systemic alkalinizers such as sodium bicarbonate and sodium lactate. It has been suggested that blindness can be prevented by administering small doses of ethyl alcohol. Since the same enzyme metabolizes both ethyl alcohol and methyl alcohol, administration of ethyl alcohol is thought to utilize part of the available enzymes and thereby slow down the metabolism of the methanol. This, in turn, slows production of the toxic metabolites of methanol—especially formaldehyde, believed responsible for retinal damage.

THERAPEUTIC EFFECTS OF ETHYL ALCOHOL

Applied locally, ethyl alcohol has many therapeutic uses. It may be used in a sponge bath to increase evaporation and lower body temperature. The same drying effect may be useful in the treatment of otitis externa. Topical alcohol has been used for its antiseptic, astringent, cleansing, and rubefacient properties. Injected close to nerves or nerve ganglia, alcohol may be used as a local anesthetic for the relief of pain.

Alcohol may also be used therapeutically for its systemic effects. Small doses may be useful for sedation and relief of tension. The "appetizer" effect of having an alcoholic drink before meals is thought to result more from the sedation effect and relief of anxiety than from stimulation of the gastrointestinal tract. Cancer patients may receive an intravenous infusion of alcohol to relieve pain and to provide energy. Intravenous infusions of alcohol have also been used in obstetrics for the relief of postpartum pain and for preventing premature labor.

REFERENCES

Gelperin, Abraham, and Gelperin, Eve. "The Inebriate in the Emergency Room." *American Journal of Nursing 70*:1494, July 1970.

Kimmel, Mary E. "Antabuse in a Clinic Program." *American Journal of Nursing 71*:1173, June 1971.

Rodman, Morton J. "Drugs in Alcoholism Management." *RN 30*:51, December 1967.

APPLICATION QUESTIONS

I. *True-False*

For each statement below, write **a** if the statement is true or **b** if it is false.

_____ 1. Alcohol is a stimulant when taken in small quantities.

_____ 2. The presence of food in the stomach does not slow the absorption of alcohol.

_____ 3. A person in an alcoholic coma is usually severely hypoglycemic.

_____ 4. Sudden death from circulatory collapse can occur when a patient is in delirium tremens.

_____ 5. Dehydration occurs with delirium tremens due to severe diaphoresis and vomiting.

_____ 6. Wrist and leg restraints should be placed on the patient with delirium tremens to prevent him from injuring himself.

_____ 7. Pathological changes in the chronic alcoholic result entirely from malnutrition and not directly from the alcohol.

_____ 8. Heavy drinkers may develop cirrhosis of the liver.

_____ 9. Because of the liver's regenerative properties, much liver damage can be reversed when the alcoholic stops drinking.

_____ 10. Alcohol may have a direct toxic effect on the myocardium, causing cardiac irregularities.

_____ 11. If alcohol is taken with disulfiram (Antabuse), the person will experience much discomfort, but no potentially fatal reactions will occur.

_____ 12. Disulfiram (Antabuse) is contraindicated for patients with heart disease.

_____ 13. Disulfiram (Antabuse) inhibits the absorption of drugs such as diphenylhydantoin (Dilantin), isoniazid, and anticoagulants such as coumarin.

_____ 14. One gram of alcohol produces more energy than an equal amount of protein or carbohydrate.

II. *Multiple Choice*

For each of the following questions, indicate the letter providing the *best* answer.

_____ 1. Where does most of the absorption of alcohol take place? (a) stomach (b) beginning of small intestine (c) lower portion of small intestine (d) large intestine

_____ 2. Which of the following drugs would be given to increase the respiratory rate of a person in an alcoholic stupor? (a) caffeine sodium benzoate (b) insulin (c) paraldehyde (d) chlorpromazine (Thorazine)

_____ 3. Which of the following drugs, when used to treat alcoholic excitement, is most likely to cause a severe fall in blood pressure? (a) paraldehyde (b) chlordiazepoxide (Librium) (c) diazepam (Valium) (d) chlorpromazine (Thorazine)

_____ 4. Which of the following would best treat hallucinations during alcoholic withdrawal? (a) paraldehyde (b) phenothiazines (c) barbiturates (d) minor tranquilizers

_____ 5. Which of the following drugs would be used to relieve cerebral edema, if present during alcoholic withdrawal? (a) paraldehyde (b) diphenylhydantoin (Dilantin) (c) urea (d) chlorpromazine hydrochloride (Thorazine)

_____ 6. Neurological complications in the alcoholic are due to a deficiency of which of the following nutrients? (a) thiamine (b) ascorbic acid (c) amino acid (d) glucose (e) vitamin A

_____ 7. What is the common symptom of Korsakoff's psychosis? (a) ocular muscle paralysis (b) disturbance in memory (c) numbness and tingling (d) lack of muscular coordination

_____ 8. What complication of chronic alcohol ingestion is characterized by eye muscle paralysis, lack of coordination, and confusion? (a) Wernicke's disease (b) Korsakoff's psychosis (c) polyneuropathy (d) cirrhosis

9. In addition to blindness, which of the following complications is likely to occur following the ingestion of methyl alcohol? (a) deafness (b) acidosis (c) alkalosis (d) renal shutdown (e) respiratory arrest

10. If it takes one hour for the body to metabolize completely 10 cc. of alcohol, how long would it take to metabolize completely two cocktails with 2 ounces of alcohol in each? (a) 2 hours (b) 4 hours (c) 6 hours (d) 12 hours

III. *Matching*

Match each effect of locally applied alcohol to the situation demanding the effect.

_____ 1. evaporation

_____ 2. rubefacient

_____ 3. disinfecting

_____ 4. solvent

(a) backrub

(b) swimmer's ear

(c) contact with poison ivy

(d) presurgical scrub

Dopermine – a drug found in brain –
Schizos are considered

Blood-spectrum neuroleptics

Promazine
Levomepromazine
Clopenthixol
chlor prothixene
Thioridazine
Chlorpromazine
Reserpine
Haloperidol
Trifluoperazine
Perphenazine
Fluphenazine
Thiopropazate
Thioproperazine .

Long term neuroleptics

anti depressants

tricyclics   (BLAVIL)

Drugs That Affect Mental and Emotional Function and Behavior

SECTION TWO

6

Sedative-Hypnotics and other Antianxiety Drugs

There are three major classifications of drugs used for sedation and the relief of anxiety: (1) the barbiturates; (2) the nonbarbiturate sedative-hypnotics; and (3) the minor tranquilizers or antianxiety agents. The physician must endeavor to determine the underlying cause of anxiety, but while such determinations are being made, medications may be used to provide symptomatic relief.

BARBITURATES AND NONBARBITURATE SEDATIVE-HYPNOTICS

The barbiturate drugs vary in the duration of their action and in the length of time before the onset of action. Sodium thiopental (Pentothal) is an *ultra short acting* barbiturate. When administered intravenously, it acts immediately and lasts for only a few minutes. The major use for this drug is for anesthesia or induction of anesthesia; it is discussed in more detail in Chapter 13. Sodium secobarbital (Seconal) and sodium pentobarbital (Nembutal) are *short acting* barbiturates. These drugs act in about fifteen minutes and last about four hours. Because of their short onset and duration, these drugs are often administered in hypnotic doses of 100 mg at bedtime to help bring about sleep. Amobarbital (Amytal) and sodium butabarbital (Butisol) are *intermediate acting* drugs. These drugs act in about thirty minutes; their action lasts up to eight hours. Sodium phenobarbital (Luminal) is a *long acting* barbiturate that acts within sixty minutes and lasts up to ten hours. The last two categories of barbiturates are more likely to be used in smaller, sedative doses to provide prolonged sedation than in hypnotic doses to relieve insomnia.

Nonbarbiturate sedative-hypnotics include chloral hydrate (Noctec), ethchlorvynol (Placidyl), flurazepam hydrochloride (Dalmane), glutethimide (Doriden), methaqualone (Quaalude), methyprylon (Noludar), and paraldehyde (Paral).

Insomnia

Anxiety and discomfort can often keep a person from getting the rest and sleep he needs. Since hospitalization in itself may be an anxiety-provoking situation, a sedative-hypnotic drug may be ordered to help the hospitalized patient get to sleep. These drugs are considered to produce "natural" sleep, since they do not induce such a stupor that the patient cannot readily be aroused. Habitual use of barbiturates and most other sedative-hypnotics may alter normal sleep patterns and may lead to dependence on these drugs.

If a patient is unable to fall asleep or awakens soon after falling asleep, it is most important that the nurse endeavor to determine *why* the patient is not sleeping. Patients in pain do not respond well to the administration of a hypnotic alone; in fact, pain may seem more intense when these drugs are used without analgesics. Some patients, especially the elderly, exhibit a paradoxical excitement response to sedative-hypnotic drugs, instead of the expected calm. The nurse may help the patient fall asleep without medication by straightening the bedclothing, providing adequate ventilation in the room, offering the patient a soothing backrub or a warm snack, or just by sitting with the patient and offering reassurance by being present.

People vary in their requirements for sleep. Occasional loss of sleep by an otherwise healthy person has no serious consequences. It may be best for a person who cannot sleep to find constructive ways to use the hours of wakefulness rather than worrying about his insomnia. If a patient has a prescription for a sleeping medication, he should be told to take it only when necessary and to keep it out of the reach of children. Preferably, these drugs should not be stored within easy reach of the bed where an already sedated patient might easily take them in overdose.

Preoperative Sedation

The short acting barbiturates or other sedative-hypnotics are often ordered to be given the night before surgery to insure a good night's sleep. The dose may then be repeated approximately one hour before surgery. The patient thus arrives in the operating room calm and sedated, which facilitates induction of anesthesia. To insure safety when hypnotic doses are given, it is best to put the side rails up on the bed and remind the patient not to get up without assistance. The patient should also be instructed not to smoke unattended after these drugs are given, as he could easily fall asleep while holding a lighted cigarette.

THE MINOR TRANQUILIZERS

The minor tranquilizers include drugs such as chlordiazepoxide hydrochloride (Librium), diazepam (Valium), hydroxyzine hydrochloride (Vistaril), and meprobamate (Equanil). These drugs can calm an anxious patient without causing the degree of drowsiness caused by the barbiturates. These antianxiety agents act more specifically on the limbic system, whereas the barbiturates act on the reticular activating system. Small sedative doses of the barbiturate drugs, however, may be just as effective as the minor tranquilizers, cause about the same degree of depression, and cost much less. The newer antianxiety agents are claimed to be more effective than the barbiturates for relieving muscular tension and tremors. Some authorities argue, however, that this action occurs only when the antianxiety agents are given parenterally in high doses.

SIDE EFFECTS AND CAUTIONS OF THE SEDATIVE-HYPNOTIC AND ANTIANXIETY AGENTS

Many of the sedative-hypnotics and antianxiety drugs have similar side effects, cautions, and contraindications. Patients taking any of these drugs for daytime sedation should be cautioned against driving an automobile or operating machinery. This should be observed at least for the first few days of treatment, until the degree of depression the drug will cause the patient can be established. Patients should be warned against drinking alcoholic beverages when taking these drugs, since the combined depressant effects of even small doses can be dangerous and possibly fatal. Additive depressant effects also occur when two depressant drugs are administered simultaneously. Therefore, if a minor tranquilizer is given with a barbiturate or narcotic, the dosage must be decreased accordingly.

One advantage that the newer depressant drugs have over the barbiturates is their wider margin of safety between a hypnotic dose and a lethal dose. An accidental or deliberate overdose of a minor tranquilizer may produce stupor or coma, but death is rare. With an overdose of barbiturates, death from respiratory or cardiovascular failure is common. Nonprescription products promoted for producing sleep also have a wide safety margin in the degree of CNS depression they cause. They are not free of toxic effects, however, and *can* cause death from causes other than CNS depression if taken in massive overdose. These products may combine drugs such as antihistamines, anticholinergics, and possibly a mild analgesic. Because of the action of these drugs, overdose can cause bizarre symptoms resulting mainly from their central excitatory effects.

Although taking sedative-hypnotic or antianxiety drugs for temporary relief of insomnia will not usually produce dependence, it must be remembered that *all* of these drugs are capable of producing dependence if taken regularly over a long period of time. Most of the drugs can cause physical as well as psychological dependence. They should be used most cautiously with alcoholic patients and other dependence-prone patients.

REFERENCES

DISTASIO, MARCIA NAWROM. "Methaqualone." *American Journal of Nursing* 73:1922, November 1973.

FASS, GRACE. "Sleep, Drugs, and Dreams." *American Journal of Nursing* 71:2316, December 1971.

MORGAN, ARTHUR J. "Minor Tranquilizers, Hypnotics, and Sedatives." *American Journal of Nursing* 73:1220, July 1973.

RODMAN, MORTON J. "Drugs for Treating Anxiety." *RN* 36:57, September 1973.

APPLICATION QUESTIONS

I. *True-False*

For each statement below, write **a** if the statement is true or **b** if it is false.

1. The minor tranquilizers act specifically on the limbic system.

2. The barbiturate drugs act specifically on the reticular activating system.

3. Cautions about operating machinery or ingesting alcohol need to be given only to the person taking a barbiturate drug and not to the person taking a minor tranquilizer.

Table 6–1. Sedative-hypnotics and other antianxiety drugs.

Generic Name	Trade Name	How Supplied	Route	Usual Dose	Comments
sodium pentobarbital	Nembutal	capsules 30 mg., 50 mg., 100 mg.	P.O.	30 mg. P.O. t.i.d. or q.i.d. for sedation; 100 mg. P.O. for hypnotic effect	
		sustained release suppositories 30 mg., 60 mg., 120 mg., and 200 mg.	rectal	adult dose 120 mg. to 200 mg. for hypnotic effect	
		elixir 20 mg./5 cc. teaspoonful	P.O.	20 mg. P.O. t.i.d. or q.i.d.	
		ampuls 100 mg./2 cc. 250 mg./5 cc.	I.V., I.M.	100 mg. I.V. 150–200 mg. I.M.	
		vials 20 cc., 50 cc. 50 mg./cc.	I.V., I.M.	100 mg. I.V. 150–200 mg. I.M.	
		sustained release tablet 100 mg.	P.O.	100 mg.	
sodium amobarbital	Amytal	elixir 22 mg./5 ml. in 16 fl. oz. bottle; 44 mg./5 ml. in 16 fl. oz. and gallon bottles	P.O.	30–50 mg. b.i.d. or t.i.d. for sedation	
		tablets 15 mg., 30 mg., 50 mg., 100 mg.	P.O.	100–200 mg. P.O. h.s. for hypnotic effect	
		capsules 65 mg., 200 mg.	P.O.	65 mg. to 200 mg. h.s.	
		ampuls (dry powder) 60 mg., 125 mg. 250 mg., 500 mg.	I.M., I.V.	I.M. 65 mg.–0.5 Gm. I.V. dose determined by patient response.	Subcutaneous injections may be painful and may produce abscess. I.V. not to exceed 1 cc. of 10% solution/ minute. Ampul should be rotated to facilitate solution of powder—do not shake.
sodium phenobarbital	Luminal	tablets 15 mg., 30 mg., 60 mg., 120 mg.	P.O.	15–60 mg. up to four times a day for sedation	I.V. use only when other administration routes not feasible. Dose should not exceed 10 gr. in 24 hours.
		ampuls (powder) 120 mg.	I.M., I.V.	100–320 mg. for hypnotic effect	
		ampuls 1 cc. 120 mg./cc.			
chloral hydrate	Noctec	capsules 250 mg., 500 mg. syrup 500 mg./5 cc.	P.O.	500 mg. to 1 Gm. P.O. h.s. for hypnotic effect 250 mg. P.O. t.i.d. p.c. for sedative effect	Single or daily dose not to exceed 2 Gm.

Generic Name	Trade Name	How Supplied	Route	Usual Dose	Comments
paraldehyde *sedative-hypnotic*	Paral	capsules 1 Gm. ampuls 2 cc., 5 cc., 10 cc. 1 Gm./cc.	P.O. rectal I.M., I.V.	Dosage varies according to patient need	May be dissolved in oil as a retention enema for rectal administration.
chlordiazepoxide hydrochloride *minor tranquilizer*	Librium	capsules 5 mg., 10 mg., 25 mg. tablets 5 mg., 10 mg., 25 mg. ampuls 100 mg. powder with 2 cc. diluent for I.M. use	P.O. I.M. I.V.	5–100 mg. t.i.d. P.O. parenteral doses individualized	Up to 300 mg. daily may be administered. Use with caution during pregnancy.
hydroxyzine pamoate *minor tran.*	Vistaril	capsules 25 mg., 50 mg., 100 mg. oral suspension 25 mg./5 cc.	P.O.	25–100 mg. P.O. t.i.d. or q.i.d.	
hydroxyzine hydrochloride		vials 10 cc. 25 mg./cc. vials 2 cc. 50 mg./cc. disposable syringe 1 cc. 25 mg./cc. 50 mg./cc. disposable syringe 2 cc. 50 mg./cc.	I.M.	50–100 mg. stat., and q. 4–6h. p.r.n.	Not for I.V. use.

_a_ 4. The dosage of a barbiturate is higher for a hypnotic effect than for a sedative effect.

_b_ 5. Hypnotic drugs are not considered to produce natural or restful sleep.

_b_ 6. Nonprescription medications for sleep do not cause dangerous or lethal effects from overdosage.

_a_ 7. Barbiturates should be used cautiously with elderly persons, as they may cause a paradoxical excitement response.

_b_ 8. The sedative-hypnotic and antianxiety drugs may cause psychological dependence but do not cause physical dependence.

II. *Multiple Choice*

For each of the following questions, indicate the letter providing the *best* answer.

_b_ 1. What is the classification used to denote drugs that are sleep-producing? (a) sedatives (b) hypnotics (c) anti-anxiety agents (d) tranquilizers

_d_ 2. Which of the following drugs is a barbiturate? (a) Placidyl (b) Doriden (c) paraldehyde (d) Seconal

_d_ 3. Which of the following drugs is *not* a barbiturate? (a) sodium phenobarbital (b) Nembutal (c) Luminal (d) meprobamate (e) Amytal

_d_ 4. At 9:30 PM a hospitalized patient appears to be in moderate to severe pain. If no pain medication has been ordered for this patient, which of the following would you do *first*? (a) administer the barbiturate hypnotic that has been ordered p.r.n., h.s. (b) offer warm fluids or a light snack (c) give the patient a backrub (d) call the doctor to obtain an order for pain medication

_b_ 5. How would the average single adult dose of a narcotic be changed if a patient is receiving diazepam? (a) increased dosage (b) decreased dosage (c) no alteration (d) omission of the narcotic

_a_ 6. Which of the following is a long acting barbiturate? (a) sodium phenobarbital (b) sodium pentobarbital (c) amobarbital (d) butabarbital sodium

C   7. If phenobarbital was given at 9:00 PM, what is the expected time of the onset of action? (a) 9:15 (b) 9:30 (c) 10:00 (d) 11:00

III. *Calculations*

1 of 16 mg.   1. A medication order is written for phenobarbital gr. ¼, P.O. In the medicine cabinet, you notice phenobarbital tablets in strengths of 16 mg.; 32 mg.; and 64 mg. How many tablets of which strength will you give?

0.4 cc   2. 2 mg. of Valium is ordered I.M. Injectable Valium is supplied in a 2 cc. ampul labeled 10 mg./2 cc. How many cc. will you give?

15 cc   3. Amobarbital elixir is supplied in a bottle labeled "440 mg./100 cc. (2 gr. per fl. oz.)" How much elixir would you pour to administer 60 mg. of amobarbital?

7

Drugs Used in the Management of Mental Illness

Psychotherapeutic drugs do not cure psychotic patients, but their ability to control symptoms makes it easier for patients to benefit from other forms of treatment such as psychotherapy. This chapter deals primarily with two types of drugs used in the treatment of serious psychiatric disorders: (1) the major tranquilizers, which are used to control the symptoms of schizophrenia and other psychoses marked by agitation and withdrawal; and (2) the antidepressant drugs, which are used to aid depressed patients. The use of lithium salts is also briefly discussed.

THE MAJOR TRANQUILIZERS

The major tranquilizers include the following four classifications: (1) the phenothiazine derivatives; (2) the butyrophenone derivatives; (3) the thioxanthine compounds; and (4) the rauwolfia alkaloids.

The Phenothiazine Derivatives

Promethazine hydrochloride (Phenergan) was one of the first phenothiazines used in medicine. It was introduced as an antihistaminic agent for the treatment of allergic symptoms but was later found to have sedative and antiemetic effects. The apparent versatility of the phenothiazines led to the introduction of more drugs in this class. These derivatives can be divided into three chemical subgroups: (1) the aliphatic subgroup, including chlorpromazine hydrochloride (Thorazine), promazine hydrochloride (Sparine), and triflupromazine hydrochloride (Vesprin); (2) the piperazine subgroup, which includes prochlorperazine (Compazine), perphenazine (Trilafon), and trifluoperazine hydrochloride (Stelazine); and (3) the

piperidyl subgroup, which includes mesoridazine (Serentil), piperacetazine (Quide), and thioridazine hydrochloride (Mellaril). Although all the phenothiazines are similar to the prototype drug, chlorpromazine hydrochloride, in their effectiveness as antipsychotic agents, the three classes of phenothiazines differ from one another in their potency and in the side effects they tend to produce. The drugs of the piperazine subclass, for example, are effective in doses of a few milligrams, while drugs of the other two subclasses require doses of hundreds of milligrams. The piperazines are more likely to cause extrapyramidal motor side effects, while the other two subclasses are more likely to cause side effects of oversedation and hypotension.

Pharmacological Effects of the Phenothiazines. The phenothiazines have sedative effects, antipsychotic effects, antiemetic effects, potentiating effects, and autonomic blocking effects. The autonomic blocking effects occur more commonly with the aliphatic and piperazine subgroups. These effects, which result in undesirable symptoms, will be discussed later in the section on adverse reactions. The antiemetic effects of the phenothiazines—mainly the piperazine subgroup—are discussed in Chapter 37. The phenothiazines are able to prolong and intensify the actions of other depressant drugs, including the narcotics and the barbiturates. Although this action may be useful for the relief of pain and for preanesthesia, it could prove dangerous if the dosage of the narcotic or barbiturate were not decreased accordingly.

The phenothiazines produce sedation of a different quality from that produced by the barbiturates, other sedative-hypnotics, and the minor tranquilizers. After taking these drugs, patients become indifferent to exciting stimuli without demonstrating severe mental and motor impairment. They do not go through any preliminary excitement phase before becoming calm, as sometimes occurs when alcohol or barbiturates are used. Large doses of these drugs do not cause stupor, coma, and respiratory distress as other central depressants do. And, because there is no euphoric release of inhibitions, psychological dependence rarely occurs.

Clinical Indications for the Use of the Phenothiazines. Phenothiazines may be used in the treatment of agitation, withdrawal, and mild to moderate anxiety. Patients with acute schizophrenic reactions of all types respond rapidly to the sedative effects of the phenothiazines, especially drugs of the aliphatic subgroup. These drugs are also useful for quickly controlling the excitement and disturbed behavior of patients showing a toxic reaction to LSD and those in acute alcoholic intoxication. The manic phase of manic-depressive psychosis may be brought under control with one of the more sedating phenothiazines. The slower acting lithium salts are administered simultaneously in this situation, and the phenothiazines are often discontinued when an effective level of lithium is attained. The restlessness, confusion, and excitement of chronic brain syndrome and the excitement that may occur in mentally retarded children may also be controlled with the phenothiazines.

Drugs of the piperazine subgroup are often preferred in the treatment of schizophrenic withdrawal to counteract bizarre catatonic posturing and mutism. Chlorpromazine hydrochloride may be just as effective in these situations, however. Lethargic patients respond poorly to the phenothiazines if their state results from one of the depressive syndromes rather than from schizophrenia. Mentally depressed patients who show signs of agitation, however, may profit from the addition of a phenothiazine such as perphenazine (Trilafon) to their antidepressant medication.

Adverse Effects of the Phenothiazines. Side effects of the phenothiazines may result from excessive action on the central nervous system or from inhibition of nerve impulse transmission in the autonomic nervous system. Endocrine imbalances and side effects resulting from allergic hypersensitivity may also occur. Photosensitivity may occur as a side effect, leading to severe sunburn if the patient has prolonged exposure to the sun. The patient may experience drowsiness, dizziness, weakness, faintness, and postural hypotension, especially with drugs of the aliphatic subgroup. In men, temporary reduction in sex drive or impotence may occur when the phenothiazines are administered; women may experience signs similar to pregnancy, such as delayed menses, breast enlargement, and gain in weight. A sudden severe sore throat may indicate the development of a blood dyscrasia such as agranulocytosis, and jaundice may indicate the development of liver involvement. Frequent blood studies

and liver function tests are recommended for patients receiving long-term therapy with these drugs. Motor activity may be reduced when phenothiazines are administered, or the patient may develop signs similar to those characteristic of Parkinson's disease. Drug-induced pseudoparkinsonism is reversible when the drug dosage is reduced or the drug is discontinued. It should also be noted that the phenothiazines may make epileptic patients more susceptible to seizures.

A patient may become alarmed when side effects occur, particularly if they are of such a nature that he feels the symptoms of his disorder are returning. The nurse must assure the patient that the side effects are a temporary result of his medication and should be prepared to educate outpatients in precautionary areas, such as avoiding overexposure to sunlight.

The Butyrophenone Derivatives

There are two drugs in this chemical class. Droperidol (Inapsine) is a neuroleptic drug used chiefly as an adjunct to anesthesia. Haloperidol (Haldol) resembles the piperazine subgroup of phenothiazines in its actions; it is used to control severely agitated manic states in schizophrenia and in manic-depressive psychosis. Haloperidol may also be used to control hostility and confusion in elderly patients with organic brain damage and to control excitement in mentally retarded children.

The most common side effect of haloperidol is pseudoparkinsonism. Such symptoms may be controlled by administering antiparkinsonism drugs such as benztropine mesylate and trihexyphenidyl hydrochloride to minimize toxicity. The initially high doses of haloperidol used to control acute psychotic symptoms are gradually reduced to lower maintenance levels.

The Thioxanthene Compounds

There are two drugs available in this chemical class: chlorprothixene (Taractan), which is similar to the aliphatic subgroup of phenothiazines; and thiothixene (Navane), which is similar to the piperazine subgroup of phenothiazines. Both drugs are used primarily in treating acutely and chronically ill schizophrenic patients. The use and side effects of these drugs are similar to those of the phenothiazines.

The Rauwolfia Alkaloids

Reserpine was one of the first tranquilizers used in psychiatry. However, it and other derivatives of the rauwolfia plant are less effective and less convenient to use than the phenothiazines; as a result, they are reserved for those few patients who are hypersensitive to synthetic antipsychotic chemicals. Reserpine and related drugs are more useful for treating hypertension than for treating schizophrenia. These drugs are discussed in more detail in Chapter 20.

THE ANTIDEPRESSANT DRUGS

There are two main classes of antidepressant drugs: (1) the tricyclic type and (2) the monoamine oxidase (MAO) inhibitor type. Both classes of antidepressant drugs are thought to act by helping to overcome a deficiency of monoamines in the brain. The MAO inhibitors interfere with the breakdown of catecholamines, and the tricyclics increase the amount of free norepinephrine.

Tricyclic Antidepressants

The tricyclic antidepressants include amitriptyline hydrochloride (Elavil), desipramine hydrochloride (Norpramin), doxepin hydrochloride (Sinequan), imipramine hydrochloride (Tofranil), nortriptyline hydrochloride (Aventyl), and protriptyline hydrochloride (Vivactil). These drugs are usually administered first for the treatment of patients with moderate to severe depression, because they are less likely than MAO inhibitors to cause dangerous side effects. If the patient does not respond to treatment with the tricyclic drugs, he can be quickly transferred to treatment with the MAO inhibitors. The reverse is not true. The tricyclic drugs cannot be safely administered until at least two weeks after the MAO inhibitors are discontinued.

Some of the tricyclics are said to possess advantages in treating particular types of depressed patients. Nortriptyline hydrochloride (Aventyl) and amitriptyline hydrochloride (Elavil), for example, have sedative or tranquilizing effects that may be useful in treating psychomotor depression. Doxepin hydrochloride (Sinequan) is claimed to be particularly effective for patients with symptoms of anxiety as well as retardation. If anxiety or agitation is severe, however, it is desirable to administer a phenothiazine drug along with an antidepressant. Protriptyline hydrochloride (Vivactil) is a tricyclic compound with no sedative or tranquilizing effect; the patient may overcome feelings of fatigue through a surge of energy, thus becoming less withdrawn after the drug is administered.

Adverse Effects and Contraindication of the Tricyclics. It is important to observe a depressed patient very

carefully as he becomes more alert and active during drug therapy, because he may also become better able to marshal his energies for a suicide attempt at this time.

As previously mentioned, the tricyclic antidepressants may affect the central nervous system to produce symptoms of either excitement or drowsiness. Other side effects of these drugs result from actions on the autonomic nervous system. They include mouth dryness, blurred vision, constipation, nausea and vomiting, headache, difficulty in voiding, postural hypotension, localized sweating, and impotence and delayed ejaculation in men. Motor overstimulation may result in muscle twitching and tremors, hyperreflexia, and possibly in convulsions. Sensory signs such as tinnitus and parasthesia may also occur. Hypersensitivity reactions may include obstructive jaundice, agranulocytosis, and skin eruptions.

Massive overdosage of the tricyclics may result in cardiac arrhythmias, including fatal fibrillations or asystole.

The tricyclic compounds should be used with caution for patients with glaucoma, prostatic hypertrophy, or cardiovascular disease. These drugs should not be administered together with drugs of the MAO inhibitor class, because this combination would tend to potentiate the central stimulation and autonomic blocking effects of the tricyclics.

Monoamine Oxidase Inhibitor Antidepressants

The MAO inhibitor drugs include isocarboxazid (Marplan), nialamide (Niamid), phenelzine sulfate (Nardil), and tranylcypromine (Parnate). These drugs are usually reserved for treating patients who do not respond to the safer tricyclic drugs. They are beneficial for patients who suffer from psychoneurotic or reactive depression. Some schizophrenic patients with depressive symptoms may, however, respond better to a combination of an MAO inhibitor drug with one of the phenothiazines than to treatment with the tricyclics.

Adverse Effects of MAO Inhibitor Drugs. Postural hypotension may occur when MAO inhibitor drugs are administered. More dangerous, however, are episodes of *hyper*tension that may result in hypertensive crisis, leading to fatal cerebral hemorrhage. Because of this danger, MAO inhibitor drugs are used with caution for patients with cerebrovascular disease and hypertension. Tranylcypromine (Parnate), the most potent drug of this class, is not ordinarily administered to any patients more than sixty years old.

Side effects like those of atropine—mouth dryness, blurred vision, constipation, and difficulty in voiding —may occur with the MAO inhibitor drugs. Delayed ejaculation or impotence and localized sweating may also occur. Central side effects include an initial feeling of euphoria, which may progress to manic hallucinations, delirium, and convulsions. Hypersensitivity reactions may also occur with these drugs.

A patient taking a MAO inhibitor drug should be warned against taking *any* other medication without checking first with his physicians. Severe drug interactions occur when MAO inhibitors are combined with many other drugs—some of which can be found in proprietary preparations. Drug interactions may occur with other antidepressant drugs, sedatives, analgesics, antiparkinsonism drugs, sympathomimetics, amphetamines, antihypertensive agents, diuretics, antihistamines, and some anesthetics. Foods with a high tyramine content also cause a severe reaction when taken in combination with the MAO inhibitors. Patients taking these drugs, then, should be warned not to eat such foods as cheese (particularly strong or aged cheese), sour cream, wine, beer, pickled herring, chicken livers, canned figs, raisins, chocolate, or soy sauce. The patient should be particularly reminded to avoid alcoholic beverages and depressant drugs such as the barbiturates and narcotics.

Patients maintained on MAO inhibitor drug therapy should have periodic liver function tests; the drugs should not be used if there is a history of liver disease. These drugs are considered contraindicated for patients with glaucoma, prostatic hypertrophy, hyperthyroidism, epilepsy, angina pectoris, and pheochromocytoma.

USE OF LITHIUM SALTS

Lithium salts such as lithium carbonate (Lithonate) may be useful in the treatment of manic-depressive psychosis. This drug does not seem useful in other depressive syndromes or for control of mania or depression in schizophrenic patients. Lithium salts may be used to control acute manic episodes without leaving the patient lethargic. Low, prophylactic doses of lithium salts may also be used along with a tricyclic antidepressant to reduce the relapse rate of acute manic and depressive episodes.

The nurse should observe for signs of toxicity such as anorexia followed by nausea, vomiting, and diarrhea. Other signs of toxicity include drowsiness, muscle weakness, and lack of motor coordination. If signs of impending lithium toxicity occur, the drug must be discontinued.

To prevent lithium toxicity, serum lithium levels should be determined frequently during early dosage and periodically during prolonged maintenance therapy.

REFERENCES

DAVIES, A. L., and O'LEARY, J. "The Use of Chlorpromazine in Schizophrenia." *Nursing Times* 69:1694, December 1973.

KICEY, CAROLYN. "Catecholamines and Depression: A Physiological Theory of Depression." *American Journal of Nursing* 74:2018, November 1974.

KLINE, NATHAN S., and DAVIS, JOHN M. "Psychotropic Drugs." *American Journal of Nursing* 73:54, January 1973.

RODMAN, MORTON J. "Drugs for Managing Mood Disorders." *RN* 33:43, December 1970.

Table 7–1. Drugs used in the management of mental illness.

Generic Name	Trade Name	How Supplied	Route	Usual Dose	Comments
promethazine hydrochloride	Phenergan	tablets 12.5 mg., 25 mg., 50 mg.	P.O.	12.5 mg.–25 mg. 25–50 mg.	
		syrup 6.25 mg./5 cc.			
		concentrate 25 mg./5 cc.			
		suppositories 25 mg., 50 mg.	rectal		
		ampuls 1 cc. 25 mg./cc. 50 mg./cc.	I.V. I.M.	25–50 mg.	50 mg./cc. ampuls are for I.M. use only.

Generic Name	*Trade Name*	*How Supplied*	*Route*	*Usual Dose*	*Comments*
chlorpromazine hydrochloride	Thorazine	tablets 10 mg. 25 mg., 50 mg. 100 mg., 200 mg.	P.O.	10–100 mg. t.i.d. or q.i.d.	Maximum dosage seldom exceeds 1000 mg. q.d.
		sustained release capsules 30 mg. 75 mg., 150 mg., 200 mg., 300 mg.			
		syrup 10 mg./5 cc. in 4 fl. oz. bottle			
		concentrate 30 mg./cc. in 4 fl. oz. bottles and 1 gallon bottles 100 mg./cc. in 8 fl. oz. bottles			
		suppositories 25 mg., 100 mg.	rectal	25–100 mg. q. 6–8h., p.r.n.	
		ampuls 1 cc., 2 cc. 25 mg./cc.	I.M. I.V.	25–50 mg. t.i.d. or q.i.d.	Subcutaneous injection not advised. Avoid injecting undiluted Thorazine into vein. I.V. route only for severe hiccups or for surgery.
		multiple dose vials 10 cc. 25 mg./cc.			
perphenazine	Trilafon	tablets 2 mg., 4 mg., 8 mg., 16 mg.	P.O.	2–16 mg. b.i.d. or t.i.d.	
		sustained release tablets 8 mg.			
		syrup 2 mg./5 cc. in 4 fl. oz. bottle			I.V. given very rarely —maximum dose 5 mg. Injection should not be given to patients in coma or severely depressed states. I.M. not to exceed 15 mg. in ambulatory and out-patients or 30 mg. in hospitalized patients.
		concentrate 16 mg./5 cc. in 4 fl. oz. bottle			
		ampuls 1 cc. 5 mg./cc.	I.M.	5 mg. I.M. q. 6h.	
		multiple dose vials 10 cc. 5 mg./cc.			
thioridazine hydrochloride	Mellaril	tablets 10 mg., 15 mg., 25 mg., 50 mg., 100 mg., 150 mg., 200 mg.	P.O.	10–100 mg. b.i.d., t.i.d. or q.i.d.	Not intended for children under two years of age.
		concentrate 30 mg./cc. in 4 fl. oz. and 1 pint bottles.			Daily dose in excess of 300 mg. reserved for use only in severe neuropsychiatric cases.

Generic Name	Trade Name	How Supplied	Route	Usual Dose	Comments
haloperidol	Haldol	tablets 0.5 mg., 1 mg., 2 mg., 5 mg. concentrate 2 mg./cc. in 15 cc. and 120 cc. bottles	P.O.	0.5–5.0 mg. b.i.d. or t.i.d.	Dosage is based on severity of the symptoms.
		ampuls 1 cc. 5 mg./cc.	I.M.	3–5 mg. I.M. q. 4–8h.	Doses higher than 15 mg. seldom required.
amitriptyline hydrochloride	Elavil	tablets 10 mg., 25 mg., 50 mg.	P.O.	25–50 mg. b.i.d., t.i.d., or q.i.d.	Not recommended for children under twelve years of age.
		vials 10 cc. 10 mg./cc.	I.M.	20–30 mg. q.i.d.	
tranylcypromine	Parnate	tablets 10 mg.	P.O.	10–30 mg. q.d.	Not to be administered to anyone beyond sixty years of age. Many drug and food interactions possible.
lithium carbonate	Lithonate	capsules 300 mg.	P.O.	300–600 mg. t.i.d.	Not recommended for children. Serum lithium levels should be determined regularly.

APPLICATION QUESTIONS

I. *Multiple Choice*

For each of the following questions, indicate the letter providing the *best* answer.

a 1. Which of the following antidepressant drugs is a monoamine oxidase inhibitor type drug? (a) isocarboxazid (Marplan) (b) nortriptyline hydrochloride (Aventyl) (c) imipramine hydrochloride (Tofranil) (d) amitriptyline hydrochloride (Elavil)

d 2. The nurse should be observant for which of the following if a patient is being treated with a tricyclic antidepressant? (a) hypertension (b) excessive salivation (c) urinary frequency (d) suicidal attempt

b 3. What is the most important observation the nurse should make to detect toxic effects of an MAO inhibitor? (a) daily weights (b) frequent blood pressure readings (c) frequent hematology reports (d) frequent checking of pulse rate

c 4. Which of the following clinical situations would not be treated with phenothiazines? (a) acute alcoholic intoxication (b) manic phase of manic-depressive psychosis (c) affective depression (d) chronic brain syndrome (e) schizophrenic withdrawal

 5. Which is the safest and most widely used group of antidepressant drugs? (a) MAO inhibitors (b) rauwolfia alkaloids (c) phenothiazines (d) tricyclics

b 6. If a patient being maintained on one of the phenothiazine drugs complains of a sore throat, which of the following actions would be most appropriate for the nurse? (a) check his blood pressure (b) check the results of recent hematology tests (c) observe for yellow discoloration of sclera (d) check the recent urinalysis report

b 7. Which of the following groups of drugs have reduced the need for electroshock therapy? (a) major tranquilizers (b) antidepressants (c) antipsychotics (d) neuroleptics

a 8. Which of the following drugs is not a phenothiazine? (a) Haldol (b) Thorazine (c) Trilafon (d) Mellaril

b 9. Of the three phenothiazine subgroups, which generally requires the lowest dosage? (a) aliphatic (b) piperazine (c) piperidyl

d 10. Which of the following is *not* an effect of the phenothiazine drugs? (a) antiemetic (b) potentiating the effect of narcotics (c) reducing motor ability (d) euphoria *d* 11. Which of the following is *not* considered an adverse effect of tricyclic antidepressants? (a) blurred vision (b) excessive excitement (c) drowsiness (d) tearing and excessive salivation

a 12. Which of the following is the *most dangerous* side effect of the MAO inhibitor drugs? (a) hypertension (b) hypotension (c) nausea (d) euphoria

d 13. Which of the following would be an appropriate teaching area for a patient receiving MAO inhibitor drugs? (1) self-medication with other drugs (2) dietary restrictions (3) prescribed exercise regimen (4) limiting alcoholic intake.
(a)1, 2, 3 (b) 1, 3, 4 (c) 2, 3, 4 (d) 1, 2, 4

d 14. Which of the following conditions may be treated with the phenothiazines? (1) schizophrenic agitated depression (2) chronic brain syndrome (3) schizophrenic reactions (4) restlessness with mental retardation
(a) 1, 3, 4 (b) 2, 3, 4 (c) 1, 2, 3 (d) 1, 2, 3, 4

d 15. Which of the following is indicative of phenothiazine toxicity? (a) metrorrhagia (b) menorrhagia (c) hypertension (d) syncope

a 16. In treating a patient with moderate depression, what is the desired course of action if the tricyclics are ineffective? (a) quickly transfer him to an MAO inhibitor drug (b) wait two weeks before starting an MAO inhibitor drug (c) quickly transfer him to a phenothiazine drug (d) wait six weeks before starting any other drug therapy

a 17. Which of the following statements support the advantages of the phenothiazines over the barbiturates? (1) patients are more readily awakened (2) patients do not go through an initial excitement phase before becoming calm (3) psychological dependence rarely develops (4) susceptibility to seizures is reduced in epileptic patients
(a) 1, 2, 3 (b) 1, 3, 4 (c) 2, 3, 4 (d) 1, 2, 4

II. *Calculation*

13 cc 1. In a psychiatric hospital, a patient is ordered to receive Thorazine concentrate 400mg q. 6 h. If the concentrate is 30 mg./cc., how much would you pour for one dose?

Psychomotor and Other Central Stimulants

Central nervous system stimulants are classified according to their primary action site. Thus they are classified as (1) psychomotor or cerebral stimulants; (2) analeptics, or brain stem stimulants; and (3) convulsants, or spinal stimulants. Some central stimulants also act at peripheral sites. The amphetamines, for example, affect the heart and blood vessels by their direct action on the adrenergic neuroeffectors.

PSYCHOMOTOR STIMULANTS

Caffeine

Caffeine is the oldest of the central stimulants. It is a weak stimulant found in coffee beans, tea leaves, and kola nuts. Caffeine produces mild stimulation and helps to overcome drowsiness and feelings of fatigue. Caffeine may increase one's alertness to sensory stimuli, but there is doubt as to whether it improves learning ability or memory. In fact, caffeine-induced tremors may actually interfere with the efficiency of motor performance requiring muscular coordination.

People may become habituated to caffeine (the "coffee habit") and physical symptoms such as cardiac irregularities, gastrointestinal upsets, and restlessness may occur with overindulgence of coffee drinking. There is also evidence that withdrawal symptoms such as irritability and headache may occur when a heavy coffee drinker is deprived of coffee.

Uses of Caffeine. Caffeine may be found in two types of proprietary tablets. It is added to headache remedies such as A.P.C. tablets (aspirin, phenacetin, caffeine), although its usefulness in this preparation is questionable. Caffeine is also the main ingredient of products promoted for preventing drowsiness. Since a

cup of coffee usually contains more caffeine than one of these tablets, purchasing the tablets may be considered a waste of money.

Caffeine may be used in the treatment of acute alcoholic intoxication. An intramuscular injection of caffeine sodium benzoate may be administered to stimulate depressed respirations in this situation. However, it may be very unwise and even dangerous to encourage a person to "sober up" after consuming several alcoholic beverages by drinking coffee. Caffeine does not hasten the metabolism of alcohol or improve coordination or judgment. Thus the person may be more alert, but he is still at the same degree of intoxication, and still dangerously unfit to drive.

Amphetamines

The most commonly used psychomotor stimulants are the amphetamines. Because these drugs have been abused, their manufacture and use have been greatly decreased in recent years. The amphetamine drugs include amphetamine sulfate (Benzedrine), dextroamphetamine sulfate (Dexedrine), methamphetamine hydrochloride (Methedrine), and methylphenidate hydrochloride (Ritalin).

These drugs produce two types of effects: (1) they increase alertness and wakefulness, and (2) they elevate the mood. However, the amphetamines are not a source of energy; they only mask feelings of fatigue. When these drugs are taken to counteract fatigue and complete some project or activity, the person may become more alert, but his mental and motor abilities remain impaired. Use of amphetamines in this manner can lead to abuse and dependence. Drug abuse has been discussed in Chapter 4.

Clinical Uses of Amphetamines
(1) *Narcolepsy* is a neurological condition characterized by periods of uncontrollable drowsiness. Large doses of amphetamines—25 to 50 mg daily—may be used to prevent narcoleptic sleep paroxysms. Since individuals afflicted with narcolepsy are unable to

pursue an occupation or even a productive social life without treatment, large doses of amphetamines in this case seem worthwhile.

(2) *Hyperkinesis* is a behavioral disorder of children which may be the result of slight brain damage. It is also called *minimal brain dysfunction* or *MBD*. The hyperactivity associated with this condition may be controlled by treatment with amphetamines such as methylphenidate hydrochloride (Ritalin) or dextroamphetamine sulfate (Dexedrine). These drugs often exert a paradoxical quieting effect which enables such children to profit from school classes and psychotherapy. Other disorders caused by hyperactivity of groups of nerve cells, such as selected cases of petit mal epilepsy, may also respond to treatment with the amphetamines.

(3) *Postencephalitic lethargy* and extrapyramidal motor symptoms may also be treated with psychomotor stimulants. Amphetamines may be used to reduce parkinsonism tremors, drowsiness, and oculogyric crisis. Drug-induced dystonias may be treated with intravenous injection of caffeine sodium benzoate, instead of amphetamines.

(4) *Mild mental depression* may sometimes be counteracted by small doses of an amphetamine. Patients with more severe degrees of mental depression are *not* treated with amphetamines. This is because the insomnia and anorexia caused by these drugs may be harmful to patients who are already sleeping and eating poorly.

(5) *Weight reduction* programs may include amphetamines, on a temporary basis, for their anorexigenic properties. It is believed that the usefulness of these drugs in weight reduction results primarily from their mood-elevating action, which helps the obese person adhere to a low calorie diet despite its discomforts. After four to eight weeks of use, tolerance may develop to the effects of the amphetamines; at this time it is desirable to discontinue the drug for a time rather than increasing the dosage. Raising the dosage may lead to cardiovascular side effects or to abuse of the drug. After a few weeks of abstinence from the drug, the patient may lose his tolerance to its effects. He may then begin treatment again with the original dose, if the drug is still needed. Efforts have been made to find safer, more effective anorexic agents, but those introduced so far are all chemically related to the amphetamines. The newer anorexic agents, such as diethylpropion hydrochloride (Tenuate) and phendimetrazine tartrate (Bacarate), are claimed to be less likely to cause central stimulation and adrenergic cardiovascular effects. All the "nonamphetamine" appetite suppressants available, however, are capable of causing these effects and must be used with the same cautions as the amphetamines. The drug fenfluramine (Pondimin) has sedative properties which may make it more useful for people who have insomnia and tend to eat heavily late at night. On the other hand, drowsiness is a common side effect of this drug.

Side Effects, Cautions, and Contraindications of Psychomotor Stimulants

Side effects resulting from central stimulation when psychomotor stimulants are taken include nervousness, restlessness, irritability, anorexia, insomnia, headache, and dizziness. Continued use of these drugs may lead to anxiety, tension, difficulty in concentrating, and confusion; eventually, their use may result in delirium, hallucinations, and toxic psychosis with paranoid delusions. Peripheral side effects include adrenergic symptoms such as cardiac palpitations, tachycardia, chest pains, hypertension, dryness of the mouth, constipation, nausea, vomiting, excessive sweating, and dilated pupils resulting in blurred vision. These drugs should not be used by patients with a history of cardiovascular disease, or drug abuse. Drug interactions may occur when a psychomotor stimulant is administered simultaneously with drugs such as guanethidine, any of the monoamine oxidase inhibitors, coumarin-type anticoagulants, diphenylhydantoin, or phenylbutazone.

ANALEPTICS

Analeptics are drugs which stimulate the nerve cells of the respiratory center and the centers that influence consciousness. Unfortunately, when these drugs are administered in the doses needed to produce clinically desirable effects, they can also cause undesirable effects such as vomiting, convulsions, and cardiovascular or respiratory difficulties.

Uses of Analeptics

Depressant Drug Intoxication. Analeptics may be employed to counteract the effects of overdosage of barbiturates or other central nervous system depressants. Pentylenetetrazol (Metrazol) is a rapid acting stimulant with a short duration of action; picrotoxin is a stimulant with a slower onset and more prolonged action. Both drugs are capable of causing convulsions when administered to patients who are only in relatively light stupor. These drugs may also bring about recovery of the vomiting reflex, without full consciousness, and thereby increase the risk of aspiration pneumonia from the regurgitation of stomach contents.

Postanesthetic Respiratory Depression. Following anesthesia, nurses encourage patients to turn, cough, and breathe deeply to prevent development of atelectasis. Recently, some anesthesiologists have suggested that analeptic drugs might be useful for stimulating deep breathing and hastening the recovery of productive coughing. Doxapram hydrochloride (Dopram), the newest analeptic drug, has reportedly helped to prevent postoperative respiratory complications when infused intravenously for thirty-minute periods.

Chronic Obstructive Lung Disease. Analeptic drugs cannot reverse the underlying cause of hypoventilation in chronic respiratory diseases such as emphysema, but they may help to overcome some of the complications that result from rapid and shallow labored breathing. Drugs such as ethamivan (Emivan)

Table 8-1. Psychomotor and other central stimulants.

Generic Name	Trade Name	How Supplied	Route	Usual Dose	Comments
dextroamphetamine sulfate	Dexedrine	tablets 5 mg. sustained release capsules 5 mg., 10 mg., 15 mg. elixir 5 mg./5 cc. in 16 fl. oz. bottles	P.O.	5 mg. b.i.d.	Not usually given after 4:00 P.M. to avoid insomnia.
caffeine		available in many combination drugs and solutions.	P.O. I.M. I.V. Rectal	0.2-0.5 Gm. p.r.n.	Up to 500 mg. may be given as a respiratory stimulant. Solutions containing caffeine may be given rectally.
methylphenidate hydrochloride	Ritalin	tablets 5 mg., 10 mg., 20 mg.	P.O.	10-15 mg. b.i.d. or t.i.d.	Should not be used with children under six.
phendimetrazine tartrate	Bacarate	tablets 35 mg.	P.O.	1 tablet b.i.d. or t.i.d. a.c.	Not recommended for children under twelve.
pentylenetetrazol	Metrazol	tablets 100 mg. syrup 100 mg./5 cc. in 1 pt. bottles. ampuls 1 cc. of 10% solution 100 mg./cc. vials 30 cc. of 10% solution 100 mg./cc.	P.O. I.V. I.V.	100 mg.-200 mg. t.i.d. P.O. 100-500 mg.	Parenteral route used for diagnosis and treatment of drug-induced depression or coma.
doxapram hydrochloride	Dopram	vials 20 cc. 20 mg./cc.	I.V.	(recommended maximums) 24 mg./kg. q.d. duration 2 days total dose 3.0 Gm.	Maintenance infusion given I.V. at the rate of 1-3 mg./minute. Not recommended for children under twelve.

and doxapram hydrochloride (Dopram) may be used to increase the depth of respiration and to improve ventilation.

CONVULSANT DRUGS

Convulsant drugs stimulate the motor areas of the central nervous system so strongly that muscle groups are forced into violent contractive or convulsive spasms. Substances such as strychnine have no real clinical usefulness; they are best not even used in rodent poisons because of the danger of accidental poisoning.

Convulsant drugs such as flurothyl (Indoklon) and pentylenetetrazol (Metrazol) may be used to produce convulsions in treating psychiatric patients with psychotic depression or certain schizophrenic reactions. Today, however, if convulsive therapy is required, electroshock therapy rather than chemoshock therapy is preferred.

REFERENCES

CASKEY, KATHRYN, et al. "The School Nurse and Drug Abusers." *Nursing Outlook* 18:27, December 1970.

DIPALMA, JOSEPH R. "Drugs for the Hyperactive Child." *RN* 35:61, May 1972.

LEIDIG, RUTH M. "Narcolepsy: Jody's Story." *American Journal of Nursing* 73:491, March 1973.

RODMAN, MORTON J. "Use and Abuse of the Amphetamines." *RN* 33:55, August 1970.

APPLICATION QUESTIONS

I. *True-False*

For each statement below, write **a** if the statement is true or **b** if it is false.

_b_   1. Caffeine is useful in improving the driving ability of a person who has been drinking alcoholic beverages.

_a_   2. Caffeine is useful as a respiratory stimulant in treating acute alcoholic intoxication.

_a_   3. A cup of coffee contains more caffeine than one of the proprietary tablets for preventing drowsiness.

_b_   4. Amphetamines should not be used to treat patients with mild depression, but rather reserved for those severely depressed and withdrawn.

_b_   5. Amphetamines counteract feelings of fatigue and provide a source of energy.

_b_   6. Amphetamines are useful in treating depression, as an adjunct to the MAO inhibitor drugs.

II. *Multiple Choice*

For each of the following questions, indicate the letter providing the *best* answer.

_d_   1. Caffeine may be given by which of the following routes? (1) intravenous (2) oral (3) intramuscular (4) rectal
(a) 1, 2 (b) 1, 3 (c) 1, 2, 3 (d) 1, 2, 3, 4

_b_   2. Which of the following statements about the use of amphetamines for fatigue are true? (1) amphetamines are a source of energy (2) amphetamines have a euphorigenic effect (3) amphetamines may mask the symptoms of fatigue (4) amphetamines allow a task to be completed with no impairment in ability
(a) 1, 4 (b) 2, 3 (c) 1, 2, 3 (d) 2, 3, 4

_d_   3. Amphetamines are *not* indicated in which of the following situations? (a) to treat the symptoms of narcolepsy (b) for short-term obesity control (c) for treating hyperkinesis in children with minimal brain dysfunction (d) to increase motor coordination in the presence of fatigue

_a_   4. What is the intended main action of an analeptic drug? (a) to stimulate respiration (b) to decrease appetite (c) to control vomiting (d) to decrease involuntary muscle activity

_b_   5. Which of the following is a principal danger in administering an analeptic drug to counteract barbiturate overdosage? (a) acid-base imbalance (b) aspiration pneumonia (c) respiratory depression (d) hypotension

_c_   6. What action should be taken if a patient develops a tolerance to the pharmacological effect of an amphetamine drug five weeks after beginning treatment for obesity? (a) reduce the drug dosage (b) increase the drug dosage (c) discontinue the drug for a few weeks (d) supplement the drug with another stimulant

_d_   7. Which of the following are clinical indications for analeptic drugs? (1) postanesthesia (2) barbiturate poisoning (3) epileptic disorders (4) chronic obstructive lung disease
(a) 3 (b) 2, 3 (c) 2, 4 (d) 1, 2, 4

_a_   8. Metrazol is used for which of the following pharmacological effects? (1) as an analeptic (2) as a convulsant (3) in conjunction with electroconvulsive therapy (4) in the treatment of epilepsy
(a) 1, 2 (b) 1, 4 (c) 2, 3 (d) 1, 2, 3

III. *Matching A*

Match each classification of stimulant drugs to its primary site of action.

<u>b</u> 1. analeptics

<u>a</u> 2. psychomotor

<u>c</u> 3. convulsants

(a) cerebrum

(b) brain stem

(c) spinal cord

IV. *Matching B*

Match each drug to its classification.

<u>b</u> 1. Ritalin

<u>b</u> 2. Dexedrine

<u>b</u> 3. caffeine

<u>c</u> 4. strychnine

(a) analeptic

(b) psychomotor stimulant

(c) convulsant

Drugs Used in Neurological and Musculoskeletal Disorders

SECTION THREE

9

Neurospasmolytic Agents

This chapter deals with neurospasmolytic muscle relaxants. Muscle relaxants are used in the treatment of many conditions associated with spasms or spasticity. Spasms are acute muscle cramps originating and occurring in the *musculoskeletal* areas as a result of injury or irritation. Spasticity originates within the *nervous system*, causing involuntary, abnormal muscle movements in response to injury or irritation. In these instances, a neuromuscular blocking agent or a local anesthetic might be used for direct action on the muscles; or, a general anesthetic, barbiturate, or other depressant might be used as a centrally acting muscle relaxant. A major advantage of neurospasmolytic drugs over other centrally acting muscle relaxants is that the neurospasmolytics relieve pain and spasm by more selective action; they do not, therefore, produce the excessive sedation or respiratory depression common to the barbiturates and other central depressants.

Neurospasmolytic agents include drugs such as diazepam (Valium), carisoprodol (Soma), methocarbamol (Robaxin), orphenadrine citrate (Norflex), and meprobamate (Equanil). These drugs are most effective when administered by injection in moderately high doses. Small oral doses have little antispasmotic effect but may be useful because of the mild sedative or antianxiety effect most of them exert.

MUSCULOSKELETAL DISORDERS

Neurospasmolytic agents may be used in the treatment of musculoskeletal disorders such as muscle strains or sprains, whiplash injuries, low back syndrome, cervical root syndromes, and dislocations or fractures. Diazepam, methocarbamol, and carisoprodol act by reducing the responsiveness of spinal interneurons to incoming sensory impulses; this, in turn, prevents initiation of motor responses. These drugs are often used in conjunction with physical and mechanical measures for relieving muscle spasms, such as heat, massage, traction, and bed rest.

NEUROLOGICAL DISORDERS

Neurological disorders characterized by spasticity, such as cerebral palsy, multiple sclerosis, muscular dystrophy, hemiplegia following stroke, and quadriplegia following spinal cord injuries, may be treated with spasmolytic drugs. These disorders result in blocking of upper motor neurons which usually exert an inhibitory influence. Corresponding excitatory neurons, which are not blocked, are responsible for spasticity. The neurospasmolytic drugs are thought to depress the excitatory interneurons and thus restore the balance between inhibitory and excitatory influences.

The improvement caused by neurospasmolytic drugs is temporary and purely symptomatic, since they do not treat or remove the underlying cause. They may, however, permit the patient to benefit more fully from other therapy. For example, children with cerebral palsy may sleep better because of the sedative effect of the neurospasmolytics, and because the drugs reduce involuntary movements. The children can also exercise more easily, with less risk of developing cramps and contractures, because of the reduction of painful muscle cramps. A spastic limb may be easier to manipulate during physiotherapy if involuntary movements and rigidity are reduced with drug therapy. The patient with multiple sclerosis, a disease characterized by emotional lability and periods of depression and anxiety, may benefit from the calming and antianxiety effects of the drugs.

Tetanus

Tetanus is an acute, potentially fatal, emergency disorder requiring very skilled intensive-care nursing. The disease is characterized by severe convulsive spasms which may persist for weeks. The barbiturates, once the only drugs available for treating the exhausting symptoms of this disease, occasionally caused further respiratory and circulatory depression. Today, injectable diazepam can be used to control the movements of the disease without causing dangerous depression of respiration and circulation.

ADVERSE EFFECTS

The neurospasmolytic drugs have a wide margin of safety, especially if taken in small oral doses. They may cause some gastrointestinal upsets, such as nausea, vomiting, hiccups, and epigastric distress. Although excessive sedation is less likely to occur with these drugs than with other central depressants, drowsiness is the most common side effect. Patients should be cautioned against driving a car or operating machinery while taking these drugs. They must also be warned about the additive depressant effects of drinking alcohol or taking barbiturates, narcotics, or other central depressant drugs while receiving a neurospasmolytic. Overdosage can lead to respiratory and cardiac depression and coma.

Cardiovascular side effects of these drugs are usually limited to flushing and variations in the pulse rate (either bradycardia or tachycardia). Hypotension, syncope, and shock can occur, however. These adverse reactions can often be prevented if intravenous infusions are given slowly, with the patient lying down.

Carisoprodol has, on occasion, caused an idiosyncratic reaction after the first dose of the drug, characterized by extreme muscle weakness, transient quadriplegia, and temporary blindness. Methocarbamol may cause thrombophlebitis when given intravenously; it is a very painful medication to give intramuscularly. Orphenadrine citrate has mild anticholinergic action and a tendency to cause blurred vision and dry mouth. When a patient is taking this drug, the nurse should be aware of the side effects, cautions, and contraindications associated with anticholinergic drugs (see Chapter 16).

Hypersensitivity reactions may occur with neurospasmolytic agents. The most common hypersensitivity reaction is a skin rash, although histamine-type reactions may occur. Anaphylactic shock is very rare. Most neurospasmolytic drugs are capable of producing psychological dependence, but their ability to produce physical dependence is questionable. They should, however, be used with caution for patients who are prone to dependency.

Table 9–1. Neurospasmolytic agents.

Generic Name	Trade Name	How Supplied	Routes	Usual Dose	Comments
carisoprodol	Soma	tablets 350 mg. capsules 250 mg.	P.O.	350 mg. t.i.d. and h.s. Children over five: 250 mg. b.i.d. or t.i.d.	Safe use of this drug in pregnancy or lactation has not been established. Not recommended for children under five.
methocarbamol	Robaxin	tablets 500 mg., 750 mg. ampuls 1 Gm./10 cc.	P.O. I.M. I.V.	1–2 tablets q.i.d. 1–3 ampuls daily for not more than 3 days (maximum dosage rate for I.V. 3 cc./minute)	Not recommended for children under twelve unless for use in tetanus. Injectable form should not be administered to patients with known or suspected renal pathology. Should not be used in women who are or may become pregnant. This drug not recommended for subcutaneous administration.
orphenadrine citrate	Norflex	tablets 100 mg. ampuls 2 cc. 30 mg./cc.	P.O. I.M. I.V.	2 tablets b.i.d. 1 ampul	Not recommended for children.
diazepam	Valium	See Chapter 11.			

REFERENCE

RODMAN, MORTON J. "Drugs for Neuro-muscular Pain and
Spasm." *RN 29:62*, May 1966.

APPLICATION QUESTIONS

I. *True-False*

For each statement below, write **a** if the statement is true or **b** if it is false.

a 1. Small oral doses of neurospasmolytic drugs have little antispasmotic activity.

b 2. A patient should not receive physical therapy while under treatment with a neurospasmolytic agent.

a 3. Injectable diazepam (Valium) causes less respiratory and circulatory depression than the barbiturates.

a 4. Methocarbamol (Robaxin) should be administered intravenously with much caution, because it is likely to cause thrombophlebitis.

a 5. Intramuscular injection of methocarbamol (Robaxin) may be painful.

a 6. The patient should be lying down during intravenous administration of a neurospasmolytic drug, to reduce the cardiovascular depressant effect.

a 7. The patient should be cautioned against drinking alcohol when taking diazepam (Valium).

b 8. Blood dyscrasias are the most common side effect of neurospasmolytic agents.

a 9. Most neurospasmolytic drugs can cause psychological dependence.

a 10. Spacticity results from injury within the nervous system.

II. *Multiple Choice*

For each of the following questions, indicate the letter providing the *best* answer.

c 1. As muscle relaxants, neurospasmolytic drugs have an advantage over barbiturates for which of the following reasons? (1) they do not cause physical or psychological dependence (2) they do not ordinarily produce excessive drowsiness (3) in therapeutic doses, they do not produce respiratory depression (4) they are more specific in their physiological action
(a) 1, 3 (b) 1, 4 (c) 2, 3, 4 (d) 1, 2, 3, 4

d 2. Which of the following actions may relieve muscle spasms? (1) application of heat (2) massage (3) traction (4) rest
(a) 1, 2, 3 (b) 1, 2, 4 (c) 2, 3, 4 (d) 1, 2, 3, 4

b 3. If spasms occur, where is the lesion or injury causing them? (a) within the nervous system (b) within the musculoskeletal area (c) in the cerebral cortex (d) in the spinal nerve roots

b 4. Diazepam (Valium) and methocarbamol (Robaxin) are thought to relieve spasms by inhibiting which of the following neurons? (a) sensory (b) excitatory motor (c) inhibitory motor

c 5. Which of the following drugs exert anticholinergic effects? (a) diazepam (b) carisoprodol (c) orphenadrine citrate (d) meprobamate

10

Antiparkinsonism Drugs

Parkinson's disease is a degenerative disease of the basal ganglia, which are part of the extrapyramidal system. This motor tract is responsible for actions that, although voluntary, are carried out automatically without much conscious thought. These automatic functions include activities requiring muscle tone, such as balance, walking, and spontaneous facial expressions. Characteristic symptoms of Parkinson's disease include muscle rigidity, tremors, bradykinesia, masklike facies, and propulsive gait. Even short periods of inactivity can exaggerate the muscle rigidity and lead very quickly to joint immobility and contractures. It is of utmost importance to keep all joints of the patient with Parkinson's disease moving in their full range of motion. The patient should not be kept on bedrest unless absolutely necessary, and tasks he can do for himself should not be done for him. Memory and intelligence are not necessarily impaired with the disease, although the nurse or family may tend to interpret the lack of facial expression as a sign of mental dullness. Because of this, the nurse should make every effort to support the patient and alleviate his discouragement. Symptoms may be increased in stressful situations but may be decreased with purposeful movement or control.

TREATMENT WITH LEVODOPA

Patients with parkinsonism have been found to be lacking dopamine, a neurochemical in the basal ganglia. Many patients have demonstrated remarkable improvement of symptoms when the lack of dopamine was corrected. Levodopa is the drug of choice for treating Parkinson's disease. It is a precursor of dopamine which is converted to the necessary neurochemical in the brain. Because dopamine does not pass the blood-brain barrier it is not used in the treatment of parkinsonism.

Most patients are treated initially with small doses of levodopa; the dosage is gradually increased to an optimum level. Adjusting a patient's dosage may take weeks or even months. The patient should be aware that maximum improvement will not occur until several weeks after the optimal dose level has been reached.

The nurse must be aware of safety factors when assisting a patient with Parkinson's disease. Because of his propulsive gait and tendency to shuffle his feet, he is subject to falls. After starting treatment with levodopa, the patient may try to get up from bed too quickly and may fall because of orthostatic hypotension. Some patients, after beginning treatment with levodopa, become so enthusiastic about their improvement that they attempt activities beyond their abilities. The resulting fatigue, falls, and injuries may change enthusiasm to discouragement.

Side Effects

Many patients experience gastrointestinal upsets when taking levodopa and are therefore advised to take the medication with meals. In addition to gastrointestinal disturbances and orthostatic hypotension, other side effects of the drug may include heart palpitation, weakness, dizziness, increased sex drive, and changes in behavior such as hallucinations or depression. Hypertension may occur if a patient who is taking levodopa also receives adrenergic drugs or MAO inhibitor drugs. It has been found that vitamin B_6 (pyridoxine) tends to reduce the effectiveness of levodopa; therefore, if the Parkinson's patient requires a multiple vitamin, he must take one with no pyridoxine, such as Larobec.

OTHER TYPES OF TREATMENT

Parkinson's disease may be treated symptomatically with antihistamine and anticholinergic drugs to block the effects of acetylcholine. The antihistamines have less potent antiparkinsonism activity than the anticholinergics, but also have fewer side effects. Refer to Chapter 32, for more information about antihistamines.

The anticholinergic drugs, such as atropine sulfate, trihexyphenidyl hydrochloride (Artane), and benztropine mesylate (Cogentin), block the action of acetyl-choline and thus inhibit the passage of motor impulses to the muscles. These drugs may cause uncomfortable side effects such as dry mouth, blurred vision, heart palpitations, tachycardia, facial flushing, constipation, and difficulty in voiding. The patient with Parkinson's disease may require such high doses of these drugs to combat disease symptoms that the side effects can be quite intolerable. Anticholinergic drugs should be used with caution for patients with glaucoma, asthma, or prostatic hypertrophy. Refer to Chapter 16 for a more complete discussion of anti-cholinergic drugs.

Table 10-1. Antiparkinsonism Drugs.

Generic Name	Trade Name	How Supplied	Routes	Usual Dose	Comments
levodopa	Larodopa	tablets 0.1 Gm., 0.25 Gm., 0.5 Gm. capsules 0.25 Gm., 0.5 Gm.	P.O.	Individualized: Initially, 0.5 Gm. –1 Gm./day divided in two or more doses with food. Then increased gradually in maximum increments of 0.75 Gm. every three to seven days.	Therapeutic response may not be reached for six months. The safety of this drug in children under twelve has not been established. Maximum daily dosage should not exceed 8 Gm.
benztropine mesylate	Cogentin	tablets 0.5 mg., 1 mg., 2 mg. ampuls 2 cc. 1 mg./cc.	P.O. I.V. I.M.	Lowest dose that provides optimum relief with minimum of side effects. Not to exceed 6 mg./day.	
trihexyphenidyl hydrochloride	Artane	elixir 2 mg./5 cc. in 16 fl. oz. bottles tablets 2 mg., 5 mg. sustained release capsules 5 mg.	P.O.	Individualized.	
biperiden	Akineton	tablets 2 mg. ampuls 1 cc. 5 mg./cc.	P.O. I.V. I.M.	1 tablet t.i.d. or q.i.d.	
diphenhydramine hydrochloride	Benadryl	elixir 12.5 mg./5 cc. capsules 25 mg., 50 mg. vials 10 cc., 30 cc. 10 mg./cc. 10 cc., 50 mg./cc. disposable syringe 50 mg./cc. ampuls 50 mg./1 cc.	P.O. I.V. I.M.	2–4 tsp. t.i.d. or q.i.d. Adult: 50 mg. t.i.d. or q.i.d. 10–50 mg. I.V. or deeply I.M. Maximum daily dosage 400 mg.	
amantadine hydrochloride	Symmetrel	syrup 50 mg./5 cc. in 1 pt. bottles capsules 100 mg.	P.O.	Adult: 100 mg. b.i.d. Child: age 1–9: 2–4 mg./lb.; age 9–12: 100 mg. b.i.d.	

REFERENCES

CARINI, ESTA, and OWENS, GUY. *Neurological and Neurosurgical Nursing.* ed. 6. St. Louis: C. V. Mosby, 1974.

COTZIAS, GEORGE; VAN WOERT, MELVIN H.; and SCHEFFER, LEWIS M. "Aromatic Amino Acids and Modification of Parkinsonism." *The New England Journal of Medicine* 276:374, Feb. 16, 1967.

DIPALMA, JOSEPH R. "L. Dopa, New Hope for C.N.S. Disease." *RN* 34:63, March 1971.

FANGMAN, ANNE, and O'MALLEY, WILLIAM E. "L-Dopa and the Patient with Parkinson's Disease." *American Journal of Nursing* 69:1455, July 1969.

RODMAN, MORTON J. "Advances in Treating Parkinsonism." *RN* 32:59, November 1969.

APPLICATION QUESTIONS

I. *True-False*

For each statement below, write **a** if the statement is true or **b** if it is false.

_a_ 1. Atropine is an anticholinergic drug.

_b_ 2. Levodopa is used to treat Parkinson's disease if the patient has glaucoma, in which case the anticholinergics are contraindicated.

_a_ 3. Any antiparkinsonism drug must be used with caution in patients with prostatic hypertrophy.

_b_ 4. To prevent accidental falls and injury, the patient with Parkinson's disease should be encouraged to stay in bed when beginning treatment with levodopa.

_b_ 5. Artane and Cogentin help maintain muscle tone and contractibility.

II. *Multiple Choice*

For each of the following questions, indicate the letter providing the *best* answer.

_d_ 1. Which of the following symptoms do *not* usually occur with Parkinson's disease? (a) tremor (b) masklike facies (c) bradykinesis (d) mental impairment

_d_ 2. How should the activity of a patient receiving levodopa be altered? (a) It should be increased to prevent urinary retention. (b) It should be decreased to prevent hypertension. (c) It should be decreased to promote tissue healing. (d) It should not be changed from pretherapy, but he should be observed to prevent fainting, falls, and fatigue.

_b_ 3. Which of the following would be the *best* guide in caring for a patient with Parkinson's disease? (a)

Keep him quiet, with external stimuli reduced to a minimum. (b) Keep him physically independent as long as possible. (c) Keep him stimulated physically and emotionally. (d) Build up his resistance against infection.

_c_ 4. What is the primary action of levodopa? (a) reducing the effectiveness of acetylcholine (b) acting directly on the basal ganglia to block their inhibitory mechanism (c) converting to dopamine in the body

_b_ 5. Which of the following is *not* a side effect of the anticholinergic drugs? (a) blurring of vision (b) excessive salivation (c) constipation (d) difficulty in voiding

_c_ 6. Why are antihistamines not widely used for the treatment of Parkinson's disease? (a) dangerous side effects (b) high cost (c) weak antiparkinsonism activity (d) rapid development of tolerance

_a_ 7. What is the most common side effect of levodopa? (a) gastrointestinal upset (b) increased libido (c) hallucinations (d) postural hypotension

_d_ 8. Patients taking levodopa who also require a vitamin supplement should take a multiple vitamin preparation that does *not* contain which of the following? (a) thiamine (B_1) (b) riboflavin (B_2) (c) niacin (B_5) (d) pyridoxine (B_6)

III. *Situation A*

Assume that each of the following orders is written by a physician for a patient with Parkinson's disease. Write **a** if you would question the order or **b** if you would not question the order.

_a_ 1. Complete bed rest with bed bath.

_b_ 2. Cogentin 2 mg. qd. h. s.

_a_ 3. L-Dopa 4 mg. q.i.d.

_b_ 4. To Physical Therapy t.i.d.

IV. *Situation B*

Assume that each of the following orders is written by a physician for a patient with Parkinson's disease, *taking levodopa.* Write **a** if you would question the order or **b** if you would not question the order.

_b_ 1. Blood pressure standing and lying b.i.d.

_a_ 2. Multiple vitamin q.d.

_a_ 3. Epinephrine .5 mg. I.M. q 6h p.r.n.

_b_ 4. Neostigmine .5 mg. I.M. p.r.n. urinary retention

_b_ 5. Milk of Magnesia oz. 1 h.s.

_a_ 6. Kaopectate 30 ml. q.d.

V. *Calculations*

—— 1. A patient is to receive Artane elixir 3mg t.i.d. The elixir strength is 2 mg/5cc. How many cc. will he receive for each dose? How many teaspoons would you tell the patient to take for each dose when he goes home?

—— 2. A patient is to receive 2.6 Gm of levodopa in one dose. Tablets are available in strengths of 0.1 Gm, 0.25 Gm, and 0.5 Gm. How many tablets of which strengths would you take to the patient?

11

Anticonvulsants

Seizures are sudden, abnormal discharges of electrical energy from abnormally functioning brain cells, which result in transient disturbances of cerebral functions. Seizures may be symptomatic, indicating a lesion in the brain, such as a tumor; they may be acquired as sequelae following head trauma; or they may be idiopathic, meaning that the underlying cause is unknown. The majority of patients who experience seizures have recurrent episodes and are diagnosed as having epilepsy.

Epilepsy is considered a chronic illness because patients are usually required to take medication daily for the rest of their lives. Epilepsy may interfere with a patient's normal daily patterns. Sometimes this interference is justified, depending on the severity of the seizures, and particularly if they cannot be completely controlled. Often, however, the interference with daily living is caused more by public ignorance and fear, which have attached a stigma to the disease.

TYPES OF SEIZURES

Seizures can be classified in many ways. For the purpose of discussion here, the following classification will be used: (1) major motor; (2) petit mal; (3) minor motor; and (4) psychomotor.

Major Motor Seizures

Included in this category are seizures of the grand mal type and those of the focal or Jacksonian type. The typical grand mal seizure includes an aura, a tonic phase, a clonic phase, and a postictal phase. The focal, or Jacksonian, seizure is similar to the clonic phase of the grand mal seizure. It differs from the grand mal seizure in that seizure activity is usually unilateral and the patient does not lose consciousness.

Treatment. Drugs of choice for major motor seizures are sodium phenobarbital (Luminal), primidone (Mysoline), and diphenylhydantoin sodium (Dilantin). These drugs may be used alone or in combination. The objective of drug therapy is to render the patient seizure free with no adverse reactions from the anticonvulsant.

Phenobarbital is the safest drug for long-term use, because it does not cause the organ toxicity or bone marrow damage that might be seen with other anticonvulsants. Side effects of normal anticonvulsant dosage of phenobarbital are generally limited to drowsiness and headache.

Early treatment with primidone is often accompanied by drowsiness, headache, and ataxia. These side effects may cease as the patient becomes more tolerant of the drug. Other side effects that may occur with primidone are skin rash, nausea, vomiting, and blood changes such as leukopenia or megaloblastic anemia. Pregnant women maintained on primidone may need to take vitamin K for one month prior to delivery to avoid hemorrhages in the baby. Nursing mothers who use this drug may find that their babies become quite drowsy; some adjustment in drug therapy or feeding patterns should be made. Serious toxicity with primidone is not common.

Side effects of diphenylhydantoin may include lethargy, nystagmus, diplopia, nausea, vomiting, ataxia, dizziness, and blood changes such as megaloblastic anemia. Occasionally, a more serious blood dyscrasia may develop. Gingival hyperplasia may occur with diphenylhydantoin therapy, so the patient should be encouraged to follow thorough mouth hygiene and to make routine visits to the dentist. The patient taking diphenylhydantoin should be warned against taking other medication without checking with a physician. Certain drugs, such as disulfiram, warfarin, and isoniazid, may retard the destruction of diphenylhydantoin, leading to toxicity even when normal doses are taken.

Both diphenylhydantoin and phenobarbital can be administered by intramuscular or intravenous injection in emergency situations or if the patient is unable to swallow. Primidone is not available for parenteral use.

Petit Mal Seizures

This classification includes only the classic or absence type seizure, usually seen in children. Such seizures, characterized by a brief blank stare, may occur many times a day. The drug of choice for treating petit mal seizures is ethosuximide (Zarontin). Trimethadione (Tridione) is also effective but is potentially more toxic than ethosuximide.

Side Effects of Drug Therapy. Side effects occurring with ethosuximide may include anorexia, hiccup, nausea, vomiting, drowsiness, and lack of motor coordination. Although serious hematological, hepatic, and renal reactions are rare, periodic blood, liver, and kidney tests are advised.

Side effects occurring with trimethadione may include drowsiness, gastrointestinal disturbances, photophobia, and skin rash. Because of the possibility of exfoliative dermatitis or erythema multiforme, any skin rash should receive prompt attention; if necessary, the drug may be discontinued until the rash is cleared. Blood tests should be observed closely for a continuing decrease in white cells and neutrophils. Blood dyscrasias such as leukopenia, neutropenia, thrombocytopenia, pancytopenia, agranulocytosis, hypoplastic anemia, and even fatal aplastic anemia have occurred with trimethadione therapy. Hepatic and renal disturbances have occurred with this drug; liver and kidney function tests should be observed carefully. Trimethadione should be used with extreme caution by pregnant women.

Minor Motor Seizures

This category includes two additional types of seizures very similar to classical petit mal seizures: *akinetic* and *myoclonic.* Both types are of very short duration and, like the absence or stare type petit mal, may occur many times a day. Both occur primarily in children. Myoclonic seizures are characterized by brief clonic activity of muscles; akinetic seizures are characterized by brief, complete loss of muscle tone.

Drug Therapy. These seizures respond to treatment with the same drugs used for the classic petit mal seizures—ethosuximide (Zarontin) and trimethadione (Tridione). They also respond to the drugs used for major motor seizures, diphenylhydantoin (Dilantin), phenobarbital (Luminal), and primidone (Mysoline). Children who have minor motor seizures do not respond as easily as adults to treatment with the petit mal drugs. However, diazepam (Valium) is reported to be effective for treatment of myoclonic seizures in children.

Psychomotor Seizures

These seizures are characterized by changes in behavior. The activities that may take place during these seizures are extremely varied. The behaviors appear purposeful but cannot be interrupted and are usually not appropriate for the time and place; the patient has no memory of the events. Drugs used to control these seizures are the same as those used for major motor seizures: primidone (Mysoline), phenobarbital (Luminal), and diphenylhydantoin (Dilantin).

STATUS EPILEPTICUS

This condition presents a life-threatening situation for the epileptic patient. The usual cause of this condition is the abrupt discontinuance of prescribed anticonsulvant medication. When status epilepticus occurs, the patient has one major seizure after another; he remains unconscious, has inadequately oxygenated blood and poorly perfused tissues. His vital signs may all be severely affected. The drug commonly used in this situation is diazepam (Valium), given intravenously. Diphenylhydantoin may also be given intravenously, but this drug is more likely to cause cardiac arrhythmias or even cardiac arrest if injected too rapidly. Diazepam is faster acting and safer.

THE NURSE'S RESPONSIBILITY

In general, when caring for any epileptic patient, the nurse needs to inform him and his family that anticonvulsant drugs may cause some drowsiness at first. The patient should consequently be cautious when operating machinery or performing activities requiring alertness. This drowsiness may lessen as drug therapy continues.

The nurse must observe for skin rashes and be alert to abnormal results from blood, liver, and kidney tests. Both the nurse and the patient should watch for any sore throat or infectious illness that could indicate leukopenia. Encourage the patient to see his physician and dentist regularly and to discuss any questions about the disease or the drugs openly with the physician or nurse. Stress the importance of taking medications regularly, and inform the patient of the dangers of not taking the medication. Explain to the patient the importance of informing close friends and co-workers about his condition and of being safety conscious in situations in which a seizure might be dangerous. Also explain the importance of checking with the physician before taking any medication, to be sure it will not interact with the anticonvulsant. Remind him to notify any physician who might be

Table 11–1. Anticonvulsants.

Generic Name	Trade Name	How Supplied	Routes	Usual Dosage	Comments
sodium diphenylhydantoin	Dilantin	capsules 30 mg., 100 mg. tablets 50 mg. powder 1 oz. bottles oral suspension 30 mg./5 cc. and 125 mg./5 cc. in 8 fl. oz. bottles ampuls 2 cc., 5 cc., 50 mg./cc.	P.O. I.M. I.V.	Adult: 100 mg. P.O. t.i.d. Child: 5 mg./kg./day not to exceed 300 mg. daily I.V. 150–250 mg. administered slowly, followed by 100–150 mg. 30 minutes later, if necessary.	Also available in combination with phenobarbital. Must be administered slowly, not to exceed 50 mg./minute I.V. When reconstituting powder for parenteral injection, warm the solution to dissolve the powder.
sodium phenobarbital	Luminal	tablets 16 mg. (1/4 gr.); 32 mg. (1/2 gr.) ampuls 1 cc., 130 mg./cc. (2 gr./cc.)	P.O. I.M. I.V.	Adult: 16–32 mg. P.O. t.i.d. or q.i.d. not to exceed 600 mg./24h. Child: Dosage adjusted to individual situation.	I.V. administration should be limited to situations where other routes are not possible.
primidone	Mysoline	tablets 50 mg., 250 mg. suspension 250 mg./5 cc. in 8 fl. oz. bottles	P.O.	Adult: 250 mg. P.O. t.i.d. or q.i.d. not to exceed 2 Gm. Child: Approx. 1/2 adult dose.	
ethosuximide	Zarontin	capsules 250 mg.	P.O.	250 mg. P.O. b.i.d.	
trimethadione	Tridione	capsules 300 mg. chewable tablets 150 mg. concentrated solution 1.2 Gm./fl. oz. in 1 pt. bottles	P.O.	Adult: 300–600 mg. t.i.d. or q.i.d. Child: according to individual situation	Should be used with extreme caution during pregnancy.
diazepam	Valium	tablets White, 2 mg.; Yellow, 5 mg.; Blue, 10 mg. ampuls 2 cc., 10 mg./2 cc. vials 10 cc., 5 mg./cc. disposable syringes 2 cc., 10 mg./2 cc.	P.O. I.M. I.V.	Adult and Child: individualized	May be used orally in conjunction with other anticonvulsants. Primarily used parenterally for control of status epilepticus. When used intravenously, it should be injected slowly, taking at least one minute for each cc. (5 mg.) given. Use with caution during pregnancy.

treating him that he is taking an anticonvulsant. The patient may choose to carry a card or wear a necklace or bracelet to alert others that he is subject to seizures.

REFERENCES

CARINI, ESTA, and OWENS, GUY. *Neurological and Neurosurgical Nursing.* ed. 6. St. Louis: C. V. Mosby, 1974.

CAROZZA, VIRGINIA J. "Understanding the Patient with Epilepsy." *Nursing Clinics of North America* 5:13, March 1970.

RODMAN, MORTON J. "Drugs for Treating Epilepsy." *RN* 35:63, September 1972.

APPLICATION QUESTIONS

I. *True-False*

For each statement below, write **a** if the statement is true or **b** if it is false.

b 1. The words *epilepsy* and *seizure* are synonyms and can be used interchangeably.

a 2. Trimethadione (Tridione) is potentially a more toxic drug than ethosuximide (Zarontin) when used for treating petit mal seizures.

b 3. It is always best to treat a patient diagnosed with epilepsy with two or more anticonvulsants, rather than only one.

b 4. The dosage of diphenylhydantoin (Dilantin) should be increased if a patient begins treatment with an antituberculosis drug such as isoniazid.

b 5. Women taking anticonvulsants should not nurse their babies.

b 6. Newborn babies of mothers who have been maintained on primidone (Mysoline) are given anticoagulants immediately following birth.

II. *Multiple Choice*

For each of the following questions, indicate the letter providing the *best* answer.

c 1. Which of the following would be a drug of choice in treating petit mal seizures of the "absence" type?
(a) diphenylhydantoin (Dilantin) (b) primidone (Mysoline) (c) ethosuximide (Zarontin) (d) phenobarbital (Luminal)

a 2. Which of the following would be a drug of choice in treating psychomotor seizures? (a) primidone

(Mysoline) (b) trimethadione (Tridione) (c) paramethadione (Paradione) (d) ethosuximide (Zarontin)

a 3. Which of the following is *not* considered a side effect of the anticonvulsant ethosuximide (Zarontin)? (a) increased appetite (b) hiccups (c) nausea and vomiting (d) drowsiness

d 4. Which of the following side effects should the nurse be alert to if a young patient is maintained on long-term anticonvulsant dosage of phenobarbital? (a) bone marrow depression (b) euphoria (c) liver toxicity (d) headache

c 5. Which of the following is *not* considered a side effect of diphenylhydantoin (Dilantin)? (a) ataxia (b) gingival hyperplasia (c) euphoria (d) megaloblastic anemia

a 6. Which of the following would be considered a common oral dose of diphenylhydantoin (Dilantin)? (a) gr. i ss. t.i.d. (b) 0.5 gm q.i.d. (c) 300 mg q.i.d. (d) gr. vii ss t.i.d.

b 7. Status epilepticus is most likely to occur in which of the following situations? (a) increasing the dosage of an anticonvulsant drug (b) abruptly discontinuing an anticonvulsant drug (c) changing from one anticonvulsant to another under a physician's supervision (d) increasing physical activities

b 8. If a patient on a maintenance dose of diphenylhydantoin (Dilantin) is started on daily doses of warfarin, which of the following should the nurse be aware of? (a) The anticonvulsant tends to increase the toxicity of the anticoagulant. (b) The anticoagulant tends to increase the toxicity of the anticonvulsant. (c) The anticoagulant destroys the molecules of the anticonvulsant, so the patient may be prone to seizures. (d) The anticonvulsant destroys the molecules of the anticoagulant, so the dosage of warfarin may need to be increased to obtain therapeutic results.

d 9. Which of the following drugs, when taken with diphenylhydantoin (Dilantin), can increase its toxicity? (a) amphetamines (b) barbiturates (c) primidone (d) isoniazid

c 10. Which of the following is of *least* importance when caring for a patient with toxic symptoms of trimethadione (Tridione)? (a) darken the room (b) have emesis basin available (c) have padded tongue blade available (d) collect urine specimens

a 11. Which of the following areas of personal hygiene needs special emphasis for the patient taking diphenylhydantoin (Dilantin)? (a) mouth care (b) skin care (c) foot care (d) nail care

III. *Calculations*

____ 1. A child weighing 88 pounds is to receive Dilantin oral suspension. The dosage is to be calculated on the basis of 5 mg./kg./day. What is the total daily dose in mg. this child will receive? If the total daily dose is divided into four equal doses, and the suspension strength is 125 mg./5 ml., how much (in cc.) will the child receive for each dose?

____ 2. A patient is to receive 7 mg. of Valium I.M. The medication strength is 5 mg./ml. How much (in cc.) will you give?

Drugs Used for the Relief and Prevention of Pain

SECTION FOUR

12

Analgesics

Relieving pain is one of the most important services that can be offered to a patient. Pain may be reduced by a soothing backrub, a change in position, straightening linens and bedclothing, providing a quiet environment, diverting attention away from the pain, and by many other nondrug measures. Drugs of many different kinds are also used in relieving pain. Drugs that relax smooth muscle spasms or reduce excessive reflex contractions of skeletal muscle may aid in the reduction of pain (see Chapter 9). Local anesthetics and general anesthetics may be used to decrease awareness of pain (see Chapter 13). Analgesics are used to relieve pain primarily by their central action, in doses that do not cause unconsciousness. Analgesics may be grouped in two classes: (1) those that relieve mild to moderate pain, and (2) those that relieve moderate to severe pain.

DRUGS THAT RELIEVE MODERATE TO SEVERE PAIN (POTENT ANALGESICS)

The potent or strong analgesics are mainly narcotic agents. They have several types of pharmacological action: analgesic, sedative, tranquilizing, hypnotic, antiperistaltic, spasmogenic, antisecretory, and antitussive. Morphine, an opium alkaloid, is the prototype potent analgesic.

Opiates act as analgesics by reducing the patient's perception of pain, changing his reaction to pain, and producing sleep despite severe pain. By reducing the anxiety that pain perception ordinarily provokes, they allow the patient to be calm and relaxed. Even though the patient may be aware of the pain, he does not seem to mind it. The ability of these drugs to quiet the patient's anxiety may be a factor in psychological dependence on them. Continued use of these drugs may also lead to tolerance and physical dependence. See Chapter 4 for a discussion of drug abuse and addiction.

Sedative-Hypnotic Effect

Narcotic analgesics can cause narcosis or stupor when taken in large doses. The hypnotic action of these drugs may be desirable if the patient requires complete rest and relaxation. Such sedation would be excessive, however, if the patient should remain ambulatory and active.

Sometimes a patient experiences a paradoxical reaction of restlessness and excitement following the administration of a narcotic, instead of the expected sedation. This reaction can be serious, particularly if the drug has been given in preparation for surgery.

Antitussive Effect

Small doses of narcotic analgesics depress the cough center and may be used to control coughing. The more potent antitussives, such as morphine sulfate, methadone hydrochloride (Dolophine), and hydromorphone (Dilaudid), are usually reserved for use in conditions characterized by both pain and coughing. These conditions include rib fracture, pleurisy, and lung cancer. Codeine and hydrocodone (Hycodan), more commonly employed to control coughing, are less potent antitussives. They are not, however, so capable of producing dependence as the more potent analgesic-antitussives.

Some available antitussives are neither narcotics nor analgesics. These drugs, typified by dextromethorphan (Romilar), may be preferred in many situations because they are less likely than opiates to cause such side effects as drowsiness, dizziness, headache, and constipation.

Spasmogenic Effect

Opiates may directly contract some visceral smooth muscles, causing spasms in the biliary tract and spasms of the urinary and rectal sphincters. The most potent opiates, such as morphine, should not be used for relief of pain associated with biliary colic, ureteral colic, or renal colic, because the spasm and pain will only be aggravated. Since the opiates may lead to difficulty in voiding, they are contraindicated for men with prostatic hypertrophy.

Antiperistaltic Effect

Constipation is a common side effect of the opiate drugs, caused by the increase in sphincter tone, decrease in intestinal peristalsis, and reduction of secretion of bile and pancreatic fluids. Immobility, of course, adds to the constipating effect of these drugs; measures to prevent constipation should therefore be instituted immediately if an immobilized patient is receiving narcotics. Refer to Chapter 37 for a more complete discussion of the treatment of constipation.

The constipating effect of the opium alkaloids may be utilized clinically in the management of diarrhea. One to two teaspoons of paregoric—an opiate—taken several times a day is the traditional treatment for dysentery. Severe diarrhea may be treated with parenteral morphine to prevent dehydration, electrolyte imbalance, and exhaustion.

Lomotil is an antidiarrheal drug containing atropine sulfate and diphenoxylate hydrochloride, a synthetic chemical related to meperidine hydrochloride (Demerol). Lomotil is often used in place of paregoric for symptomatic relief of diarrhea. Although sometimes abused, diphenoxylate hydrochloride has a lower potential for producing dependence than paregoric.

Other Central and Peripheral Effects

Skin and Mucous Membranes. The patient's skin may become flushed, sweaty, and itchy when he is receiving an opiate drug. A soothing bath not only helps to relieve the side effects of the drug, but may also increase the patient's feeling of well-being and aid in the relief of pain. The mucous membranes of the mouth and nose may also become uncomfortably dry, necessitating frequent mouth care and the application of moisturizers to the mucous membranes.

Nausea and Vomiting. Stimulation of the central vomiting mechanism often occurs following the administration of a narcotic. Nausea, vomiting, and dizziness are side effects more likely to occur in ambulatory patients.

If a patient complains of both nausea and pain, the nurse must consider the nausea and vomiting that might be caused by a narcotic before administering it for pain. Particularly if the patient has had surgery very recently, the narcotic may relieve the pain only to have the side effect of nausea and vomiting cause

further pain and discomfort. However, administering both a narcotic and an antiemetic may cause excessive depression. Good nursing judgment is required in such situations.

Respiratory Depression. Respiratory depression is the most dangerous central effect of the opiates. In doses that produce the same degree of pain relief, all potent analgesics are equal in their ability to depress respiration.

The opiates may also exert some bronchoconstriction activity. This effect, along with respiratory depression and antitussive effects, makes the narcotic drugs very dangerous for patients with bronchial asthma, emphysema, cor pulmonale, or any other chronic respiratory disease.

Retention of carbon dioxide may cause confusion and coma, and may precipitate coma in patients with liver damage. Patients with head injuries may experience increased intracranial pressure as a result of cerebral vasodilation caused by retained carbon dioxide.

Patients who have had biliary, gastric, chest, or abdominal surgery may splint their surgical incision and thereby decrease respirations. Administering a narcotic for pain may further decrease respiration and lead to serious pulmonary complications. It is important for the nurse to take advantage of the analgesic action of the drug and encourage the patient to move about, cough, and breathe deeply while the pain is decreased.

Use of Potent Analgesics

Beyond the specific situations already mentioned, narcotic analgesics may be employed whenever moderate to severe pain occurs. However, it is very important to determine the cause of acute pain before administering an analgesic. Narcotics may mask the pain and interfere with accurate localization and diagnosis. Even though potent analgesics must be used with extreme caution in many situations, the relief of pain must sometimes take precedence over the contraindication for the drug.

Pain Medications Given "p.r.n." Medications ordered to relieve acute pain should be administered promptly. Analgesics are more effective if given before pain has become severe and compounded with anxiety. Physicians often order pain medications to be given p.r.n. This order demands sound nursing judgment. P.r.n. does *not* mean that the drug should be given when and only when the patient asks for it. A patient who cannot ask for medication because he is not fully conscious may demonstrate pain by rest-lessness or by a change in vital signs. Careful observations by the nurse may indicate a need for pain medication.

Some patients, not wanting to be a "bother," will not ask for pain medication. They may assume that the nurse will know if and when they should receive medication. If the nurse does not take the time to assess the needs of such a patient, he may have to endure long hours of unnecessary suffering. Some patients believe they should be stoical, and that taking pain medication would indicate weakness. Others may fear taking narcotics because they do not want to become addicted.

If a patient is not oxygenating well or moving about because of postoperative pain, the nurse has an obligation to administer an analgesic if it has been ordered, to prevent the development of complications. The nurse should check frequently with the patient during the first day or two following surgery, as he may require pain medication around the clock for 24 to 48 hours. If, during the night, the patient requests pain medication, the nurse may find the patient apparently asleep when she brings the medication to him. If the nurse's original assessment was that the patient's pain was severe enough to warrant medication, he has probably only dozed and should probably be awakened gently and given the medication to aid him in more restful sleep. Barbiturates or other medications ordered for sleep should never be given at night if the patient is in pain, as these drugs only *increase* the patient's perception of pain.

Preoperative Use of Potent Analgesics

Opiates may be used preoperatively; for this purpose, however, the minor tranquilizers, such as hydroxyzine (Vistaril) or diazepam (Valium) may be preferred because they are less likely to cause the paradoxical reaction of excitement and the postoperative effects of nausea, vomiting, and constipation. Patients who are to undergo a relatively short procedure such as changing a massive dressing, setting a fracture, or reducing a dislocation, are best prepared with an analgesic drug that wears off relatively rapidly, such as alphaprodine hydrochloride (Nisentil).

Neuroleptanalgesia. Neuroleptanalgesia is a new form of preoperative preparation combining a neuroleptic agent with a potent analgesic. The drug Innovar contains the neuroleptic agent droperidol (Inapsine) with a new synthetic narcotic analgesic, fentanyl (Sublimaze). Fentanyl is about one hundred times as potent as morphine; its analgesic action is potentiated

by the droperidol, which induces a state of detached calmness. Because it has little adverse effect on the cardiovascular system, this drug is useful for preparing elderly and poor risk patients for surgery. The disadvantages of Innovar are that it causes respiratory depression, both directly and through skeletal muscle rigidity involving the respiratory muscles.

Nonnarcotic Potent Analgesics

The new synthetic potent analgesic agents were prepared in the hope that they would be less likely to cause dependence. Unfortunately, they are still capable of producing tolerance and dependence. These drugs include pentazocine (Talwin) and methotrimeprazine (Levoprome); they may be less addictive than the opiates, but all the same precautions for minimizing tolerance and addiction must be observed. Although hallucinations have sometimes occurred with pentazocine, it is the preferred drug for relief of chronic pain in ambulatory patients, because it is less likely than methotrimeprazine to cause drowsiness and dizziness. Pentazocine can cause respiratory depression and must therefore be used with caution in patients with bronchial asthma or depressed respiration. Overdosage of pentazocine is treated with the new narcotic antagonist, naloxone hydrochloride (Narcan).

Methotrimeprazine is a phenothiazine derivative. All the side effects, cautions and contraindications of any phenothiazine (see Chapter 7) apply to this drug. Methotrimeprazine does not cause dependence, depress respirations, or depress the cough reflex. It may be administered preoperatively to help reduce apprehension and anxiety and to potentiate the residual effects of general anesthesia. If a patient is ambulatory following the administration of methotrimeprazine, he must be observed closely for the development of orthostatic hypotension, weakness, faintness, and dizziness, which could result in falling and injury.

Narcotic Antagonists

Overdosage of the potent analgesics usually leads to severe respiratory depression, stupor, and coma. Overdose is not treated symptomatically with analeptic agents, but rather with specific antidotes which act by displacing molecules of the drug from the nerve cell receptors. The most commonly used narcotic antagonists are nalorphine hydrochloride (Nalline) and levallorphan tartrate (Lorfan). A new drug of this class, naloxone hydrochloride (Narcan) does not cause the narcotic-like depression that the other two drugs do. As a result, it can be used to determine whether a patient who has taken an overdosage has taken opiates or barbiturates. If the patient responds to naloxone with increased respirations and lightening of depression, his condition is diagnosed as opiate overdose. If the overdose is from barbiturates, his condition will not improve after administration of naloxone—*but it will not worsen either,* as it would if one of the other narcotic antagonists were used.

DRUGS THAT RELIEVE MILD TO MODERATE PAIN

The weaker analgesics are classified as salicylates and nonsalicylates; they are all referred to by their primary pharmacological actions—analgesic-antipyretics. These drugs may be taken in daily doses for long periods of time without producing tolerance or dependence. They are relatively free of serious side effects when taken in doses adequate for relief of moderate headache or moderate pain in joints, or muscles. They are relatively ineffective against pain arising in visceral organs.

Salicylates

The most commonly used class of analgesic-antipyretics are the derivatives of salicylic acid. The salicylates include sodium salicylate, methyl salicylate, and acetylsalicylic acid (aspirin). In addition to analgesic and antipyretic actions, the salicylates also exert an anti-inflammatory action.

Analgesic Effect. Aspirin is thought to relieve pain by a combination of central and peripheral actions. The effects on the central nervous system are believed to be exerted at subcortical sites such as the thalamus rather than on the cerebral cortex; as a result, psychological functioning is not affected. These drugs can decrease perception of pain without causing the drowsiness or euphoria that occurs with the potent analgesics. Salicylates are also thought to act at the point of origin of pain impulses. One theory is that they block the action upon pain receptors of an injury-released polypeptide called bradykinin.

Antipyretic Effect. The salicylates lower body temperature by their action on the heat regulating centers in the hypothalamus. This antipyretic activity treats only the symptom of fever, and not the underlying cause. Many physicians believe it is better to treat the cause of fever with antibiotics or anti-infectives and allow the temperature to decrease as the cause of the fever is eliminated.

Salicylates are still considered desirable for making the patient more comfortable by relieving the symptoms of fever. They also help to avoid the convulsions that sometimes occur when children maintain high fevers.

Anti-inflammatory effect. One of the most valuable properties of the salicylates is their ability to suppress inflammatory reactions in connective tissue. The mechanism of this anti-inflammatory action is uncertain. The salicylates are considered the safest and most effective antirheumatic drugs (see Chapter 31).

Side Effects, Cautions, and Toxicity. The most common side effect of the salicylates is gastrointestinal irritation, especially if large doses are taken. Administering the drug with a snack, such as milk and crackers, or with a teaspoon of sodium bicarbonate may decrease gastric irritation. Gastrointestinal bleeding has occurred as a result of gastric irritation, and overt hemorrhage has occurred in people with previously undetected gastric lesions such as peptic ulcer. Nonsalicylate analgesic-antipyretics are preferred for patients with a history of chronic gastritis, esophagitis, or peptic ulcer.

Although it has not been proven that aspirin products containing alkaline buffers cause less gastrointestinal irritation than plain aspirin, the buffered products are probably preferable. Enteric coated tablets which do not dissolve in the stomach may also be preferred to minimize gastric irritation, especially if large quantities of salicylates must be taken daily.

A patient may be hypersensitive to salicylates. If a patient states that he has suffered skin eruptions or breathing difficulties after receiving aspirin, he may be hypersensitive to the drug. A nonsalicylate analgesic-antipyretic should be used in such a case.

Salicylism may be an early warning of impending salicylate toxicity; it may be first detected by the development of tinnitus. Patients on large doses of salicylates should be questioned frequently about the occurrence of ringing, buzzing, or other noises in the ears.

Salicylate poisoning from the ingestion of large quantities of aspirin is the most common type of accidental poisoning in children. Salicylate poisoning is characterized by convulsions, respiratory failure, and cardiovascular failure. Electrolyte imbalance and bleeding disorders caused by hypoprothrombinemia or thrombocytopenia may also occur in salicylate poisoning.

Nonsalicylate Analgesic-Antipyretics

The nonsalicylate analgesic-antipyretic drugs include the aniline derivatives, such as acetaminophen

(Tylenol) and phenacetin, and the pyrazolon derivatives, such as phenylbutazone (Butazolidin).

The pyrazolon derivatives are too toxic for routine use as analgesic-antipyretic agents; however, because of their excellent anti-inflammatory effects, they may be used in treating some cases of rheumatic disorders. These drugs are discussed in Chapter 31.

Acetaminophen has analgesic and antipyretic effects that seem quite similar to, and as effective as, the salicylates. This drug has only a minimal anti-inflamatory effect, however, and so is not very useful in the treatment of arthritis.

The most common toxic effects seen with drugs in this class involve hemolytic anemia and kidney damage. Acetaminophen, however, has little tendency to cause *any* side effects, even when large doses are taken. This drug is much safer than aspirin for use with children. In fact, a family with small children might wisely keep *only* this product as a household remedy for minor pains and fever, and thereby eliminate the possibility of a child ingesting a large amount of aspirin and suffering salicylate poisoning.

Acetaminophen does not cause the gastric distress that aspirin does; it may also cause less interaction with anticoagulant drugs than aspirin. Acetaminophen is the preferred drug for use by patients who are sensitive to aspirin.

MANAGEMENT OF CHRONIC PAIN

Patients with nonfatal conditions involving chronic pain, such as rheumatoid arthritis, rarely receive narcotic analgesics because of the potential for addiction and tolerance. Addiction may not be regarded as a problem for the patient in pain from terminal cancer; tolerance to the drug, however, must be considered. Care must be taken to avoid such a degree of tolerance to narcotics that even large doses do not control pain. Narcotics are often held in reserve so they will be effective when the terminally ill patient needs them most.

Pain experienced by the cancer patient early in the disease is often treated with nonnarcotic analgesics such as aspirin and phenacetin for as long as possible. An antianxiety drug such as diazepam (Valium) may be added to the regimen. The addition of propoxyphene hydrochloride (Darvon) is claimed to offer more potent analgesia than aspirin given alone. When these nonnarcotic drugs fail to control the pain, a minimally dependency-producing opiate such as codeine may be employed. When codeine or hydrocodone (Hycodan) is combined with aspirin or acetaminophen, the two analgesics have additive effects, because they act in different places along the pain pathways. As further pain relief is needed, an oral preparation of the potent analgesic pentazocine (Talwin) may be given; subsequently, the drug may be given parenterally. When narcotics become necessary, they should be given at irregular intervals rather than on a regular schedule to decrease the possibility of tolerance and dependence. Nonnarcotic drugs should still be used intermittently when pain has temporarily lessened.

TREATMENT OF HEADACHE

Headache is one of the most common pains for which people seek relief. The headaches that most people experience occasionally, characterized by minor pain, are readily relieved by one of the analgesic-antipyretic drugs. People who complain of recurring headaches should consult a physician because of the possibility of organic disease. The most common kinds of recurrent headaches, however, are tension headaches and vascular headaches.

Tension Headaches

Tension headaches result from a person's unconscious reactions to stress. The muscles of the neck and scalp go into a sustained state of contraction. The same kind of muscle tension occurs in people who maintain one head position as they work. Headaches of this kind are best managed by eliminating the cause (change position, exercise and massage the neck, decrease reaction to stress) rather than by repeated use of drugs. If medication is needed, aspirin or acetaminophen is usually sufficient to give relief. For occasional tension headaches of more severity, a weak narcotic such as codeine or hydrocodone may be added to the analgesic-antipyretic drug. Other drugs which may be useful include sedative-hypnotics, antianxiety agents, skeletal muscle relaxants, and antidepressants.

Vascular Headaches

Dilation of blood vessels in the tissues surrounding the brain results in throbbing headaches that are particularly painful. Cranial vasodilation may be caused by high blood pressure or infection, in which case it can be treated. Migraine headaches, however, have a complex psychological and biochemical cause and are not as easy to explain or control.

The ergot alkaloid, ergotamine tartrate (Gynergen) is relatively specific for control of migraine attacks. At the first sign of an impending episode, the patient should take the entire amount of ergotamine that he has learned from experience will stop the episode. He should also cease his activities and lie down in a quiet, darkened room to rest. Side effects, cautions, and toxicity of ergotamine are discussed in Chapter 38.

Methysergide (Sansert), a drug chemically related to ergotamine, has been proven effective for preventing migraine attacks. Because it is potentially toxic, this drug is usually reserved for individuals suffering frequent attacks of migraine that are not relieved by safe doses of ergotamine. Gastrointestinal upset may occur with methysergide, but a more severe side effect is vasospasm in the extremities, heart, and abdominal organs. Methysergide has also caused fibrous tissue damage in the pelvic region, lungs, and elsewhere. It is recommended that methysergide be gradually discontinued toward the end of every six-month period to give the patient a drug-free period of three to four weeks.

Table 12–1. Analgesics.

Generic Name	Trade Name	How Supplied	Route	Usual Dose	Comments
morphine sulfate		tablets 8 mg., 10 mg., 15 mg., 30 mg., 60 mg. various strengths for parenteral use	P.O. I.M. I.V. Sc	8–15 mg. q. 3h. p.r.n.	Included within the jurisdiction of Control Substances Act (CSA).
codeine sulfate		tablets 15, 30, 60 mg. various strengths for parenteral use	P.O. I.M. Sc	15–60 mg. q. 3h. p.r.n.	Included within the jurisdiction of CSA.
meperidine hydrochloride	Demerol	tablets 50 mg., 100 mg. elixir 50 mg./tsp. vials 30 cc., 50 mg./cc. 20 cc., 100 mg./cc. ampuls 0.5 cc., 1 cc., 1.5 cc., 2 cc., 50 mg./cc.; 1 cc., 100 mg./cc. disposable syringe 50 mg./cc., 75 mg./cc., 100 mg./cc.	P.O. I.M. I.V. Sc	25–100 mg. q. 3h. p.r.n.	Included within the jurisdiction of the CSA. Disposable syringes may contain an additional cc. volume to enable mixing with other drugs.
pentazocine	Talwin	tablets 50 mg. multiple dose vials 10 cc., 30 mg./cc. ampuls 1 cc., 30 mg./cc. 2 cc. 30 mg./cc.	P.O. Sc I.M. I.V.	1–2 tablets q. 3–4h. p.r.n. 30 mg. I.V., I.M. and S.C. q. 3–4h. p.r.n.	Total daily dosage not to exceed 600 mg. orally, 360 mg. parenterally. Aspirin may be administered concomitantly. Not recommended for children under twelve. Doses over 30 mg. I.V. or 60 mg. I.M. or S.C. not recommended.
methotrimeprazine	Levoprome	ampuls 1 cc. 20 mg./cc. vials 10 cc. 20 mg./cc.	I.M.	10–20 mg. I.M. q. 4–6h.	May be mixed in a syringe with atropine sulfate or scopolamine hydrobromide only. When multiple injections are used, rotation of the injection site is advisable. Not to be confused with Levophed or levodopa.

Generic Name	Trade Name	How Supplied	Route	Usual Dose	Comments
acetylsalicylic acid	A.S.A.	capsules, tablets, suppositories (commonly 5 gr. tablets)	P.O. rectal	0.3–0.6 Gm. q. 3–4h. p.r.n.	Not to exceed 3 Gm. in 24 hours.
acetaminophen	Tylenol	tablets 325 mg. chewable tablets 120 mg. elixir 120 mg./5 cc. drops 60 mg./0.6 cc.	P.O.	1–2 tablets t.i.d. or q.i.d. p.r.n. children's dosage adjusted according to age	Not to be confused with Talwin. The elixir must not be confused with the drops, which are much more concentrated.
opium camphorated tincture	Paregoric	bottles of various sizes	P.O.	2–10 cc. p.r.n.	Included within the jurisdiction of C.S.A.
diphenoxylate hydrochloride with atropine sulfate	Lomotil	tablets 2.5 mg. diphenoxylate and 0.025 mg. atropine sulfate liquid 2.5 mg. diphenoxylate and 0.025 mg. atropine sulfate/ teaspoon	P.O.	2 tablets q.i.d. 2 teaspoons q.i.d.	Dosage may be decreased as desired response is reached. Used with caution in children. Do not use tablets for children under twelve. Contraindicated for children under two.
methysergide maleate	Sansert	tablets 2 mg.	P.O.	4–8 mg. q.d. with meals	There must be a three- to four-week interval free of medication after each six-month course of treatment.

REFERENCES

BICKERMAN, HYLAN. "Antitussives." *American Journal of Nursing* 63:61, April 1963.

BOYD, E. M. "The Safety and Toxicity of Aspirin." *American Journal of Nursing* 71:964, May 1971.

DIPALMA, JOSEPH R. "Aspirin, Wonder Drug or Placebo?" *RN* 37:55, January 1974.

DRAIN, CECIL B. "Innovar–a Neuroleptic Drug." *American Journal of Nursing* 74:895, May 1974.

DRAKONTIDES, ANNA B. "Drugs to Treat Pain." *American Journal of Nursing* 74:508, March 1974.

HOSKINS, LOIS M. "Vascular and Tension Headaches." *American Journal of Nursing* 74:846, May 1974.

RODMAN, MORTON J. "Drugs for Pain Problems." *RN* 34:59, April 1971.

APPLICATION QUESTIONS

I. *True-False*

For each statement below, write **a** if the statement is true or **b** if it is false.

_b_ 1. The synthetic nonnarcotic drug methotrimeprazine (Levoprome) often causes hypertension.

_b_ 2. Codeine is one of the most potent antitussives.

_a_ 3. Small doses of codeine have no adverse effects upon the patient's respiration.

_a_ 4. A common side effect of the opiates is constipation.

_b_ 5. An advantage of neuroleptanalgesia is the reduced danger of respiratory depression.

_a_ 6. Patients with chronic rheumatoid arthritis rarely receive potent analgesics for control of joint pain.

_b_ 7. Analgesics should not be administered until pain is fully developed.

_b_ 8. Potent analgesics should be given to terminally ill patients on a regular schedule.

_b_ 9. Dextromethorpan (Romilar) is a narcotic antitussive with low dependency-producing effects.

_b_ 10. Buffering substances increase the analgesic effect of aspirin.

_b_ 11. The average single adult dose of aspirin used for headache or fever is 6 grams.

_b_ 12. The salicylates lower body temperature by their action on the cerebral cortex.

_a_ 13. Migraine headache is not easy to control.

_b_ 14. Patients receiving ergotamine for migraine headaches should stay active while the drug is in effect.

_b_ 15. If possible, it is better to treat the fever from infection with an antipyretic and avoid the use of an antibiotic.

II. Multiple Choice

For each of the following questions, indicate the letter providing the *best* answer.

_b_ 1. Morphine would best be used as an antitussive in which of the following situations? (a) pneumonia (b) pleurisy (c) asthma (d) tuberculosis

_b_ 2. Which statement best describes the site of codeine's antitussive action? (a) the sensory nerve endings in the mucous membranes of the respiratory tract (b) the cough center in the brain (c) the sensory interpretation area of the cortex (d) the smooth muscles of the bronchi

_c_ 3. Which of the following drugs is the least likely to lead to dependence? (a) morphine (b) meperidine (c) codeine (d) heroin

_d_ 4. Which of the following are signs of central stimulation following the administration of an opiate? (1) nausea and vomiting (2) pupil dilation (3) depressed respirations (4) restlessness (a) 1, 2, 3 (b) 2, 4 (c) 2, 3 (d) 1, 3, 4

_c_ 5. Which of the following are peripheral effects of the opiates? (1) excessive salivation (2) biliary colic (3) urinary retention (4) itching skin (a) 2, 3 (b) 1, 3, 4 (c) 2, 3, 4 (d) 1, 2, 4

_c_ 6. Which of the following statements should be used as a guide for the administration of analgesics? (a) analgesics are most effective for pain control when given after pain has fully developed (b) analgesics should be administered only when the patient asks for them (c) analgesics are given only when the cause of the pain has been determined (d) potent analgesics are given routinely after surgery

_a_ 7. What is an advantage of using pentazocine (Talwin) instead of an opiate? (a) tolerance is less likely to develop (b) it does not cause dependence (c) it does not cause drowsiness (d) it does not depress respiration

_b_ 8. Opiate overdosage is best treated with which of the following? (a) amphetamines (b) naloxone (Narcan) (c) phenobarbital (d) alphaprodine (Nisentil)

_c_ 9. Place the following analgesics in the sequence in which they would most likely be used to relieve pain for a patient with terminal cancer. (1) pentazocine (Talwin) (2) aspirin and phenacetin (3) aspirin, phenacetin, and diazepam (4) oral codeine (a) 2-3-1-4 (b) 1-2-4-3 (c) 2-3-4-1 (d) 1-2-3-4

_b_ 10. Which of the following are actions of aspirin? (1) altering the mental and emotional state of the patient, resulting in euphoria (2) dulling perception of pain by a combination of central and peripheral actions (3) acting at the point of origin of the pain (4) blocking the action of bradykinin in the traumatized tissue (a) 1, 2, 4 (b) 2, 3, 4 (c) 1, 3, 4 (d) 1, 2, 3

_a_ 11. How often should Sansert be discontinued if a patient is being maintained on long-term therapy? (a) every six months for three to four weeks (b) every six weeks for two to three days (c) every year for six weeks (d) every three to four months for three to four days

_a_ 12. In which of the following situations should the nurse withhold a prescribed aspirin dose for an arthritic patient and notify the physician? (a) "I don't know why, but it seems every time you give me that aspirin I feel funny and find it hard to breathe." (b) "I'm not hurting right now, so I'll just wait and take the aspirin later . . . ." (c) "My stomach gets upset unless I take that aspirin with milk."

III. Matching A

For each situation listed below, write **a** if treatment with opiate drugs is acceptable, or **b** if the situation would be better treated with a nonopiate drug.

b   1. To control pain
     for a 24-year-old-man
     with head injuries.

b   2. To calm an 80-
     year-old lady
     whose husband has
     just died.

a   3. To control post-
     operative pain
     for a 40-year-old
     woman following
     a hysterectomy.

b   4. To control pain
     for a 60-year-old
     woman experiencing
     biliary colic.

a   5. To control phantom
     pain for a 39-
     year-old man 24
     hours after a leg
     amputation.

a   6. To control pain
     and coughing for
     a 27-year-old man
     who has broken
     ribs and a
     smoker's cough.

b   7. To control cough-
     ing for a 12-
     year-old girl
     with asthma.

(a) Could be treated
    with opiate drugs.

(b) Should be treated
    with nonopiate
    drugs.

IV. Matching B

Suppose that you found each of the following drug orders written for adult patients. Indicate whether you would question the order because the dose seems too high or too low, or whether you would give the medication with no question because the dose is within normal limits.

c   1. Meperidine 100 mg.
        I.M. q.6h. pain

a   2. Codeine 100 mg.
        P.O. q.6h. pain

c   3. Morphine gr. 1/6
        hypo q.4h.
        p.r.n. pain

c   4. Talwin 50 mg.
        P.O. q.4h. p.r.n.
        pain

b   5. Demerol 10 mg.
        I.M. q.6h. p.r.n.
        pain

(a) question the order
    because the dose
    seems too high

(b) question the order
    because the dose
    seems too low

(c) give the medication
    with no question
    because the dose is
    within normal limits

a   6. Codeine gr. ii
        p.r.n. cough

a   7. Lomotil 30 mg.
        P.O. after each
        diarrhea stool

a   8. Morphine 30 mg.
        I.V. push (slow)
        q. 6h. p.r.n. pain

V. Matching C

For each of the conditions listed below, indicate whether giving an opiate drug might increase its severity.

a   1. Biliary colic

a   2. Asthma

b   3. Diarrhea

a   4. Urinary retention

a   5. Constipation

a   6. Nausea and
        vomiting

b   7. Cough

(a) condition may be
    made worse by
    giving an opiate

(b) condition will not
    be made worse by
    giving an opiate

VI. Matching D

A patient is brought to the emergency room in a deep coma after taking an overdose of barbiturates. No information about the patient is available, however, and no one knows whether he has taken an opiate or a barbiturate. There are two narcotic antagonists available; indicate which response would occur in this patient with each of the narcotic antagonists.

b   1. Nalorphine

c   2. Naloxone

(a) respiration would
    increase; depression
    would lighten

(b) respiration would
    decrease; depression
    would worsen

(c) no change in respira-
    atory or depression
    states

VII. Calculations

____   1. A patient is to receive 35 mg. of Demerol I.M. The medication is supplied 50 mg./cc. How many cc. will you give?

_____ 2. Levoprome 15 mg. is ordered. The medication label reads 20 mg./cc. How many cc. will you give?

_____ 3. An order is written for 10 mg. of morphine sulfate to be given by injection. The medication on hand is gr. 1/4 per cc. How many cc. will you give?

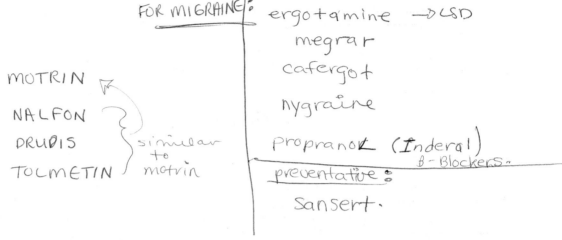

FOR MIGRAINE: ergotamine —▷ LSD
                megrar
                cafergot
                nygraine
                propranoL (Inderal)
                                β - Blockers.
                preventative:
                Sansert.

MOTRIN
NALFON   } similar
DRUDIS   to
TOLMETIN   motrin

related
chemicals {
▽ INDOMETHACIN   —▷ INDOCID
                        |
                 arthritis, gout, inflam. conditions

SULINDAC   —▽ CLINORIL

PHENYLBUTALONG —▷ BUTAZOLIDIN
                        |
        associated blood discrasias, leukemia

_____

            for migraine —

MOTRIN   METOCLOPRAMIDE (MAXERAN).

MOTRIN acetaminophen , indomethacin ,
        (TYLENOL)   (INDOCID)

phenylbutalong ; naproxen , ibuprofen
(BUTAZOLIDIN)   (NAPRESYN)   (MOTRIN)

Anesthetics

An anesthetic is a drug that renders the patient insensitive to touch or pain. Anesthetics are classified as either *general* or *local*. General anesthetics can be used to produce loss of consciousness as well as to decrease reflex movements. Local anesthetics may also affect sensory, motor, and autonomic nerves, but they exert less effect on the central nervous system, and the patient normally remains conscious. General anesthetics are commonly administered by inhalation or intravenous injection; local anesthetics are usually applied topically or injected into the areas that surround nerves.

Any patient who undergoes general anesthesia is exposed to a risk. The danger involved with general anesthesia is greater for patients with asthma, emphysema, cardiac or renal disease, or—in emergency cases—a full stomach. General anesthesia also presents danger to an unborn fetus. In all of these instances, local anesthesia would be preferred if possible.

GENERAL ANESTHESIA

The goals of general anesthesia are analgesia, unconsciousness, and skeletal muscle relaxation. General anesthetics may be classified as *potent, nonpotent,* or *basal,* according to their ability to achieve the above goals. An ideal potent anesthetic should obtain all three goals with relative safety for the patient.

Potent Anesthetics

Potent anesthetics such as ether, chloroform, cyclopropane, trichloroethylene, and halothane achieve all the goals listed above, but each may provide a threat to the patient's safety. Ether was the most widely used general anesthetic for many years; it was potent and relatively safe. It was, however, relatively slow in bringing about unconsciousness and caused very disturbing postoperative side effects. For these reasons, halothane is now more widely used. Because

of their central nervous system effects, all general anesthetics are capable of producing dangerous disturbances, especially of respiratory or cardiac function. Since there is no ideal anesthetic, most patients receive *balanced* or *combined* anesthesia. This refers to the combination of two or more types of drugs to bring about the goals of anesthesia and minimize the dangers.

Nonpotent Anesthetics

Nonpotent anesthetics such as nitrous oxide do not achieve all three of the goals of general anesthesia with safe dosages. All three may be achieved if the anesthetic is given in such high doses that toxicity occurs. Most nonpotent anesthetics are lacking in analgesic or skeletal muscle relaxing properties. They may be useful in combination with other drugs having these properties, producing balanced anesthesia.

Basal Anesthetics

Basal anesthetics such as sodium thiopental (Pentothal) produce rapid unconsciousness; they can be used for rapid induction before the use of a potent anesthetic or alone for short minor procedures. Since basal anesthetics are usually ultrashort acting barbiturates, the doses necessary for prolonged, deep anesthesia would produce severe respiratory depression.

Sodium thiopental is frequently used for induction, because it decreases the amount of inhalation anesthesia needed, and because it brings about rapid unconsciousness without the restlessness and excitement that often occur with slower induction.

Dissociative Anesthesia

Two newer drugs, ketamine hydrochloride and Innovar, are being used for anesthesia alone or in conjunction with other anesthetics. With ketamine, a nonbarbiturate injectable anesthetic, the patient appears awake although he is actually unaware of what is happening. This type of anesthesia is often called *dissociative* anesthesia. It is used with nitrous oxide and oxygen when numerous anesthetics are necessary in a short period of time, as in the treatment of burns. Care must be taken during recovery from this anesthesia to avoid undue stimulation which might lead to delirium and hallucinations.

Innovar causes neuroleptanalgesia; it is a combination drug consisting of a neuroleptic (droperidol) and a potent narcotic analgesic (fentanyl). When used alone, it produces a state of calm detachment and unconcern. If used for premedication before general anesthesia, it will reduce postoperative pain; however, any narcotic given within 24 hours after surgery must be reduced in dosage.

Adjuncts to General Anesthesia

Neuromuscular Blocking Agents. Neuromuscular blocking agents are often used when only light anesthesia is necessary, or to facilitate intubation, as with an endotracheal tube or an esophagoscope. Two types of drugs are used as neuromuscular blocking agents: competitive blockers and depolarizing blockers.

Competitive blockers, such as dimethyl tubocurarine chloride, gallamine triethiodide (Flaxedil), and pancuronium bromide (Pavulon), act by competing with acetylcholine at the receptor site of the motor end plate of skeletal muscle fibers (see Chapter 14). When acetylcholine is obstructed, the muscle fibers cannot contract, and paralysis results.

Depolarizing blockers, such as succinylcholine chloride (Anectine), actually stimulate muscles to contract until they become weak and paralyzed.

The two types of neuromuscular blocking agents produce a similar paralysis. However, overdose of a competitive blocker can be treated by administration of a cholinergic drug such as neostigmine, but overdose of a depolarizing agent must be treated symptomatically.

Succinylcholine is the preferred drug for use in conjunction with halothane, for if tubocurarine is given with this anesthetic, severe hypotension may occur. Another indication for neuromuscular blocking agents, specifically for succinylcholine, is laryngospasm, a complication which can occur during induction of or emergence from general anesthesia. If a neuromuscular blocking agent is given with an anesthetic, such as ether, which has potent muscle relaxing properties, the dosage of the blocking agent must be greatly reduced.

Preoperative and Postoperative Medication. Premedication is usually administered to help the patient stay calm and relaxed and to reduce the amount of anesthesia required. Induction of and emergence from anesthesia are easier if the patient is not fearful or apprehensive. Premedication usually consists of a hypnotic, such as a barbiturate, the night before surgery, and then injectable sedation—an antianxiety agent such as diazepam—approximately one hour before surgery. Because narcotic analgesics may depress respiration, produce postoperative vomiting, and depress the cough reflex, they should not be used routinely for preoperative medication. They should rather be reserved for patients expected to experience a great deal of postoperative pain. An anticholinergic drug such as atropine or scopolamine may be given one hour before surgery to counteract the heart-slowing effect of the vagal stimulation that halothane or organ manipulation may cause; anticholinergics are also given to reduce excessive salivary and tracheobronchial secretions.

Postoperatively, antiemetics such as the phenothiazines may be given to counteract any nausea or vomiting caused by the anesthesia. Phenothiazines are not given preoperatively because, when combined with a general anesthetic, they could cause rapid, dangerous hypotension. Cholinesterase inhibitors may also be given postoperatively to counteract abdominal distention and urinary retention caused by some anesthetics.

LOCAL ANESTHETICS

Local anesthetics are administered in one of three ways: (1) topical application to skin or mucous membranes; (2) infiltration of an area beneath the skin to affect local nerve endings; and (3) regional or conductive anesthesia, injected around the major nerves which supply the surgical field. If a specific nerve or nerves are blocked, the regional anesthesia is called *peripheral*; if the injection is close to the spinal cord, affecting a nerve or nerves as they join the central nervous system, it is called *central.*

Topical Anesthesia

Topical anesthetics such as proparacaine and benoxinate are used on the ocular mucosa when removing foreign bodies from the eye, and for procedures such as tonometry, gonioscopy, or minor eye surgery. For more complicated procedures involving the eye, such as iridectomy or cataract removal, surface anesthesia must be followed by a retrobulbar injection of a local anesthetic.

Anesthetics applied to the skin or mucous membranes decrease pain and itching associated with conditions such as poison ivy, minor burns, sunburns, and minor lacerations. They are also useful with surgical incisions such as episiotomy; fissured nipples during postpartum; pruritus ani or pruritus vulvae; and following surgical procedures such as hemorrhoidectomy. Systemic toxicity is rare with topical anesthetics applied to the skin, because they are poorly absorbed; however, allergic reactions can occur in patients who become sensitized to topical anesthetics. For this reason, it is not advisable to use such products over a long period of time. A person whose skin reacts to other chemicals, such as creams, soaps, and makeup, may become readily sensitized to topical anesthetics.

Although topical anesthetics are poorly absorbed from the skin, absorption may be very rapid through the mucous membranes of the mouth, throat, gastrointestinal tract, respiratory tract, and genitourinary tracts. It is important to keep a record of the amount of anesthesia applied to mucous membranes to avoid systemic reaction.

Infiltrated Local Anesthetics

Local infiltration may be accomplished by injecting the anesthetic directly into the operative area, or by injecting a wall of anesthesia around the operative area. The latter type of infiltration is called a *field block*.

Anesthetics infiltrated below the skin are placed systematically, first into the intradermal sites, then the subcutaneous, and finally into the intrafascial and intramuscular sites. Anesthetics injected into or under the skin will eventually be absorbed into the systemic circulation. Injecting a highly vascular area involves a greater risk of systemic toxicity than injecting a less vascular area. It is very important that the physician aspirate the needle before injecting a local anesthetic to make sure the anesthetic will not be injected directly into a blood vessel. A record must be kept of the total amount injected, and enough time must elapse for the drug's local action to take effect and for any amount of the drug systemically absorbed to be largely eliminated before further injections are made. Administering vasoconstricting drugs such as epinephrine with the anesthetic reduces the rate of absorption and thereby prolongs the anesthetizing action. Vasoconstrictors would not be used in areas of restricted or relatively terminal circulation, such as the fingers, toes, or penis; in such sites they could lead to tissue ischemia and even to gangrene.

Regional Anesthetics

Central nerve blocks include spinal anesthesia, saddle block, epidural anesthesia, and caudal block. Some patients may be fearful of having regional anesthesia because they do not wish to be awake during surgery. They may be told that they will receive premedication for sedation; they may also receive a small amount of a general anesthetic, such as Innovar, ketamine, thiopental, or nitrous oxide with oxygen, for sedation during the procedure.

Spinal Anesthesia. In spinal anesthesia, a lumbar puncture is made and the anesthetic is deposited beneath the arachnoid membrane, into the spinal fluid in the subarachnoid space. This blocks conduction in the spinal nerve routes but has little effect on the spinal cord itself. All three types of nerve fibers—autonomic, sensory, and motor—can be affected. This type of anesthesia is useful for lower extremity or abdominal surgery.

Positioning of the patient receiving spinal anesthesia is an important consideration, because of the relationship between the density of the anesthetic and that of the spinal fluid. Unless prevented by gravity, the anesthesia can diffuse upward and paralyze the intercostal muscles and the diaphragm, causing respiratory distress. To prevent or counteract respiratory distress, the patient's head and shoulders are usually elevated, if the anesthetic is heavier than spinal fluid; opposite positioning would be used if the anesthetic is lighter.

Saddle Block. A saddle block is a type of spinal anesthesia the effect of which is restricted to the sacral nerves running to the perineal area. Sensation is lost in the perineum, buttocks, and thighs—areas that would come in contact with a saddle—but the feeling and motion of the legs are unaffected. Saddle block anesthesia is useful for obstetrical, gynecological, urological, and rectal procedures.

Epidural Anesthesia. The procedure for epidural anesthesia is the same as that for spinal anesthesia. The difference is that the anesthetic is deposited in the epidural space (outside the dura), rather than in the subarachnoid space. The effect is the same as with spinal anesthesia, but there is no danger of complications involving loss or leakage of spinal fluid. Epidural anesthesia may be given continuously by leaving a catheter in place. This procedure is popular for use during labor and delivery. If the catheter is to be left in place, this should be discussed with the patient.

Caudal Block. A caudal block is a regional anesthesia in the epidural space, the effect of which is restricted to the sacral nerves. The same area is anesthetized by a caudal block as by a saddle block. Caudal blocks are difficult to administer, but they are useful in obstetrics and for rectal surgery.

CARE OF PATIENTS AFTER ANESTHESIA

Postoperative care depends not only on the procedure performed but also on the type of anesthetic used. A patient receiving a general anesthetic is unconscious and requires the care necessary for any unconscious patient until he is fully reactive. If inhalation anesthetic was used, deep breathing is especially important postoperatively, because some of the anesthetic is exhaled through the lungs. The patient who has had spinal or epidural anesthesia, though not unconscious, may be drowsy or sleeping, depending on the adjunct medications used. The patient should have been told preoperatively that loss of sensation and movement in his legs would occur, but to avoid worry or panic, the nurse should remind him postoperatively. The legs should be given gentle passive movement at intervals to prevent venous stasis until motion and sensation return. If spinal anesthesia was used, the patient may be advised to remain flat in bed for at least six hours. He may turn from side to side and may have a small pillow under his head, if this causes him no discomfort. These precautions, in addition to forcing fluids, will help prevent headache following spinal anesthesia. Because of improved techniques in administering anesthesia, such "spinal headaches" are becoming less frequent.

Table 13–1. Anesthetics.

Name	Classification and Administration	Dose	Actions and Uses	Comments
Ether	General Potent Inhalation	Induction: concentration of ether in air of 5–7 volumes %. Maintenance: 3–5 volumes %.	Produces excellent analgesia and skeletal muscle relaxation. A safe agent, rarely causing cardiac irregularities or liver damage. Irritates the respiratory mucosa and stimulates bronchial and salivary secretions. Induction is slow.	Recovery is slow. Postoperative nausea and vomiting are common. Caution is required in administering adjunctive neuromuscular blocking agents to avoid excessive paralysis.
Halothane (Fluothane)	General Potent Inhalation	Induction: 1–4% with oxygen. Maintenance: 0.5–2% with oxygen.	A rapid induction anesthesia with little excitement. Loss of consciousness in 2–10 minutes with a rapid recovery. Halothane is the anesthetic of choice for asthmatics because of its bronchodilation effects. It also provides excellent relaxation of the mouth, jaw, and uterus. Often given in combination with other agents for relaxation. Halothane may produce hypotension bradycardia.	Postoperative nausea and vomiting are rare. Intense shivering and a fall in body temperature are sometimes observed in the recovery room. Atropine is the preoperative drug of choice to counteract the bradycardia. Unexplained fever postoperatively is reason to check liver function, since damage may occur if this anesthetic is given repeatedly over short periods of time.

Name	Classifi- cation and Administration	Dose	Actions and Uses	Comments
Cyclopropane (Trimethylene)	General Potent Inhalation	Analgesia: continuous inhalation of 1–2% Induction: 50% inhalation vapor. Maintenance: 10–20 % inhalation; 4 liters needed for 1 hour anesthesia.	A rapid potent anesthetic with a rapid, pleasant induction and recovery. Provides loss of consciousness in 1–3 minutes. Considerable margin of safety.	Postoperative nausea and vomiting are less frequent than with ether and some other anesthetics. Explosive in the presence of oxygen. Postoperative headache and delirium may occur. Cardiac arrhythmias and respiratory depression are possible.
Nitrous Oxide	General Nonpotent Inhalation	Analgesia: 20% nitrous oxide, 80% oxygen. Induction: 80% nitrous oxide, 20% oxygen. Maintenance: 70% nitrous oxide, 30% oxygen.	A nonpotent, nontoxic anesthesia with good analgesic properties, especially useful in labor or short surgical procedures. Has no adverse effect on vital organs. Not a potent anesthetic or a muscle relaxant; therefore, often combined with other anesthetics, hypnotics, and relaxants.	Postoperative nausea and vomiting are rare. At least 20% oxygen must be administered in conjunction with this drug to prevent hypoxia. This agent should be used cautiously in patients with conditions such as pneumothorax, pneumoencephalogram, etc., as it will increase the pressure in these areas.
Thiopental sodium (Pentothal)	General Basal Rectal I.V.	Induction: 2–4 cc. of 2.5% solution injected intermittently every 30–60 seconds. Maintenance: 0.5–2 cc. of 2.5% solution or 0.3% continuous drip. Rectal anesthesia: 10% solution.	An ultrashort acting agent used for brief procedures. Also widely used for induction, in conjunction with other anesthetics. Easily administered with a 30–60 second smooth induction. Recovery short and comfortable. Respiratory depressant. Used in some convulsant disorders and in psychiatric procedures.	Postoperative nausea and vomiting are rare. This drug should not be used for asthmatics, persons with allergies to barbiturates, or when shock or intracranial pressure is present. Endotracheal intubation equipment and oxygen should be readily available. Avoid extravasation, because sloughing may occur. Recovery is short and comfortable, with infrequent complications.

Name	Classifi-cation and Administration	Dose	Actions and Uses	Comments
Ketamine hydrochloride	Dissociative I.V. I.M.	I.V. induction: 1–4.5 mg./kg. of body weight given over 60 seconds. Maintenance: 50–100 percent of induction dose. I.M. induction: 10 mg./kg. of body wt. (6.5–13 mg./kg.) for 12–25 minutes of anesthesia.	Rapid acting nonbar-biturate anesthetic. Used as a sole anesthesia for short minor surgical and diagnostic procedures. Does not provide adequate analgesia or muscular relaxation for abdominal surgery. Hypertension may occur upon administration.	Erratic behavior accompanied by vivid, unpleasant dreams may occur in the recovery room; therefore the environment should be quiet, and the patient should not be stimulated. Concurrent use of barbiturates or narcotics may result in prolonged recovery. This drug should be used with caution in alcoholics. Directions for dilution of prepara-tions must be carefully followed.
Lidocaine hydrochloride (Xylocaine)	Local	Topical: 2% solution, maximum 10 cc. Infiltration: 25–60 cc. of 0.5% solution. Nerve block: 30 cc. of 1% solution. Spinal: 1–1.5 cc. of 5% solution. Regional: 30–50 cc. of 0.5% solution.	Most versatile of the local anesthetics: used topically and for infiltration, nerve block, spinal, and regional anesthesia. Its properties include rapid onset and long duration. For use in minor surgery, 1:500,000 –1:100,000 of epinephrine hydrochloride should be included to enhance duration of the anesthesia and reduce systemic absorption.	The effects of CNS and cardiovascular depressing drugs may be enhanced when used simultaneously with this drug. Maximum dose should not exceed 400 mg. at 2-hour intervals. As with all local anesthetics, patients should be observed for vomiting, hypertension and cardiac arrest.
Procaine hydrochloride (Novocain)	Local Infiltration Nerve block Spinal	Infiltration: field block up to 200–300 cc. of 0.25% solution; peripheral block up to 25 cc. of 1–2% solution. Epidural: 25 cc. of 1.5% solution.	Short acting anesthetic used for infiltration, nerve block, and spinal anesthesia. Often used in combination with epinephrine, which exerts vasoconstrictor effects. May be used I.V. for relief of pain, but has many side effects when used in this manner. I.V. use may correct certain abnormal heart rhythms; however, other agents are thought to be superior for this use.	If sensitivity is suspected, a small dose should be given first to test tolerance. Maximum single dose for adults is 1 gram.

Name	Classification and Administration	Dose	Actions and Uses	Comments
Succinylcholine chloride (Anectine)	Adjunct to general anesthesia Neuromuscular blocking agent Depolarizing blocking agent I.V.	Normal: 30 mg. Range: 10–40 mg. or 0.4–0.8 mg./kg. of body weight.	Rapid onset (1 minute); short duration (5 minutes). Used for brief relaxation procedures or prolonged relaxation in major surgery. Respiratory depressant.	Careful supervision of the infusion and control of respiration are necessary to avoid hypoxia. Cholinesterase inhibitors will intensify and prolong neuromuscular block; therefore they should be discontinued 2–4 weeks before surgery. This agent potentiates the effects of digitalis preparations. Hypoxia and apnea may occur.
Tubocurarine chloride	Adjunct to general anesthesia Neuromuscular blocking agent Competitive or nondepolarizing blocking agent I.V.	6–9 mg. followed by 3–6 mg. in 5 minutes if needed.	Used as preparation for surgery to increase muscular relaxation with other agents. Also used in convulsive disorders, electric shock therapy, and diagnosis of myasthenia gravis. Respiratory depressant.	Injection should be made over a 30- to 90-second period. Dose is substantially reduced when ether is used. Acidosis potentiates this drug; it should be used with caution in patients with renal disease. Hypoxia and apnea may occur.

REFERENCES

CLARK, MARGARET. "Ketalar—a Children's Anesthetic." *Nursing Times* 69:310, March 1973.

DRAIN, CECIL B. "Innovar—a Neuroleptic Drug." *American Journal of Nursing* 74:895, May 1974.

RODMAN, MORTON J. "Drugs Used In Anesthesia." *RN* 33:53, July 1970.

TWIST, PAMELA. "Reduction of Fractures—the Valium and Pethidine Technique." *Nursing Times* 69:344, March 1973.

APPLICATION QUESTIONS

I. *True-False*

For each of the statements below, write **a** if the statement is true or **b** if it is false.

_a_ 1. Inhalation anesthetics produce progressive depression of the central nervous system.

_b_ 2. Nitrous oxide is a potent anesthetic.

_b_ 3. When used as premedication prior to anesthesia, narcotic analgesics tend to decrease postoperative nausea and vomiting.

_b_ 4. Atropine is administered preoperatively to reduce the drying effect of many anesthetics.

_a_ 5. Sodium thiopental is a barbiturate.

_a_ 6. When anesthesia is induced with a short acting barbiturate, excitement is rarely seen.

_b_ 7. Basal anesthesia keeps the patient in deep surgical anesthesia for a prolonged period.

_b_ 8. The patient who has had ketamine anesthetic requires frequent stimulation in the recovery room.

_a_ 9. Neostigmine counteracts the paralysis caused by acetylcholine blocking agents.

_b_ 10. Local anesthetics are sometimes used to produce unconsciousness.

_a_ 11. Long-term use of topical anesthetics can lead to sensitivity and allergic reactions.

a 12. Patients whose skin is predisposed to react to chemicals may not be able to use any topical anesthetics.

b 13. To produce spinal anesthesia, local anesthetic is deposited between the dura and arachnoid membranes.

a 14. Phenothiazine-type tranquilizers are effective as postoperative antiemetics.

II. *Multiple Choice*

For each of the following questions, indicate the letter providing the *best* answer.

d 1. Why are anticholinergic drugs used as premedication when halothane is used as an anesthetic? (a) for skeletal muscle relaxation (b) to reduce postoperative nausea and vomiting (c) to counteract stimulation of tracheobronchial secretions (d) to counteract the effects of vagal stimulation.

c 2. The goals of general anesthesia include which of the following? (1) analgesia (2) unconsciousness (3) skeletal muscle relaxation (4) depression of heart rate and blood pressure (a) 1, 2 (b) 2, 3 (c) 1, 2, 3 (d) 2, 4 (e) all of the above

b 3. Halothane is now more popular than ether for which of the following reasons? (1) it produces unconsciousness more rapidly (2) it causes less postoperative discomfort (3) it is nonexplosive (4) it produces excellent skeletal muscle relaxation (a) 1, 2, 3, 4 (b) 1, 2 (c) 2, 3 (d) 4

d 4. Which of the following drugs are used to counteract the disadvantages of general anesthetics? (1) sedative-hypnotics (2) antianxiety drugs (3) neuroleptics (4) antiemetics (a) 1, 2, 4 (b) 1, 3, 4 (c) 2, 3 (d) 1, 2, 3, 4

a 5. When ether is the anesthetic, how should the dose of neuromuscular blocking agents be altered? (a) markedly reduced (b) slightly increased (c) diluted with barbiturates (d) greatly increased

a 6. What is the greatest danger to the patient receiving a neuromuscular blocking agent? (a) hypoxia and apnea (b) nephrotoxicity (c) hepatotoxicity (d) hypertension

d 7. What is the drug antidote for neuromuscular blocking agents of the depolarizing type? (a) neostigmine (b) atropine (c) sodium thiopental (d) there is no antidote

d 8. Which of the following are reasons why ketamine has been found useful as an anesthetic? (1) it is a nonbarbiturate (2) it has strong muscle relaxant properties (3) it is a potent analgesic (4) it produces a dissociative state useful for minor procedures (5) it can be used alone for major surgical procedures

(a) 1, 3, 5 (b) 2, 3, 4 (c) 2, 4, 5 (d) 1, 3, 4 (e) all of the above

a 9. Which of the following local anesthetics is very short acting? (a) procaine (Novocain) (b) tetracaine (Pontocaine) (c) lidocaine (Xylocaine) (d) benzocaine (Anesthesin)

b 10. Which of the following is *not* a toxic reaction which may occur with local anesthetics? (a) cardiac arrest (b) hypertension (c) convulsions (d) vomiting

a 11. Systemic toxicity is more likely to occur if a local anesthetic is infiltrated into which of the following body areas? (a) scalp (b) sole of foot (c) back (d) kneecap

c 12. Which of the following local anesthetics is versatile enough that it can be used for every kind of local anesthesia? (a) procaine (Novocain) (b) tetracaine (Pontocaine) (c) lidocaine (Xylocaine) (d) benzocaine (Anesthesin)

c 13. You are recording the total amount of lidocaine a patient is receiving while the surgeon is suturing multiple scalp wounds. The lidocaine has been mixed with epinephrine. Which of the totals listed below would be the point at which you would inform the physician that he was approaching the maximum recommended amount of the drug? (a) 100 mg. (b) 200 mg. (c) 400 mg. (d) 800 mg.

c 14. Why would a vasoconstrictor drug be added to an injectable local anesthetic? (1) to increase the rate of absorption (2) to prolong local action (3) to reduce toxicity (4) to provide space for drug volume (5) to reduce anxiety (a) 1, 4 (b) 2, 3 (c) 2, 4 (d) 3, 4 (e) 1, 3, 5

c 15. Combining a vasoconstrictor with a local anesthetic would be indicated in which of the following local body areas? (a) ear (b) penis (c) face (d) finger

d 16. What is the best position for a patient during abdominal surgery if a heavy spinal anesthetic is used? (a) lying flat on his back (b) semi-Fowler's (c) Trendelenburg's (d) head and shoulders elevated

d 17. Which of the following nursing actions would be appropriate in the six to twelve hours immediately following spinal anesthesia? (1) turn side to side (2) passive range of motion to legs (3) check sensory level with pinprick (4) keep in semi-Fowler's position (a) 1, 2 (b) 2, 4 (c) 3, 4 (d) 1, 2, 3 (e) 2, 3, 4

III. *Matching A*

Match each general anesthetic with its usual mode of administration.

_a_ 1. nitrous oxide   (a) Inhalation

_b_ 2. sodium thiopental   (b) I.V.
         (Pentothal)

_a_ 3. halothane

IV. *Matching B*

Match each site with the appropriate means of administration of local anesthetic.

_b_ 1. along the line of   (a) topical
       surgical incision
                               (b) infiltration
_a_ 2. nerve endings in
       mucous membranes   (c) conduction
_c_
___ 3. injection into
       a nerve or nerve
       group

V. *Matching C*

Match the description of each local anesthetic with its classification.

_c_ 1. Blocking spinal   (a) spinal anesthesia
       nerves without
       penetrating   (b) saddle block
       the dura
                               (c) epidural anesthesia
_b_
___ 2. Depositing an   (d) caudal anesthesia
       anesthetic in the
       subarachnoid
       space, blocking
       only the sacral
       nerves that go
       to perineal area

_a_ 3. Blocking spinal
       nerve roots
       by depositing
       anesthetic into
       spinal fluid

_d_ 4. Blocking nerves
       of the perineum
       and abdominal
       muscles without
       entering the
       subarachnoid space

VI. *Discussion*

What is the rationale for using a local anesthetic rather than a general anesthetic in each of the following situations?

1. A patient with emphysema

2. An elderly patient

3. A patient requiring emergency surgery who has just eaten a large meal

4. A woman in labor

Drugs Acting on Autonomic Neuroeffectors

SECTION FIVE

14

The Autonomic Nervous System

The autonomic nervous system (ANS) is an involuntary system composed of two branches: the sympathetic system and the parasympathetic system. Because this is a difficult subject, this chapter presents a brief review of the action of the ANS and a brief overview of the action of drugs upon it. If necessary, the basic understanding this chapter offers can be enlarged by consulting a more detailed physiology textbook. The next two chapters will deal specifically with drugs that influence the functioning of the autonomic nervous system.

BASIC PHYSIOLOGY OF THE ANS

One of the unique features of the autonomic nervous system is that it is composed of a two-neuron chain. The first neuron, apparently arising from within the central nervous system, ends in a group of nerve cell bodies called the *ganglion*. The second neuron, beginning at the ganglion, ends at the action site. In contrast, the central nervous system is a one-neuron system: the same neuron arises in the central nervous system and ends at the action site. The two-neuron chain adds to the complexity of pharmacological action on the ANS, because there are more sites at which drugs can act. Drug action may occur on the preganglionic fibers, on the postganglionic fibers, at the ganglion, at the junction between the postganglionic fibers and the receptor sites, or directly on the receptor sites.

When a nerve impulse reaches the ending of a nerve cell fiber, a chemical substance is needed to carry the impulse across the synapse, or gap, to the second nerve cell or to the receptor site. A chemical which fulfills this role is called a neurohormone. The neurohormone acting between the sympathetic postganglionic fibers and the receptor sites is norepinephrine. The neurohormone acting between the parasympa-

thetic postganglionic fibers and the receptor sites is acetylcholine. Acetylcholine is also the neurohormone acting at all the synapses in the ganglia—both sympathetic and parasympathetic—as well as at the junction of the somatic nerve cells of the central nervous system and the voluntary skeletal muscles they influence.

After a neurohormone has been released at a nerve ending and after the impulse has passed, the neurohormone must be eliminated. Allowing either acetylcholine or norepinephrine to accumulate at synaptic junctions can cause undesirable effects. Acetylcholine is destroyed by the enzyme acetylcholinesterase, which is also released at the nerve ending. Some of the norepinephrine is destroyed in the liver and other organs by enzymes such as monoamine oxidase; however, much of the norepinephrine is taken back into the nerve endings that originally released it.

OVERVIEW OF THE AUTONOMIC NERVOUS SYSTEM

The sympathetic system is the "fight or flight" system which acts to provide energy; the parasympathetic system is concerned with conserving energy and counteracting the fatiguing effects of the sympathetic system.

Actions of the Sympathetic System

Imagine yourself in a lonely dark alley, suddenly confronted by a person pointing a gun at you. The sympathetic nervous system responds, for the most part, by activating those body responses you need at this time, and by inhibiting functions you do not need.

First, the sympathetic system stimulates the adrenal gland to release epinephrine and to begin hormonal responses that will help sustain the body if the stress is prolonged. You may need to run in this situation, so the sympathetic system causes dilation of appropriate vessels to provide the skeletal muscles with adequate blood. You will need energy, so the liver is stimulated to increase available blood glucose (glycogenolysis). Because you will need oxygen and a good supply of blood circulating to meet all these demands, the bronchial muscles dilate and the heart rate increases. The coronary vessels also dilate to provide blood to the hard-working heart muscle. The pupils dilate to enable you to see better. The sympathetic system constricts the peripheral blood vessels to increase peripheral resistance and thereby increase blood pressure. This constriction also shunts the available blood to the major organs of the body where it is needed—you do not *need* a rosy complexion.

In this situation you really do not need the processes of digestion or elimination. The sympathetic system, therefore, inhibits salivation, gastric secretion, and motility, relaxes the gallbladder, contracts the rectal and urethral sphincters, and relaxes the muscles of the urinary bladder.

Actions of the Parasympathetic System

Many of the actions of the parasympathetic system are opposite to actions of the sympathetic system. The parasympathetic system is concerned with saving energy. Energy stores are built up by digesting nutrients; therefore, the parasympathetic system stimulates digestion by increasing gastric motility, increasing gastric acid secretion, increasing salivation, and causing the gallbladder to contract. When digestion is increased, elimination must also be increased; the parasympathetic system increases the muscle tone of the intestines and the urinary bladder and relaxes the rectal and urethral sphincters. The parasympathetic system counteracts the fatiguing cardiovascular effects of the sympathetic system by decreasing the heart rate and causing generalized vasodilation in order to lower the blood pressure. In opposition to the sympathetic system, the parasympathetic system causes the pupils to constrict. The parasympathetic system also stimulates generalized sweating. Although the sympathetic system increases localized sweating, as on the palms of the hands, influence over the sweat glands is generally discussed in terms of the parasympathetic system.

Interaction of the Sympathetic and Parasympathetic Systems

The above discussion should not be interpreted to mean that the autonomic nervous system responds only in emergency or stress situations. It carries out its stimulating and inhibiting effects continually to maintain body homeostasis and to aid in adjusting to the little crises as well as the big ones. Not all receptor sites are equally receptive to both parasympathetic and sympathetic impulses; thus the two systems do not always exert exactly opposite effects on the receptor organs.

Stimulation of one branch of the autonomic nervous system usually stimulates the other branch to act also. An individual's response to prolonged stress may be dominated either by the sympathetic system or the parasympathetic system. For example, some individuals respond to stress by becoming anorexic (sympathetic action), whereas others respond by eating to excess (parasympathetic action); some become constipated (sympathetic action), whereas others experience diarrhea (parasympathetic action); and some become more alert (sympathetic action), but others faint (parasympathetic action).

The action of drugs on the ANS is difficult to comprehend, partly because of the complex ways in which this system interacts with the central nervous system and the endocrine system. In addition, each branch of the ANS can be further classified according to the types of reactors and neurohormones involved. The following is a brief discussion of the divisions of each branch of the ANS, as well as some of the specific properties of each branch.

PHYSIOLOGY OF THE SYMPATHETIC SYSTEM

The sympathetic system is sometimes referred to as thoracolumbar or adrenergic. The term *thoracolumbar* is used because the first nerve cell bodies (preganglionic fibers) are located in the thoracic and lumbar sections of the spinal cord. The term *adrenergic* (derived from "adrenalin") is used because the neurohormone involved at the synapse at the receptor site is norepinephrine or epinephrine (Adrenalin). Actually, norepinephrine is the neurohormone for the sympathetic system, and epinephrine is a hormone secreted by the adrenal medulla; but since epinephrine can occupy the same sites as norepinephrine and thus have the same effects, the two are often considered together.

It should be noted that norepinephrine is the neurohormone at the synaptic site between the postganglionic fibers and the receptor site. It is *not* the neurohormone at the synapse in the ganglion.

Alpha and Beta Receptors

Receptors in the sympathetic system are classified as *alpha* receptors or *beta* receptors. Smooth muscle cells containing mostly receptors of the alpha type respond by contracting. For example, alpha adrenergic receptors are located in the muscles of the peripheral blood vessels and in the sphincters of the gastrointestinal and genitourinary systems. Smooth muscles containing mostly receptors of the beta type usually respond by relaxing. Beta adrenergic receptors are located in the muscles of the skeletal blood vessels, in the bronchial muscles, and in the musculature of the gastrointestinal and genitourinary systems. An exception to the rule that beta receptors cause relaxation is the heart muscle. The heart contains mainly beta adrenergic receptors, but it responds to sympathetic stimulation by beating more forcefully and rapidly.

PHYSIOLOGY OF THE PARASYMPATHETIC SYSTEM

The parasympathetic system is also referred to as craniosacral or cholinergic. The term *craniosacral* indicates that some of the preganglionic fibers of this system are located in the cranium (including some of the cranial nerves, such as the vagus); the other preganglionic fibers are located in the sacral portion of the spinal cord. The term *cholinergic* indicates that the neurohormone involved in the parasympathetic synaptic junctions is acetylcholine.

Muscarinic and Nicotinic Effects

Not only is acetylcholine the neurohormone involved at the parasympathetic postganglionic synapses, but it is also involved at all ganglionic junctions in both the sympathetic and parasympathetic systems, and at the myoneural junctions of the voluntary skeletal muscles. Actions related only to the postganglionic cholinergic fibers—that is, strictly parasympathetic actions—are referred to as *muscarinic*. Actions related to the preganglionic cholinergic fibers, either sympathetic or parasympathetic, or to the somatic motor neuron fibers of the skeletal muscles are referred to as *nicotinic*.

CLASSIFICATION OF PHARMACOLOGIC ACTION

Drugs acting on the autonomic nervous system can be placed in four broad categories. (1) *Sympathomimetic* drugs enhance (or "mimic") the actions of the sympathetic system. These drugs are also referred to as adrenergic agents. (2) *Sympatholytic* drugs block or inhibit the actions of the sympathetic system. These drugs are also referred to as sympathetic blocking agents or adrenergic blocking agents. (3) *Parasympathomimetic* drugs enhance or "mimic" the actions of the parasympathetic system. These drugs may also be called cholinergic agents. "Cholinergic" is probably

the more accurate term, because most of these drugs act by influencing the action of acetylcholine, which is involved in other systems besides the parasympathetic system. (4) *Parasympatholytic* drugs block the actions of the parasympathetic system. These drugs may also be called parasympathetic blocking agents or cholinergic blocking agents.

The actions of drugs on the ANS can be classified in more detail, and to complicate matters, drugs are often referred to in terms of their specific actions. However, each of the drug classifications discussed below is actually a subclassification of one of the four mentioned above.

Classification of Sympathetic Drugs

Some drugs acting on the sympathetic nervous system have a generalized effect; others are specific for either the beta adrenergic receptors or the alpha adrenergic receptors. Thus drugs with specific actions on the sympathetic system may be classified as *alpha adrenergic stimulants, alpha adrenergic blocking agents, beta adrenergic stimulants,* or *beta adrenergic blocking agents.*

Classification of Parasympathetic Drugs

Drugs acting on the parasympathetic nervous system may have specifically muscarinic effects, specifically nicotinic effects, or both. On this basis, parasympathetic drugs may be classified as *muscarinic* or *nicotinic*. In addition, since acetylcholine is destroyed by acetylcholinesterase, parasympathetic drugs may act directly on either acetylcholine *or* acetylcholinesterase. This gives four subclasses of drugs: *cholinergic; anticholinergic; cholinesterase;* and *anticholinesterase.* Cholinergic and anticholinesterase drugs are both parasympathomimetic; anticholinergic and cholinesterase drugs are both parasympatholytic.

Because the neurohormone involved in the autonomic ganglia is acetylcholine, drugs that act there are discussed with the cholinergic drugs. Since they affect both sympathetic and parasympathetic fibers, however, they may be referred to when discussing either the sympathetic or parasympathetic drugs. Although drugs which stimulate ganglionic sites are referred to as cholinergic drugs, those which inhibit ganglionic action are often called *ganglionic blocking agents.*

UNDERSTANDING THE TERMINOLOGY

The next two chapters deal with specific drugs which act on the autonomic nervous system. Since those two chapters use the terminology introduced in this chapter, and since terminology is one of the difficulties in studying these drugs, it is important to become familiar enough with the terminology to complete successfully the questions at the end of this chapter before proceeding to the chapters which follow.

The following chapters group the sympathomimetic drugs with the parasympatholytic drugs, and the parasympathomimetic drugs with the sympatholytic drugs. Many organs have both sympathetic and parasympathetic fibers, one kind causing stimulation and the other kind causing inhibition. Stimulating the fibers of one system has a similar effect to inhibiting the fibers of the other system, especially with regard to side effects to the drugs. The drugs are grouped in this manner because of their similar actions and side effects. However, it should not be assumed that drugs within each group are used for the same indications or that they can be used interchangeably.

APPLICATION QUESTIONS

I. *True-False*

For each statement below, write **a** if the statement is true or **b** if it is false.

_____ 1. The autonomic nervous system is not influenced by the cerebral cortex.

_____ 2. The autonomic nervous system cannot usually be controlled by an act of will.

_____ 3. Fibers from the autonomic nervous system pass directly from the central nervous system to the organs they innervate.

_____ 4. Ganglia are cell bodies packed together in various locations outside the central nervous system.

_____ 5. The sympathetic system is also known as the craniosacral system.

_____ 6. Some parasympathetic fibers run in cranial nerves such as the vagus.

_____ 7. The autonomic nervous system functions only as an emergency mechanism.

_____ 8. Both divisions of the autonomic nervous system exert equal powers over all organs.

_____ 9. Neurohormones are substances stored in nerve endings.

_____ 10. The response of an organ to sympathetic nerve impulses depends on which kind of adrenergic receptors it contains.

_____ 11. Adrenergic receptors of the alpha type respond primarily by relaxing.

_____ 12. Drugs that block the action of acetylcholine are called parasympathomimetics.

_____ 13. Cholinergic transmission occurs only in the autonomic nervous system.

II. *Multiple Choice*

For each of the following questions, indicate the letter providing the *best* answer.

_____ 1. Most of the excess norepinephrine remaining after message transmission is removed by what process? (a) recapture by the nerve endings that released it (b) destruction by acetylcholinesterase (c) excretion through the kidney (d) return for storage in the adrenal medulla

_____ 2. Drugs that initiate cholinergic transmission act on which of the following? (1) parasympathetic postganglionic neuroeffectors (2) autonomic ganglia (3) skeletal muscle fibers (4) adrenergic receptors
(a) 1 (b) 2, 3 (c) 1, 2, 3 (d) 1, 2, 3, 4

_____ 3. Norepinephrine is released by which of the following kinds of nerve endings? (a) preganglionic sympathetic (b) preganglionic parasympathetic (c) postganglionic parasympathetic (d) postganglionic sympathetic

_____ 4. During cholinergic transmission, how would the function of acetylcholine be classified? (a) neutralizing force (b) chemical mediator (c) potentiator (d) enzyme antagonist

_____ 5. Once cholinergic transmission has taken place, which of the following acts to destroy any remaining acetylcholine? (a) acetylcholinesterase (b) epinephrine (c) monoamine oxidase (d) nicotinic acid

_____ 6. The parasympathetic system is responsible for which of the following effects? (a) constricted pupils (b) decreased gastrointestinal movement (c) constricted peripheral vessels (d) dilated bronchial passages

_____ 7. What two neurohormones are released by postganglionic autonomic nerves? (1) acetylcholinesterase (2) acetylcholine (3) norepinephrine (4) epinephrine
(a) 1, 2 (b) 2, 3 (c) 2, 4 (d) 1, 3

III. *Matching A*

Match each type of nerve fiber with its parasympathetic effects.

_____ 1. postganglionic cholinergic fibers

_____ 2. preganglionic cholinergic fibers

_____ 3. somatic motor fibers

(a) muscarinic effects

(b) nicotinic effects

IV. *Matching B*

Match each tissue with the type of adrenergic receptors it contains.

—— 1. blood vessels in the skin

—— 2. large skeletal muscle vessels

—— 3. bronchial muscle

—— 4. heart muscle

—— 5. sphincters in the gastrointestinal tract

(a) alpha adrenergic receptors

(b) beta adrenergic receptors

V. *Definitions*

Define or explain each of the following terms.

1. autonomic nervous system

2. sympathetic system (Give examples of its function)

3. parasympathetic system (Give examples of its function)

4. two-neuron chain

5. ganglion

6. neurohormone

7. acetylcholine

8. norepinephrine

9. epinephrine

10. acetylcholinesterase

11. thoracolumbar system

12. craniosacral system

13. synapse

14. alpha adrenergic receptors (Give examples of their location)

15. beta adrenergic receptors (Give examples of their location)

16. adrenergic

17. cholinergic

18. muscarinic

19. nicotinic

20. sympathomimetic

21. anticholinesterase

22. cholinesterase

24. ganglionic blocking agent

23. parasympatholytic

25. somatic motor neuron fibers

Block Parasympathetic

    Probanthine

Beta i   Heart & Lung (Stimulatin)
1. adrenaline
2. isuprez
3. Dopanine

Beta ii   (Heart)
1. Salbutamal
2. Ventozin
3. Acupent

15

Parasympathomimetic and Sympatholytic Drugs

Drugs used to mimic the parasympathetic system or to block the sympathetic system result in predominantly parasympathetic actions. These actions include a decrease in heart rate, vasodilation and decrease in blood pressure, increase in gastric secretion and gastrointestinal motility, increased tone of the urinary bladder, relaxation of the urethral and gastrointestinal sphincters, and constriction of the pupils (miosis). These actions suggest use of parasympathomimetic or sympatholytic drugs in conditions such as tachycardia, hypertension, peripheral ischemic diseases, paralytic ileus, urinary retention, and glaucoma.

However, because the sympathetic and parasympathetic systems do not exert precisely equal or opposite effects, and because of the specific attraction of certain drugs for specific receptors, each of the conditions listed above is better treated with one or the other classification of drugs. For example, although the parasympathomimetic drugs do cause a reduction in blood pressure, generalized vasodilation, and a slowing of the heart rate, the sympatholytic drugs are preferred for treating hypertension, peripheral ischemic diseases, and cardiac tachyarrhythmias. This is because the sympatholytic drugs have more specific and predictable responses for these conditions. On the other hand, the parasympathomimetic drugs are preferred for treating conditions involving decreased motility or paralysis of the gastrointestinal or urinary tract, and in the treatment of glaucoma.

The parasympathomimetic drugs can be classified as either *cholinergic* or *anticholinesterase* drugs. The cholinergic drugs are the true parasympathomimetic drugs, exerting only muscarinic effects. The anticholinesterase drugs have both muscarinic and nicotinic

effects; they are used primarily for their nicotinic action on skeletal muscle in the treatment of myasthenia gravis.

SIDE EFFECTS OF PARASYMPATHOMIMETIC AND SYMPATHOLYTIC DRUGS

Muscarinic

It is useful to discuss sympatholytic, cholinergic, and anticholinesterase drugs together since patients taking any of them must be observed for the same types of side effects. Any of these drugs may cause severe bradycardia or hypotension. Gastrointestinal symptoms such as nausea, vomiting, epigastric distress, abdominal cramping, and diarrhea are probably the most common complaints of patients taking any of these drugs; for this reason most of these drugs are contraindicated or used with extreme caution for patients with peptic ulcer. Most of these drugs are also contraindicated for patients with bronchial asthma, because of the side effect of bronchospasm. Increased sweating and increased salivation are two more muscarinic side effects the nurse should be aware of.

Nicotinic

In addition to muscarinic side effects, anticholinesterase drugs can produce nicotinic side effects. These actions are primarily limited to the skeletal muscles. Initially, side effects would include those associated with increased nerve impulse transmission: fasciculations, twitching, and muscle cramps. If overdose and toxic reactions occur, acetylcholine accumulates at the myoneural junction, and impulse transmission is inhibited rather than increased. Toxic effects, then, include muscle fatigue, weakness, and paralysis. The most serious of these effects would be paralysis of the muscles of respiration, leading to respiratory distress and failure.

SYMPATHOLYTIC DRUGS (ADRENERGIC BLOCKING AGENTS)

These drugs are classified as adrenergic neuron blocking agents, alpha adrenergic blocking agents, or beta adrenergic blocking agents. The adrenergic neuron blocking agents are used primarily for their effect on the heart and blood vessels in the treatment of hypertension. These drugs are discussed fully in Chapter 20. The primary effect of the alpha adrenergic blocking agents is relaxing the muscles of the peripheral blood vessels. These agents are used in treating ischemic peripheral vascular diseases; they are discussed in Chapter 21. The beta adrenergic blocking agents are used principally for their specific action on the heart muscle. They are used mainly as antiarrhythmic drugs, and are discussed in Chapter 18.

PARASYMPATHOMIMETIC (CHOLINERGIC) DRUGS

Cholinergic Drugs and the Gastrointestinal and Urinary Systems

The major indication for use of cholinergic drugs on the gastrointestinal and urinary systems is postoperative atony and distention of the abdomen or bladder. These drugs may also be used for treating postpartum urinary retention, bladder atony resulting from prolonged use of an indwelling catheter, or neurogenic atony of the bladder in patients with spinal cord injuries. Bethanechol chloride (Urecholine) is the preferred drug in the above situations because its effects are largely limited to the smooth muscles. Neostigmine, an anticholinesterase drug, may be used, but it causes both nicotinic and muscarinic actions and thus may be accompanied by many side effects.

Cholinergic Drugs in the Treatment of Glaucoma

Cholinergic drugs applied directly to the eye cause contraction of the iris, which results in miosis, or pupil constriction. This action is useful in the long-term treatment of chronic (wide-angle) glaucoma, and for preoperative preparation for the patient with acute (narrow-angle) glaucoma. Acute glaucoma requires immediate surgery (iridectomy) to relieve intraocular pressure. Short acting cholinergic eye drops, such as pilocarpine hydrochloride, and short acting anticholinesterase drops such as physostigmine are used preoperatively. Long acting anticholinesterase eye drops are never used for acute glaucoma, because they may increase intraocular pressure.

Chronic glaucoma is treated first with pilocarpine hydrochloride; tolerance tends to develop, however, and higher doses become necessary to produce therapeutic effects. The higher doses may cause local irritation and allergic conjuctivitis. If resistance develops, the patient may be transferred to carbachol or to the anticholinesterase drug physostigmine. Carbachol is less effective than pilocarpine, and physostigmine is more irritating. Using one of the latter drugs for a time may restore responsiveness of the eye to safe, nonirritating doses of pilocarpine. If the patient cannot be maintained on the short acting drugs mentioned above, he may be treated with longer acting anticholinesterase drugs such as demecarium bromide, echothiophate iodide, or isoflurophate. The action of these drugs may last as long as twelve hours or even several days, but because they have nicotinic as well as muscarinic actions, many side effects may occur.

When patients begin treatment with any miotic drug, they may complain of browaches, headaches, pain and redness of the eye, and blurring or dimming of vision. To encourage the patient to continue the medication, the nurse should explain that most of these discomforts will disappear within a week to ten days. Children treated with topical miotics may develop cysts along the pupillary margin of the iris. Elderly patients being maintained on one of the anticholinesterase drugs should be observed for development of lens opacities.

Any of the side effects related to parasympathetic action mentioned at the beginning of the chapter may develop from systemic absorption of these drugs. Systemic absorption may be avoided if the patient is taught how to instill the drops properly. The drops should be placed in the everted lower lid; the lids should then be kept apart for several seconds, and pressure applied to the inner canthus to occlude the lacrimal ducts and prevent the drops from running into the respiratory tract. Instruct the patient to close the lids gently rather than squeezing them together.

All equipment used for administering eye drops must be sterile. Care must be taken not to touch the eye with the dropper; not only would this risk injury to the eye, but it would also contaminate the rest of the bottle of solution when the dropper is replaced. If physical changes such as clouding or coloring occur in the solution, it may be ineffective and should be discarded.

Parasympathomimetic Drugs in Insecticides

Parathion is a very potent organophosphate cholinergic chemical used in agricultural insecticides. It has both muscarinic and nicotinic effects. Malathion is a cholinergic chemical used in insecticides for home gardens. Cholinergic toxicity may occur if either of these insecticides is ingested, inhaled, or permitted contact with the skin. Atropine, an anticholinergic drug, is the antidote for cholinergic poisoning, but it relieves only the muscarinic effects. If the nicotinic effects have caused paralysis of the respiratory muscles, a respirator is necessary to sustain life. Pralidoxime chloride (Protopam) is another antidote used for treating poisoning caused by the organophosphorus-type chemicals. Pralidoxime chloride reactivates the inactivated acetylcholinesterase, allowing it to destroy the accumulated free acetylcholine.

Anticholinesterase Drugs in the Treatment of Myasthenia Gravis

Myasthenia gravis is a chronic disease caused by defective neuromuscular nerve impulse transmission; it is characterized by extreme weakness and fatigue. The anticholinesterase drugs are preferred for treating this condition because of their nicotinic effects. Small doses of these drugs can increase muscle strength by increasing impulse transmission. Large doses, however, may cause an accumulation of acetylcholine at the myoneural junction and thus bring about severe loss of muscle strength and even paralysis.

Edrophonium chloride (Tensilon), an anticholinesterase drug with a very rapid onset and very short duration, is used for diagnosis of myasthenia gravis. A small dose is injected intravenously and the patient is observed. Immediate, dramatic improvement in muscle strength occurs only if the patient has myasthenia gravis.

Neostigmine (Prostigmin) is preferred for the treatment of the disease. Although it is longer acting than edrophonium, it still requires frequent administration, and since patients tend to become resistant to its effects, the dosage must be raised periodically to gain results. Pyridostigmine bromide (Mestinon) is a longer acting drug, particularly useful for administration at bedtime. A patient maintained only on neostigmine must awaken in the middle of the night to take the medication, or else take the chance that he will be too weak to get up and take his medication in the morning, or will be unable to swallow the drug because of dysphagia. Pyridostigmine bromide, taken at bedtime, permits the patient to get a full night's sleep and wake up with the ability to take his next dose of medication.

The nicotinic effects of the anticholinesterase drugs are, of course, desirable in the treatment of myasthenia gravis, but their muscarinic action can cause all the discomforting side effects mentioned at the beginning of this chapter. It is rare that the myasthenic patient can be maintained free of symptoms; therefore, the inevitable result of therapy is a middle ground between the disabling effects of the disease and the discomforting effects of the drugs. Some physicians administer the anticholinergic drug atropine along with anticholinesterase drugs to decrease the muscarinic effects. Other physicians believe it is better to allow the side effects, because an increase in their severity would draw attention to a possible overdose or an insidious cholinergic crisis. Myasthenia gravis may have periods of remission and exacerbation; periodic evaluation and readjustment of drug dosage is therefore required.

Myasthenic and Cholinergic Crises. Myasthenic patients may experience either of two crises: myasthenic crisis or cholinergic crisis. Myasthenic crisis may be caused by an exacerbation of the disease along with inadequate medication, whereas cholinergic crisis is caused by overdosage of the drug. It can be a medical dilemma to determine which crisis the patient is experiencing, since they are both characterized by respiratory depression or even respiratory failure. Cholinergic crisis requires treatment with an anticholinergic drug; myasthenic crisis requires treatment with an anticholinesterase drug. The danger of inaccurate diagnosis is that treatment with a drug having effects opposite to those needed may lead to an exaggeration of symptoms, including further respiratory depression. Edrophonium chloride is sometimes used for diagnosis because of its short action and duration. If the patient is in myasthenic crisis, he will show some improvement even from a very small dose. If he is in cholinergic crisis, his symptoms may be exaggerated, but vital functions can usually be maintained and an anticholinergic drug such as atropine can be given immediately.

Table 15–1. Parasympathomimetic and sympatholytic drugs.

Generic Name	Trade Name	How Supplied	Routes	Usual Dose	Comments
bethanechol chloride	Urecholine	tablets 5 mg., 10 mg., 25 mg.	P.O.	5–30 mg. P.O. t.i.d. or q.i.d.	Should not be given I.M. or I.V. Oral doses may be given with milk.
		ampuls 1 cc. 5 mg./cc.	Sc	2.5–10 mg. Sc t.i.d. or q.i.d.	
pilocarpine hydrochloride		in solution with castor oil for ophthalmic use. In aqueous solution in various strengths	ophthalmic	0.5–6 percent solution 1–6 times daily	
		ampuls	P.O. or Sc	5 mg.	
physostigmine salicylate	Antilirium	ampuls 2 cc. 1 mg./cc.	I.M. I.V.	0.5–2 mg. I.M. or I.V.	
echothiophate iodide	Phospholine Iodide	vials with solvent to prepare 5 cc. of the following solutions: 0.03% 0.06% 0.125% 0.25%	ophthalmic	individualized doses 0.03 percent solution 1 gtt. b.i.d.	Not indicated when uveitis and iridocyclitis are present.
edrophonium chloride	Tensilon	vials 10 cc. 10 mg./cc. ampuls 1 cc. 10 mg./cc.	I.V.	10 mg. I.V.	Short duration; used to differentiate between myasthenia crisis and cholinergic crisis.
neostigmine bromide	Prostigmin	ophthalmic solution 5% tablets 15 mg.	ophthalmic P.O.	individualized doses 150 mg. over 24 hrs.	Contraindicated in patients with mechanical bowel obstruction or urinary tract infection.
neostigmine methysulfate		ampuls 1 cc. 0.25 mg./cc. 0.5 mg./cc. 1 mg./cc. vials 10 cc. 0.5 mg./cc. 1 mg./cc.	I.M. Sc	0.5 mg. several times daily	Contraindicated in patients with mechanical intestinal or urinary obstruction.
pyridostigmine bromide	Mestinon	tablets 60 mg. sustained-release tablets (180 mg.) syrup 60 mg./5 cc.	P.O.	highly individualized doses. 1–25 tablets or 1–10 t. syrup daily, or 1–3 sustained release tablets q.d. or b.i.d.	
		ampuls 2 cc. 5 mg./cc.	I.M. or I.V. (very slowly)	individualized doses.	

REFERENCES

ABRAMS, J. D. "The Nature of Glaucoma." *Nursing Times* 68:767, June 1972.

DiPALMA, JOSEPH R. "Cholinergic and Anticholinergic Drugs." *RN* 37:83, May 1974.

GORLICK, HERTHE. "Glaucoma: The Fight for Sight." *RN* 31:44, February 1968.

LONG, KEITH R. "Pesticides—An Occupational Hazard on Farms." *American Journal of Nursing* 71:740, April 1971.

STACKHOUSE, JOAN. "Myasthenia Gravis." *American Journal of Nursing* 73:1544, September 1973.

APPLICATION QUESTIONS

I. *True-False*

For each statement below, write **a** if the statement is true or **b** if it is false.

b 1. Observation of patients receiving cholinergic drugs may be minimal because of the limited number of side effects.

b 2. Miosis is dilation of the iris.

a 3. Chronic or wide-angle glaucoma can be treated readily with cholinergic miotics.

a 4. Pilocarpine is the least toxic miotic.

b 5. The more potent long acting anticholinesterase-type miotics are used for the more serious acute or narrow-angle glaucoma.

a 6. A patient may become resistant to the effects of pilocarpine eye drops.

a 7. Atropine is an antidote for symptoms of the muscarinic type.

a 8. Cataracts may develop after long-term use of anticholinesterase miotics.

a 9. Anticholinesterase drugs have both muscarinic and nicotinic effects.

a 10. Adrenergic blocking agents prevent epinephrine and norepinephrine from exerting their effects.

a 11. One effect of alpha adrenergic blocking agents is dilation of the peripheral arterioles.

b 12. Beta adrenergic blocking agents are used to speed the heart rate.

II. *Multiple Choice*

For each of the following questions, indicate the letter providing the *best* answer.

b 1. Muscarinic side effects occurring with parasympathomimetic or sympatholytic drugs include which of the following? (1) urinary retention (2) constipation (3) bradycardia (4) hypotension (a) 1, 2 (b) 3, 4 (c) 1, 2, 3 (d) 1, 2, 3, 4

c 2. Cholinergic and sympatholytic drugs would be contraindicated in which of the following conditions? (1) bronchial asthma (2) peptic ulcer (3) hypotension (4) tachycardia (a) 1, 3 (b) 2, 4 (c) 1, 2, 3 (d) 1, 2, 3, 4

b 3. Which of the following drugs is an antidote for poisoning by organophosphate insecticides? (a) neostigmine (b) pralidoxime chloride (c) malathion (d) parathion

b 4. Cholinergic drugs have which of the following effects on the eye? (a) dilation of the pupil (b) contraction of the iris (c) opening of the tear duct (d) decrease in the sensitivity of the cornea

d 5. Which of the following discomforts occur initially with miotics? (1) browaches and headaches (2) dimming of vision (3) blurring of vision (4) eye pain (a) 1, 4 (b) 3, 4 (c) 1, 2, 3 (d) 1, 2, 3, 4

c 6. Which of the following is *not* a sign of systemic absorption of the miotics? (a) diarrhea (b) wheezing (c) tachycardia (d) sweating

a 7. Which of the following should be taught to patients who will be giving themselves miotic eye drops? (1) finger pressure at the inner canthus for a minute or two following instillation (2) closing the lids immediately after instillation (3) dropping the solution on the eye at the outer canthus (4) heating solution before using (a) 1 (b) 1, 3 (c) 2, 3, 4 (d) 1, 2, 3, 4

d 8. Which of the following anticholinesterase drugs is used primarily for diagnosis of myasthenia gravis? (a) pyridostigmine bromide (Mestinon) (b) neostigmine (Prostigmin) (c) ambenonium chloride (d) edrophonium chloride (Tensilon)

a 9. Which of the following would prevent disturbing gastrointestinal side effects when administering bethanechol chloride? (a) give with milk (b) give immediately after a meal (c) give concurrently with atropine (d) give at bedtime rather than in the morning

b 10. A toxic dose of an anticholinesterase medication would produce which of the following symptoms? (1) muscle spasm (2) respiratory depression (3) dysphagia (4) restlessness (a) 1, 4 (b) 2, 3 (c) 1, 2 (d) 1, 2, 3, 4

b 11. Myasthenic crisis may be distinguished from cholinergic crisis by which of the following tests? (a) paraffin test of the fingertips (b) small dose of edrophonium chloride (c) complete blood count (d) arterial blood gas studies b 12. What drug would be used to treat a patient with myasthenia gravis who was in myasthenic crisis? (a) atropine (b) neostigmine (c) pyridostigmine bromide (d) pralidoxime chloride

c 13. What is the advantage of using pyridostigmine bromide (Mestinon) in the treatment of myasthenia gravis? (a) it has only nicotinic actions (b) it does not cause insomnia (c) it is long acting (d) it is more potent than neostigmine

d 14. Bethanechol chloride (Urecholine) is the drug of choice for treating which of the following conditions? (a) urinary incontinence (b) chronic glaucoma (c) peptic ulcer (d) postoperative abdominal distention

III. *Matching*

Match each classification of sympatholytic drugs with the condition it is indicated for.

c 1. adrenergic neuron blocking drugs

a 2. beta adrenergic blocking drugs

b 3. alpha adrenergic blocking drugs

(a) arrhythmias

(b) peripheral ischemic diseases

(c) hypertension

IV. *Drug Use—Drug Action*

Each of the following statements gives a use for a cholinergic drug and the specific drug action involved in that use. Write **a** if both the use and the action are correct and related; **b** if both the use and action are incorrect; **c** if the use is correct, but the action is incorrect; or **d** if the use is incorrect, but the action is correct.

Therapeutic uses and pharmacological actions of cholinergic drugs:

a 1. Used for postoperative abdominal distention *because* it increases gastrointestinal motility.

d 2. Used in treating mechanical obstruction of the urinary bladder *because* it relaxes the trigone and

b   sphincter.

___ 3. Used in treating bradycardia *because* it increases the heartbeat.

c 4. Used to reduce intraocular pressure in treating glaucoma *because* it relaxes the sphincter muscle of the iris.

b 5. Used in treating bronchial asthma *because* it dilates bronchioles and decreases mucus secretions.

V. *Calculation*

.02 cc 1. An order is written for Urecholine 3.5 mg. S.C. stat. The medication is labeled 5 mg./cc. How many cc. will you give?

Sympathomimetic and Parasympatholytic Drugs

The sympathomimetic drugs, which mimic the impulses of the sympathetic system, and the parasympatholytic drugs, which block parasympathetic impulses, tend to act in ways that are predominantly sympathetic. However, the uses, actions, and side effects of these drugs vary widely; they are not so similar as the parasympathomimetics and sympatholytics discussed in the previous chapter.

This chapter will first compare the actions of the sympathomimetic and parasympatholytic drugs, and then discuss the principal indications for each type.

COMPARISON OF THE SYMPATHOMIMETIC AND PARASYMPATHOLYTIC DRUGS

In general, the drugs that act on the sympathetic impulses are used mainly for their effects on the heart and blood vessels; those that act on parasympathetic impulses are used primarily for their action on the gastrointestinal system.

Cardiac Effects

Although drugs in both classifications can be used to increase the heart rate, the parasympathetic blocking agents act specifically on the vagus nerve, whereas the sympathomimetic agents act directly on the heart muscle. Thus parasympatholytic drugs are useful only in bradycardia resulting from excessive stimulation of the vagus nerve. They are used in treating bradycardia associated with anesthesia, partial heart block, or carotid sinus syndrome. The sympathomimetic drugs can be used for treating more serious conditions of bradycardia, such as cardiac arrest and Stokes-Adams syndrome resulting from complete heart block. The

sympathomimetics are *not* used in the treatment of ventricular fibrillation.

Most drugs in both classifications are capable of producing such side effects as heart palpitations and tachycardia. The sympathomimetic drugs may also produce other cardiac arrhythmias, because they may increase cardiac irritability. Drugs of both types are contraindicated for patients with coronary artery disease such as angina, because coronary insufficiency may occur from the tachycardia.

The sympathomimetic drugs are sometimes used to *slow* the heart rate, which may seem inconsistent with the action of these drugs. Actually, intravenous injection of an alpha adrenergic drug such as phenylephrine hydrochloride (Neo-Synephrine) has no direct effect on the heart muscle. However, vasoconstriction causes such a rapid rise in blood pressure that the vagus nerve is stimulated by a compensatory reflex action to slow the heart rate. This action is specificially useful in the treatment of paroxysmal supraventricular tachycardia.

Vasomotor Action

The parasympatholytic drugs have virtually no action on the muscles of the blood vessels and rarely influence blood pressure. However, the vessels within the skin may dilate to cause flushing as a side effect or as a manifestation of toxicity.

Sympathomimetic drugs, on the other hand, are widely used in the treatment of hypotension. The vasopressors are adrenergic drugs that cause vasoconstriction, resulting in higher blood pressure.

Gastrointestinal, Genitourinary, and Biliary Actions

Both sympathomimetic and parasympatholytic drugs act to decrease gastrointestinal motility, decrease gastrointestinal and genitourinary smooth muscle tone, and increase bladder sphincter tone. Drugs of either class may be used to treat conditions such as dysmenorrhea, nocturnal enuresis (bedwetting), biliary or ureteral colic, and to decrease spasms of the gastrointestinal tract. Parasympatholytic drugs are preferred in treating peptic ulcer because their additional antisecretory action results in a decrease in gastric acid. These drugs are contraindicated for men with prostatic hypertrophy because the constriction of the urinary sphincter would compound voiding difficulties.

Ocular Effects

Drugs of both classes cause mydriasis (pupil dilation) by decreasing the muscle tone of the sphincter of the iris. Drugs of either type can be used topically to facilitate ophthalmoscopic examination. The sympathomimetic drugs (such as epinephrine) have no effect on the ciliary muscles, and would therefore be used when only mydriasis was desired. The parasympatholytic drugs (atropine sulfate, homatropine hydrobromide, cyclopentolate hydrochloride) inhibit the ciliary muscles and cause *cycloplegia,* or paralysis of accommodation. Thus parasympatholytic eye drops are useful if measuring for errors of refraction is part of the eye examination. The sympathomimetic drugs, when applied to the eye, have an additional action of local vasoconstriction; they may, therefore, be given in combination with parasympathomimetic eye drops such as pilocarpine to reduce intraocular pressure in treating chronic glaucoma. It must be remembered that all of these drugs can cause systemic side effects if, because of improper instillation, they are allowed to be absorbed.

If a patient is to have his eyes dilated for an examination, the nurse should explain that he will have blurred vision for a while. If possible, the patient should be told this before he comes for the examination, so he can arrange for someone else to drive a car if necessary. The patient should also be told to bring dark glasses, because the paralysed iris will not constrict when he goes into bright sunlight, and photophobia may occur. The nurse should assist elderly patients, or those who have difficulty with walking and balance, particularly in going up or down stairs.

Respiratory Tract Effects

The sympathomimetic drugs are very effective bronchodilators; they are used in treating diseases such as bronchial asthma, emphysema, and chronic bronchitis. The parasympatholytic drugs are weak bronchodilators which also cause a reduction in respiratory tract secretions, resulting in more viscoid mucus. The parasympatholytic drugs are contraindi-

cated for patients with asthma or chronic lung disease, because the thickened mucus may be difficult to cough up, and thus air passages may become blocked with hardened mucus.

Drugs of either classification may be used in treating the common cold or hay fever. Sympathomimetic drugs such as phenylephrine hydrochloride (Neo-Synephrine) are used as nasal decongestants; they are applied topically to the mucus membranes by means of drops or sprays to cause local vasoconstriction and to shrink swollen membranes. The parasympatholytic drugs, which inhibit mucus production, are usually given orally for their drying effects on nasal secretions.

Glandular Effects

The only gland significantly affected by the sympathomimetic drugs is the liver. Sympathomimetic drugs increase glycogenolysis and thus raise blood sugar levels. These drugs should be used with caution in patients with diabetes mellitus.

The parasympatholytic drugs decrease gastrointestinal and respiratory tract secretions. They also inhibit sweating. Although administering a parasympatholytic drug as a therapeutic measure to decrease perspiration may seem a bit drastic, it may be done in extreme instances.

The nurse should be aware that dryness of the mouth always occurs when anticholinergic drugs are given. She may suggest that the patient suck on hard candy or chew gum to relieve this discomfort. If atropine is used as a preoperative medication, the patient should be given good mouth care in the recovery room as well as when he returns to the clinical unit.

Central Nervous System Effects

The sympathomimetic drugs may cause an increase in central nervous system activity and bring about anxiety, nervousness, tremor, and insomnia. The parasympatholytic drugs, however, are not consistent in their actions on the central nervous system. Atropine sulfate, for example, causes a slight central nervous system stimulation when taken in therapeutic doses. Scopolamine hydrobromide, another anticholinergic drug, may have sufficient depressant effects to cause drowsiness and sleep. A toxic dose of either of these anticholinergics can cause excitement, restlessness, delirium, and disorientation. All of the anticholinergic drugs depress abnormal skeletal muscle tone; thus they may be used in the treatment of Parkinson's disease (see Chapter 10).

SYMPATHOMIMETIC (ADRENERGIC) DRUGS

Treatment of Cardiovascular Conditions

The two sympathomimetic agents which act most powerfully on the heart are epinephrine (Adrenalin) and isoproterenol hydrochloride (Isuprel). Both are mainly beta adrenergic stimulants which act on the heart in three ways: (1) they strengthen the heart beat; (2) they speed up the heart rate; and (3) they increase the rate of impulse conduction from the atria to the ventricles. These actions cause an increase in cardiac output.

The use of sympathomimetic drugs in treating cardiac arrest is discussed in Chapter 24. Use of these drugs to induce reflex slowing of the heart was discussed earlier in this chapter.

Stokes-Adams Syndrome.   Intravenous isoproterenol hydrochloride is most effective for treating the attacks of asystole that occur periodically with Stokes-Adams syndrome. Because overdosage can increase cardiac irritability and lead to arrhythmias, the infusion of the drug must be watched very closely. When a patient's pulse reaches about sixty beats per minute, the isoproterenol is usually discontinued. If the pulse rises further or if premature ventricular contractions (PVCs) occur on the electrocardiogram, the isoproterenol must be discontinued.

A sublingual tablet of isoproterenol is available for maintenance therapy if a patient requires medication several times a day. The patient should be told to allow the tablet to dissolve completely and be absorbed before swallowing his saliva. There are two oral drugs that may also be used for preventing attacks of Stokes-Adams syndrome: ephedrine sulfate and hydroxyamphetamine hydrobromide (Paredrine). Because these drugs have central effects that can cause insomnia, they are often combined with a barbiturate or some other sedative-hypnotic drug.

Today, many patients with Stokes-Adams syndrome are treated with permanently implanted electric pacemakers rather than with drug therapy.

Treatment of Hypotension (Shock).   Adrenergic drugs cause constriction of peripheral vessels and dilation of skeletal vessels. Beta adrenergic stimulants, which dilate skeletal vessels, are used in the treatment of ischemic conditions such as intermittent claudication, as discussed in Chapter 21. Alpha adrenergic drugs, which constrict peripheral vessels and thus increase blood pressure, are called *vasopressors.*

Neurogenic hypotensive shock is a condition resulting from diffuse vasodilation, leading to a decrease in peripheral resistance and an expansion of the circulatory bed. This condition can occur as a result of general or spinal anesthesia, or from an overdose of drugs such as barbiturates or the sympatholytic agents such as guanethidine or reserpine. Drugs administered to counteract this condition include phenylephrine hydrochloride, methoxamine hydrochloride, and ephedrine sulfate.

Acute hypotensive emergencies are treated with intravenous administration of one of the potent vasopressors such as levarterenol bitartrate (Levophed) or metaraminol bitartrate (Aramine). Metaraminol bitartrate may also be given intramuscularly in the patient's home or in an ambulance. When these drugs are given intravenously, the patient must be watched very closely, and his blood pressure must be taken almost continuously. The slightest variation of drip rate can cause a wide fluctuation in blood pressure. If allowed to leak into tissues, levarterenol will cause drastic local vasoconstriction, leading to tissue necrosis.

When vasoconstriction occurs in major organs, as in septic shock, beta adrenergic drugs such as isoproterenol hydrochloride and mephentermine sulfate (Wyamine), as well as alpha adrenergic *blocking* agents, may be useful. The vasodilating effect of these drugs is used to increase perfusion of the body organs. However, if vasodilators are used in the treatment of shock, it is important to correct hypovolemia *before* administering the drugs. Unless this is done, vasodilation leads to further hypotension. During treatment, the central venous pressure (cvp) must be watched closely to avoid overloading the circulatory system—specifically the left ventricle—as blood pressure is restored.

PARASYMPATHOLYTIC (ANTICHOLINERGIC) DRUGS

Most parasympatholytic agents are anticholinergic, exerting predominantly muscarinic blocking effects. The prototype agents of this classification are the belladonna alkaloids, such as atropine sulfate and scopolamine hydrobromide. Although these drugs are used in other situations, as discussed earlier in this chapter, only their use in treating peptic ulcer will be explored further.

Treatment of Peptic Ulcer

Probably the most significant clinical action of the parasympatholytic drugs is their action on the gastrointestinal tract. These drugs inhibit gastrointestinal motility directly, and also inhibit gastric acid secretion by inhibiting the vagus nerve. When an ulcer is pres-

Table 16–1. Sympathomimetic drugs.

Generic Name	Trade Name	How Supplied	Routes	Usual Dose	Comments
epinephrine	Adrenalin	solution 1:1000 (1 mg./cc.)	Sc or I.M. or by inhalation	0.2–0.5 mg.	Care must be taken when preparing these drugs for administration, as dosages vary greatly and may be easily confused.
		solution 1:10,000	topical I.V. intracardial		
		solution 1:100	inhalation	1 mg.	
		oil suspension 1:500	I.M.		
		ophthalmic 1 percent ung.	topical		
phenylephrine hydrochloride	Neo-Synephrine	ampuls 1 cc. and 5 cc. 10 mg./cc.	I.V., Sc or I.M.	Dosage should be adjusted according to pressor response needed.	
		ampuls 2 cc. 2 mg./cc.			
		ophthalmic solution (2.5 percent, 10 percent)	topical		
		ophthalmic viscous solution (10 percent)	topical		
		capsules 10 mg., 25 mg.	P.O.		
		elixir 1 mg./cc. in 1 pt. bottles			
		nasal spray (0.0125 percent, 0.25 percent, 0.5 percent, 1 percent sol.)	topical		
		nasal solution (0.25 percent, 0.5 percent)	topical		
		nasal jelly (0.5 percent)	topical		
isoproterenol hydrochloride	Isuprel	ampuls 1 cc. and 5 cc. 1:5000 (0.2 mg./cc.) 5 cc. 1 mg./cc.	I.V., I.M., Sc	Dosage should be adjusted according to the response needed.	
		solutions 1:200, 1:100	inhalation		
		mist 15 cc. 1:400		inhalations: 5–10	
		glossets 10 mg. 15 mg.	sublingual rectal		
		elixir 2.5 mg./15 cc. with other components	P.O.		
levarterenol bitartrate	Levophed	ampuls 4 cc. 0.2 percent	I.V.	Add 4 cc. of 0.2 percent solution to 1000 cc. 5 percent dextrose solution. Average maintenance dose 0.5–1 cc./min.	Infiltrate area with phentolamine (Regitine) if Levophed leaks into tissue. Rate of flow determined by response to the drug.

ent, the movements and secretions which accompany digestion can cause pain. They can also erode the ulcer to the extent that it will begin to bleed.

Anticholinergic drugs such as atropine sulfate or similar agents such as dicyclomine hydrochloride (Bentyl) and methantheline bromide (Banthine) are used in the treatment of peptic ulcer. They may be used in combination with an antacid both to decrease gastric acid secretion and to neutralize the acid that is secreted. If an ulcer is bleeding, the patient may require antacids as often as every fifteen to thirty minutes; or the antacid may be taken alternately with a milk-and-cream mixture that may contain a hemostatic powder. When the patient is convalescing, the drugs seem to be most effective if the anticholinergic drug is taken about one-half hour before meals and at bedtime, and the antacid is taken about one hour after meals and at bedtime, as well as when any pain occurs.

Antacids. Although antacids are not parasympatholytic drugs, they will be discussed here because of their use in the treatment of peptic ulcer. Antacid compounds usually contain aluminum, calcium, or magnesium. Aluminum and calcium compounds such

as aluminum hydroxide gel (Amphojel) and calcium phosphate tend to cause constipation. This action, combined with the slowing effect of an anticholinergic drug on the bowel, could lead to serious impaction complications. On the other hand, magnesium compounds such as magnesium hydroxide tend to cause diarrhea. The newer antacids, such as Gelusil, Riopan, and Maalox, are combinations of magnesium and aluminum compounds, to avoid further intestinal problems.

Toxic Reactions to Anticholinergic Drugs

Although death rarely occurs from atropine sulfate overdose, toxic reactions to the drug are very dramatic. Symptoms of toxicity have been described as "hot as a hare, blind as a bat, dry as a bone, and mad as a hatter," in reference to the excessive inhibition of sweating; mydriasis; excessive inhibition of saliva; and stimulation of the central nervous system. Care must be taken when preparing doses of atropine and related drugs, as they are ordered in very small amounts and may be ordered in either the apothecary system or the metric system.

Table 16-2. Parasympatholytic drugs.

Generic Name	Trade Name	How Supplied	Routes	Usual Dose	Comments
methantheline bromide	Banthine	50 mg. tablet 50 mg./vial	P.O. I.V. I.M.	50–100 mg. q.i.d.	
cyclopentolate hydrochloride	Cyclogyl	0.5%, 1%, and 2% solution in 2 cc., 7.5 cc. and 15 cc. containers.	ophthalmic	0.5–2% solution	
atropine sulfate		Supplied in many strengths. Most common is 0.4 mg. (gr. 1/150)/cc.	I.M. I.V. P.O. Sc	0.025–0.5 mg. parenterally or P.O.	Atropine is in many drug combinations.

REFERENCES

CHANDLER, JAMES G. "The Physiology and Treatment of Shock." *RN* 34:42, June 1971.

CRAVEN, RUTH FULK, and LESTER, JOAN. "Anaphylactic Shock." *American Journal of Nursing* 72:718, April 1972.

CUPIT, GARY, et al. "Antiacids." *American Journal of Nursing* 72:2210, December 1972.

DIPALMA, JOSEPH R. "Cholinergic and Anticholinergic Drugs." *RN* 37:83, May 1974.

GIVEN, B., and SIMMONS, S. "Care of a Patient with a Gastric Ulcer." *American Journal of Nursing* 70:1472, July 1970.

RODMAN, MORTON J. "Adrenergic Drugs and Adrenergic Blockers." *RN* 37:55, April 1974.

APPLICATION QUESTIONS

I. *True-False*

For each statement below, write **a** if the statement is true or **b** if it is false.

_b_ 1. Parasympatholytic drugs are used mainly for their effects on the heart and blood vessels.

_a_ 2. Tachycardia may be a side effect of both the adrenergic and the anticholinergic drugs.

_b_ 3. The beta adrenergic drugs are sometimes used to slow the heart rate.

_b_ 4. Either the sympathomimetic or the anticholinergic drugs may be used to treat hypotension.

__g__ 5. Constipation may be a side effect of both the sympathomimetic and the parasympatholytic drugs.

__b__ 6. Sympathomimetic eye drops produce both mydriasis and cycloplegia.

__a__ 7. Both the sympathomimetic and the anticholinergic drugs are contraindicated for patients with angina.

__b__ 8. The parasympatholytic drugs may be applied topically to the eye for the treatment of glaucoma.

__a__ 9. The anticholinergic drugs are contraindicated for patients with chronic lung disease.

__a__ 10. Sympathomimetic drugs may cause insomnia.

__b__ 11. Beta adrenergic stimulants are also called vasopressors.

__b__ 12. Antacid compounds containing aluminum have a tendency to cause diarrhea.

__d__ 13. Atropine keeps postganglionic parasympathetic nerves from exerting their full control over smooth muscles.

__b__ 14. Anticholinergic drugs are used effectively for the treatment of asthma.

__a__ 15. Epinephrine is also known as Adrenalin.

__a__ 16. The adrenergic drugs with the strongest cardiac effect are those which act mainly on the beta receptors.

__b__ 17. Stokes-Adams syndrome is usually treated with chemotherapy.

__a__ 18. Glycosuria is a side effect of the adrenergic drugs.

__b__ 19. Nasal congestion may be treated with oral adrenergic drugs.

II. *Multiple Choice*

For each of the following questions, indicate the letter providing the *best* answer.

__a__ 1. When applied to the eye, atropine produces which of the following effects? (1) constriction of the pupil (2) paralysis of accommodation (3) nystagmus (4) tearing
(a) 2 (b) 1, 2 (c) 2, 3, 4 (d) 1, 3, 4

__a__ 2. Which of the following drugs is preferred when only mydriasis is desired? (a) epinephrine (b) cyclopentolate hydrochloride (Cyclogyl) (c) homoatropine (d) atropine

__a__ 3. When administering atropine as a preoperative medication, what should the nurse tell the patient about the effect the drug will have on his vision? (a) "Your vision will be blurred after we give you your preoperative medication." (b) "You will have flashing colored lights before your eyes after this medication." (c) "Don't worry if you have blind moments after this shot." (d) "You will be able to read but if you look in the distance you will have blurring."

__d__ 4. Which of the following are signs of poisoning by belladonna alkaloids? (1) cold sweat (2) blurred vision (3) mental confusion (4) fever
(a) 2 (b) 1, 3 (c) 1, 2, 4 (d) 2, 3, 4

__a__ 5. Which of the following statements best describes the difference between the central nervous system effects of atropine and those of scopolamine? (a) atropine is a weak stimulant whereas scopolamine is a depressant (b) atropine is a weaker depressant than scopolamine (c) atropine has little effect on the central nervous system; scopolamine is a mild stimulant (d) atropine is a weak depressant whereas scopolamine is a stimulant

__b__ 6. Anticholinergic drugs have what effect on gastric secretions? (a) They increase digestive secretions (b) They decrease the flow of gastric acid (c) They neutralize the acidity of gastric fluid (d) They decrease the acidity of gastric secretions

__a__ 7. Which of the following patients should *not* receive anticholinergic drugs? (1) a 35-year-old farmer who has never had an eye examination (2) a 70-year-old man with a benign prostatic hypertrophy (3) a 25-year-old woman with cystitis (4) a young business executive with an irritable colon
(a) 2, 3 (b) 1, 2 (c) 1, 3, 4 (d) 2, 3, 4

__c__ 8. A patient receiving an anticholinergic drug to reduce perspiration should be observed for which of the following? (a) hypotension (b) hiccups (c) fever (d) tearing

__b__ 9. Which of the following statements describes the effect of anticholinergic drugs on the vagus nerve and the resulting effect on the heart rate? (a) they inhibit the vagus and thus decrease the heart rate (b) they inhibit the vagus and thus increase the heart rate (c) they stimulate the vagus to increase the heart rate (d) they stimulate the vagus to decrease the heart rate

__a__ 10. Methantheline bromide (Banthine) is often prescribed for which of the following clinical conditions? (1) nocturnal enuresis in children (2) paraplegic urinary incontinence (3) benign prostatic hypertrophy (4) narrow-angle glaucoma
(a) 1, 2 (b) 3, 4 (c) 1, 4 (d) 2, 3

__a__ 11. If a patient in bacteremic shock is receiving isoproterenol, which of the following findings would be of most concern to the nurse? (a) cvp 17–20 (b) heart beat 90 (c) blood pressure 110/70 (d) respiration 20

_b_ 12. Ocular effects of adrenergic drugs include which of the following? (1) mydriasis (2) vasoconstriction (3) cycloplegia (accommodation paralysis) (4) miosis
(a) 4 (b) 1, 2 (c) 1, 2, 3 (d) 2, 3, 4

_b_ 13. Which of the following drugs may be given _intramuscularly_ for emergency cardiogenic shock? (a) levarterenol (Levophed) (b) metaraminol (Aramine) (c) mephentermine (Wyamine) (d) isoproterenol (Isuprel)

_a_ 14. What instructions should be given to a patient receiving isoproterenol sublingually? (a) "Try not to swallow until the pill dissolves." (b) "Go ahead and swallow as the pill melts." (c) "Spit your saliva out in the emesis basin." (d) "After the pill has melted rinse your mouth out with mouthwash."

_b_ 15. Sympathomimetic drugs should be used with caution in which of the following clinical conditions? (a) hypothyroidism (b) angina pectoris (c) obesity (d) asthma

_b_ 16. What _useful_ effects does epinephrine have on the heart? (1) it increases the heart rate (2) it decreases the rate of impulses from the atria to the ventricles (3) it strengthens the heartbeat (4) it decreases cardiac irritability
(a) 1 (b) 1, 3 (c) 1, 3, 4 (d) 2, 3, 4

_c_ 17. Adrenergic drugs are _not_ appropriate in treating which of the following cardiac conditions? (a) Stokes-Adams syndrome (b) cardiac arrest (c) ventricular fibrillation (d) digitalis intoxication

_b_ 18. Which of the following statements would indicate a side effect of an adrenergic drug? (a) "I'm sleepy, nurse, come back later to talk, okay?" (b) "I guess it's just the hospital, but I feel so nervous and I'm not sleepy at all." (c) "I'm so thirsty, I can't seem to get enough to drink." (d) "I've sure had a lot of diarrhea lately."

III. _Calculation_

____ 1. Atropine, on hand, is labeled gr. 1/150 per cc. There is an order for Atropine, 0.2 mg. How many cc. will you give?

Drugs Acting on the Heart and Circulation

SECTION SIX

Digitalis

Digitalis and preparations containing it are the most widely used cardiotonic drugs. No synthetic compound is as effective as these drugs in improving the efficiency of the heart as a pump in order to prevent or treat congestive heart failure. Although digitalis may be used in treating arrhythmias such as paroxysmal tachycardia, atrial fibrillation, or atrial flutter, its principal indication is congestive heart failure.

ACTION AND USE OF DIGITALIS

The primary action of digitalis is slowing and strengthening of the heartbeat. Digitalis stimulates the vagus nerve to exert a slowing effect on the heart rate. By direct action as well as through vagal stimulation, digitalis depresses the A-V node; as a result, the ventricles do not respond to a bombardment of impulses from the S-A node (pacemaker). Digitalis lengthens the refractory period and thus allows the ventricles a longer time to fill completely with blood. According to Starling's law, then, the more stretched the elastic ventricular muscle becomes, the more forceful the contraction. This more forceful contraction yields a greater stroke volume and an increase in total cardiac output.

As cardiac output is increased, kidney function becomes more efficient. This diuretic effect is important in relieving the edema which accompanies congestive heart failure. Edema may be a severe enough threat to warrant administration of a diuretic along with the digitalis (see Chapter 19). It is important to remember that diuresis can decrease potassium and lead to hypokalemia. This condition, in turn, may sensitize the heart muscle to increased automaticity as a toxic effect of digitalis.

SIDE EFFECTS OF DIGITALIS

Gastrointestinal side effects of digitalis include anorexia, nausea, and vomiting. In addition, visual disturbances such as diplopia, flashing lights, and moving spots may develop. Gynecomastia may occur in male patients.

Digitalis Intoxication

The most severe side effect of the drug is digitalis intoxication, which may result in bradycardia or tachyarrhythmias. Anorexia, nausea, and vomiting are often the first signs of digitalis intoxication; however, they can be confused with the symptoms of congestive heart failure.

Bradycardia. Digitalis may induce bradycardia by prolonging the refractory period to such an extent that too few atrial impulses reach the ventricles. This situation could eventually lead to heart block. Treatment of bradycardia includes withholding the drug, giving drugs such as atropine or isoproterenol, and in some cases, using a temporary pacemaker.

Tachyarrhythmias. Tachyarrhythmias induced by digitalis may be manifested as ectopic beats or as premature ventricular contractions (PVCs). The patient's pulse must be observed closely. Tachyarrhythmias may occur as manifestations of the disease condition itself, indicating underdigitalization. If tachyarrhythmia is caused by digitalis intoxication, the drug should be withheld and potassium given to decrease the automaticity of the heart. Antiarrhythmic drugs such as quinidine or procainamide may be necessary (see Chapter 18). The patient must be closely observed during treatment with potassium or antiarrhythmic drugs, as these agents also tend to increase the atrial-ventricular defect, and may lead to heart block and cardiac standstill. The newer antiarrhythmic drugs lidocaine and diphenylhydantoin sodium (Dilantin) seem more effective and safer to use, because they reduce the automaticity without interfering with A-V conduction.

ADMINISTRATION OF DIGITALIS

Before any dose of a digitalis preparation is given, the nurse must carefully check the pulse. An apical pulse should be counted for one full minute. If the pulse is more than 20 points above or below the "normal," the drug should be withheld and the doctor notified. In an adult patient, for example, an apical pulse rate below 60 or above 100 warrants withholding the drug. In an infant, an apical pulse rate below 100 or above 140 would warrant withholding the drug. The nurse should also take the radial pulse before administering digitalis, and the radial pulse rate should be compared with the apical pulse rate. Any widening of the pulse deficit warrants withholding of the drug.

When therapy with digitalis is initiated, the patient must first be "digitalized." Large loading doses are given to obtain a rapid and complete tissue level of the drug. After digitalization, the daily maintenance dose is adjusted to equal the amount of digitalis excreted daily. Because large doses are used for digitalization, toxicity can occur rapidly during this time, so the patient must be observed closely.

The nurse must of course withhold digitalis if, after careful assessment, it is felt that the patient is demonstrating untoward or toxic effects of the drug. However, digitalis should never be withheld unnecessarily. If the daily maintenance dose is interrupted, the patient may need to be "re-digitalized." Often, a patient who is N.P.O. because of an impending diagnostic procedure will nevertheless be allowed to take his digitalis drug with a small amount of water, to be sure that the maintenance program is not interrupted.

DIGITALIS PREPARATIONS

Several different digitalis preparations are available; their effects are quite similar. The main difference among the preparations is the purification: small doses of highly purified glycosides give the same effect as larger doses of less purified glycosides. Table 17–1 compares onset of action, elimination, cumulative effect, and dosage range of the three major preparations: crude, powdered digitalis; digoxin; and digitoxin. Note that digoxin would be the drug best suited for emergency situations, because it acts rapidly and can be given intravenously. Since the drug names are so similar that they may easily be confused, it is of the utmost importance that care be taken to avoid errors. If 0.5 mg. of *digitoxin* were given accidentally when the physician's order was for 0.5 mg. of *digoxin*, the patient would receive *ten times* the usual dose of digitoxin.

Table 17–1. Comparison of digitalis and related cardiotonic drugs.

	digitalis	digoxin (Lanoxin)	digitoxin (Crystodigin), (Purodigin)
Onset of action	slow (25 minutes to 2 hours)	rapid (5 to 30 minutes)	slow (25 minutes to 2 hours)
Elimination	slow (2 to 3 weeks)	rapid (2 to 6 days)	slow (2 to 3 weeks)
Cumulative	more likely	less likely	more likely
Total daily digitalizing dose (usually given in divided doses)	1 to 2 Gm. P.O.	2 to 4 mg. P.O. 0.75 to 1 mg. I.V.	1 to 1.5 mg. P.O. or I.V.
Total daily maintenance dose (usually given in one dose)	100 to 200 mg.	0.25 to 1 mg.	0.05 to 0.2 mg.

REFERENCES

Gans, John A. "Digitalis Glycosides." *Nursing 73* 3:59, June 1973.

Spencer, Roberta. "Problems of Drug Therapy in Congestive Heart Failure." *RN* 35:46, August 1972.

Winslow, Elizabeth Hahn. "Digitalis." *American Journal of Nursing* 74:1062, June 1974.

APPLICATION QUESTIONS

I. *True-False*

For each statement below, write **a** if the statement is true or **b** if it is false.

_a_ 1. Digitalis preparations are used to decrease the pulse deficit.

_a_ 2. All digitalis products have similar effects on the heart.

_b_ 3. Digitalis glycosides decrease stroke volume.

_a_ 4. Hypokalemia sensitizes the heart to toxic effects of digitalis.

_a_ 5. A dosage error of only a fraction of a milligram of a pure digitalis glycoside can cause serious cardiac toxicity.

_a_ 6. Daily maintenance doses of digitalis should equal the amount of digitalis eliminated each day.

II. *Multiple Choice*

For each of the following questions, indicate the letter providing the *best* answer.

_b_ 1. What effect does digitalis have on the myocardium? (a) it shortens the refractory period (b) it causes more forceful contractions (c) it causes more rapid depolarization (d) it speeds the passage of impulses arising from the atria

_a_ 2. Which digitalis preparation would be the best to use in an emergency situation? (a) digoxin (b) digitalis leaf (c) digitoxin (d) Crystodigin

_c_ 3. After a patient begins oral digitalization, clinical improvement is indicated by which of the following pulse changes? (a) rapid drop in pulse rate into the 60s (b) extrasystolic rhythm (c) gradual decrease in pulse rate into the 70s (d) maintenance of rate with increase in quality

_b_ 4. What action should the nurse take if, prior to administering a digitalis preparation, a radial pulse rate of 60 is detected? (a) withhold the drug and notify the physician (b) check the apical pulse rate and give the drug if there is no widening of the patient's usual pulse deficit (c) check the blood pressure and withhold the drug if there is a widening pulse pressure (d) give the drug and record the pulse

_b_ 5. What is often the first indication of digitalis intoxication? (a) furry tongue (b) anorexia (c) anuria (d) a tingling sensation in the fingers

_d_ 6. Digitalis preparations may produce which of the following toxic cardiac effects? (1) ventricular bradycardia (2) premature ventricular contractions (3) increased automaticity (4) heart block (a) 4 (b) 2, 3 (c) 1, 4 (d) 1, 2, 3, 4

_b_ 7. Visual toxic effects of digitalis commonly include which of the following? (a) hemianopia (b) diplopia (c) photophobia (d) anopia

_a_ 8. What is *pulse deficit*? (a) the difference between the apical pulse and the radial pulse (b) the difference between systolic and diastolic blood pressures (c) the difference between the atrial and ventricular beats (d) the difference between the right and left radial pulses

_c_ 9. If an elderly patient who is to be discharged from the hospital expresses confusion about taking his many medications at home, which of the following approaches should the nurse use? (a) "You need to take this digitalis like the doctor told you to, Mr. Jones." (b) "What did I tell you about your medicines, Mr. Jones?" (c) "It must seem very confusing, Mr. Jones. Let's start with this one, digitalis—how often do you take these?" (d) "Don't worry, Mr. Jones, I'll just explain it to your wife."

_d_ 10. Which of the following drugs would be used to treat digitalis-induced bradycardia? (a) ouabain (b) aminophylline (c) morphine (d) atropine

_c_ 11. Digitalis-induced tachyarrhythmias may be treated with which of the following drugs? (a) sodium salts (b) isoproterenol (c) diphenylhydantoin (Dilantin) (d) magnesium sulfate

_d_ 12. Which of the following foods might the nurse recommend for a patient being maintained on digitalis, as being high in potassium and low in sodium? (1) dates (2) unsalted peanuts (3) hard candy (4) orange juice (5) bananas (a) 4 only (b) 2, 4 (c) 3, 4, 5 (d) 1, 2, 4, 5 (e) 1, 2, 3, 4, 5

III. *Matching A*

Match each digitalis preparation to its speed of onset.

_b_ 1. digitoxin (Crystodigin)

_a_ 2. digoxin (Lanoxin)

_b_ 3. digitalis (powdered leaf)

(a) rapid onset

(b) slow onset

IV. *Matching B*

Match the usual daily maintenance dose with the digitalis preparation for which it is appropriate.

_b_ 1. 100–200 mg.

_c_ 2. 0.25–1 mg.

_a_ 3. 0.05–0.2 mg.

(a) digitoxin (Crystodigin)

(b) digitalis (powdered leaf)

(c) digoxin (Lanoxin)

IV. *Discussion*

For each patient statement given below, write **a** if teaching is needed, or **b** if no teaching is indicated. If you answer that teaching is needed, outline the content you would teach.

_a_   1. "Now don't laugh at me, nurse, but I think I gotta stop taking that medicine the doc put me on—I mean, well, I must be turning into a woman—look at my breasts!"

_h_   2. "I just don't believe in taking any drug so regularly that it may become a habit, so I occasionally don't take my digitalis."

_b_   3. "I've discovered that when I eat much extra salt my digitalis doesn't seem to work as well, and my legs swell, so I try to avoid doing that."

V. *Calculation*

_____ 1. A patient is to receive digitoxin 0.05 mg by injection. The digitoxin is labeled 0.2 mg/ml. How many cc. will you give?

18

Antiarrhythmic Drugs

Cardiac arrhythmias are conditions in which the atria or the ventricles contract at an abnormal rate or with an abnormal rhythm. Arrhythmia can result from impulses arising outside the sinoatrial pacemaker (ectopic sites) or from impulses that spread through the heart by abnormal pathways. Arrhythmias may result in rapid or slow rhythms. This chapter deals with drugs used to treat rapid arrhythmias. Treatment of slow arrhythmias is discussed in Chapter 16, dealing with autonomic drugs.

ANTIARRHYTHMIC THERAPY

Many people experience occasional abnormal heartbeats that usually require no treatment. If the abnormality appears to result from anxiety and tension, a minor tranquilizer may be prescribed to control the abnormal rate or rhythm indirectly. The use of antiarrhythmic drugs is indicated when the ventricles beat so fast that cardiac output is reduced; when a minor arrhythmia (such as premature ventricular contraction) threatens to develop into a more dangerous one; or when a dangerous arrhythmia has developed which may become fatal.

Antiarrhythmic therapy has two objectives: (1) to abolish abnormal rhythm and restore normal sinus rhythm; and (2) to prevent recurrence of the arrhythmia. Although digitalis is considered an antiarrhythmic drug by some, it does not meet these objectives. Digitalis does protect the ventricles from the effects of atrial fibrillation (a bombardment of impulses on the A-V node originating from ectopic sites in the atria), but it does not convert the atria to a normal sinus rhythm.

ANTIARRHYTHMIC DRUGS

The five antiarrhythmic drugs to be discussed here include two older drugs, quinidine sulfate and pro-

cainamide hydrochloride, and three newer antiarrhythmic drugs, lidocaine hydrochloride, diphenylhydantoin sodium, and propranolol hydrochloride.

Quinidine Sulfate and Procainamide Hydrochloride

Both of these drugs suppress ectopic automaticity and prolong the effective refractory period of all parts of the heart. The first action is useful in treating such disorders as premature beats and tachycardias; the second action is useful in stopping abnormal pathways such as "circus" movements.

When toxic doses are taken, either drug may cause excessive slowing of conduction, which may result in cardiac arrest. The drugs can also depress myocardial contractions, weakening the heartbeat to such an extent as to cause heart failure.

Diphenylhydantoin Sodium $(D \cdot P \cdot H \cdot)$

Although diphenylhydantoin is not approved by the FDA for this use, it is now the preferred drug for treating arrhythmias resulting from digitalis toxicity (see Chapter 17), since it does not further depress A-V conduction as quinidine sulfate and procainamide hydrochloride do. It is important to remember that diphenylhydantoin sodium can potentiate the action of anticoagulant drugs. If a patient is receiving both drugs, the dosage of the anticoagulant must be adjusted and the patient closely observed for bleeding.

Lidocaine Hydrochloride

Quinidine sulfate and procainamide hydrochloride are still used for treating some ventricular tachyarrhythmias; however, the more serious irregularities, such as premature ventricular contractions following an acute myocardial infarction, are treated with lidocaine hydrochloride (Xylocaine hydrochloride). Lidocaine hydrochloride controls the arrhythmia without depressing cardiac conduction or reducing the contractile strength of the heart muscles.

107

Table 18–1. Antiarrhythmic drugs.

Generic Name	Trade Name	How Supplied	Routes	Usual Dose	Comments
quinidine sulfate	Quinidex	sustained release tablets 300 mg.	P.O.	2 tablets q. 8–12h.	Should be given P.O. in individualized dosage schedules. Other soluble salts are available for parenteral use.
		regular tablets 200 and 300 mg.	I.M.	adjusted as pt. needs	
quinidine hydrochloride		injection 120 mg./ml. in 1.5, 5, 10 ml. container; 800 mg./ml. in 10 ml. container	I.V.	adjusted as pt. needs	
procainamide hydrochloride	Pronestyl	capsule 250 mg., 375 mg., 500 mg.	P.O.	50 mg./kg. of body weight P.O. q. 3h.	I.V. use should be reserved for emergencies. The 500 mg./cc. potency of Pronestyl injection should be diluted prior to I.V. use.
		multiple dose vials 10 cc., 100 mg./cc. 2 cc., 500 mg./cc.	I.M. I.V.	500 mg. I.M. q. 6h. 200 mg.–1 Gm. I.V.	
diphenylhydan-toin sodium	Dilantin	vials 100 mg./2 cc. 250 mg./5 cc.	I.V. I.M.	5–10 mg./kg. of body weight I.V. 125–250 mg. I.M.	Especially useful for digitalis intoxication because it does not decrease A-V conduction. I.V. dose should not exceed 50 mg. per minute.
		tablet 50 mg. capsules 30 mg., 100 mg. suspension 30 mg./5 cc. 125 mg./5 cc.	P.O.	100–200 mg. P.O.	
lidocaine hydrochloride	Xylocaine	direct injection: ampuls 100 mg./5 cc. and 50 mg./5 cc. I.V. additives: vials 1 Gm. and 2 Gm. for dilution	I.V.	50–100 mg. I.V. 25–50 mg./minute	A second dose may be given after 5 minutes if the desired response is not produced. No more than 200–300 mg. should be administered in one hour. Xylocaine mixed with epinephrine (used for local anesthesia) should never be used for cardiac patients.
propranolol hydrochloride	Inderal	tablets 10 mg. 40 mg. 80 mg. ampuls 1 cc. 1 mg./cc.	P.O. I.V.	10–30 mg. q.i.d. 1–3 mg. I.V. not to exceed 1 mg./cc. per minute.	I.V. use reserved for life-threatening arrhythmias or those occurring under anesthesia.

(handwritten: Phenytoin D.P.H.)

Lidocaine hydrochloride has a short duration of action and is rapidly eliminated. This is an advantage because if overdosage occurs, it will last only a short time. It is a disadvantage in that to achieve the desired effects, the drug must be given in continuous slow intravenous infusion for several days. When a patient is receiving intravenous lidocaine, the nurse must be very observant to insure that the dosage is proper. The infusion equipment and the patient's blood pressure should be checked very frequently, because even the slightest increase in drip rate can cause a severe hypotensive response. The electrocardiogram should also be observed for lengthening of the P-R interval (indicating delayed conduction *to* the ventricles) or widening of the QRS complex (indicating delayed conduction *through* the ventricles, which leads to myocardial depression). Lidocaine hydrochloride can affect the central nervous system as well as the heart; patients should be watched for signs of excitement, followed by drowsiness, disorientation, dyspnea, convulsions, and coma.

Propranolol Hydrochloride

Arrhythmias may occur during anesthesia. If a patient appears to be a candidate for cardiac arrhythmias, an antiarrhythmic drug is administered before and during the induction of anesthesia. Procainamide hydrochloride or propranolol hydrochloride (Inderal) may be used in this situation. Propranolol hydrochloride is a beta adrenergic blocking agent; it is therefore useful for controlling rhythm disorders caused by excessive sympathetic nervous system activity or by adrenal medullary hormones, in addition to those caused by anesthetics such as halothane and cyclopropane.

Because of its beta adrenergic blocking effect, this drug can produce some dangerous noncardiac side effects. For example, it may depress the sympathetic nerve impulse to the bronchial smooth muscles; in an asthmatic patient, this could lead to an acute asthmatic attack. Diabetic patients who have learned to recognize hypoglycemia or insulin reaction from the epinephrine response should learn to watch for other responses instead when taking propranolol hydrochloride, as the epinephrine response will be blocked.

NURSING RESPONSIBILITIES WITH ANTIARRHYTHMIC DRUGS

Observation is the most important skill for the nurse caring for a patient receiving antiarrhythmic drugs. The nurse must monitor the patient's apical and radial pulses to detect arrhythmias and widening pulse deficit, as well as checking his blood pressure to detect hypotension. The electrocardiogram must be observed, especially for the lengthening of the P-R interval and widening of the QRS complex by more than 25 percent. The nurse should be alert for cinchonism (sensitivity to or toxicity of cinchona bark from which quinidine is derived) and be aware of the initial signs and symptoms of heart failure. The nurse must also be sure that emergency drugs and equipment for treating heart failure and cardiac arrest are readily available.

REFERENCES

Gans, John A. "Antiarrhythmics." *Nursing 73* 3:29, August 1973.

Mayer, Gloria Gilbert, and Kaelin, Patricia. "Arrhythmias and Cardiac Output." *American Journal of Nursing* 72:1597, September 1972.

Shinn, Arthur, et al. "Drug Interactions of Common CCU Medications." *American Journal of Nursing* 74:1442, August 1974.

APPLICATION QUESTIONS

I. *True-False*

For each statement below, write **a** if the statement is true or **b** if it is false.

_b_ 1. All cardiac arrhythmias require drug therapy.

_a_ 2. Some arrhythmias can be controlled with the use of mild tranquilizers.

_a_ 3. An ectopic beat is an impulse originating anywhere other than the S-A node.

_b_ 4. Quinidine sulfate enhances the conduction of impulses through the A-V node.

_b_ 5. An advantage of lidocaine hydrochloride (Xylocaine hydrochloride) for treating arrhythmias is that it affects only cardiac tissue.

_a_ 6. Propranolol tends to produce noncardiac side effects.

II. *Multiple Choice*

For each of the following questions, indicate the letter providing the *best* answer.

_C_ 1. Which of the following are potentially dangerous side effects of quinidine and procainamide? (1) heart failure (2) cardiac arrest (3) arrhythmias (4) hypertension
(a) 2 (b) 1, 4 (c) 1, 2, 3 (d) 1, 2, 3, 4

_b_ 2. What action of antiarrhythmic drugs would be useful for treating "circus" movements? (a) suppressing automaticity (b) prolonging the refractory period of the heart muscle (c) increasing A-V conduction (d) inhibiting the S-A node

_a_ 3. *Cinchonism* refers to sensitivity to which of the following drugs? (a) quinidine sulfate (b) procainamide hydrochloride (c) lidocaine hydrochloride (d) diphenylhydantoin sodium

_a_ 4. Which of the following is a property of lidocaine hydrochloride? (a) it is rapidly eliminated from the body (b) it depresses cardiac conduction (c) it has an extended duration of action (d) it reduces the contractile strength of the heart muscle

_c_ 5. The patient who develops premature ventricular contractions following an acute myocardial infarction would be treated most effectively and safely with which of the following drugs? (a) quinidine sulfate (b) procainamide hydrochloride (c) lidocaine hydrochloride (d) diphenylhydantoin sodium

_d_ 6. The nurse must carefully monitor the blood pressure of a patient receiving continuous intravenous lidocaine hydrochloride to detect which of the following side effects of the drug? (a) rapid rise in diastolic pressure (b) gradual hypertension (c) narrowing of the pulse pressure (d) rapid hypotension

_a_ 7. If a patient being treated with intravenous lidocaine hydrochloride develops a delay in conduction to the ventricles, what change occurs on his electrocardiogram? (a) longer P-R interval (b) wider QRS complex (c) extra P waves (d) inverted T waves

_a_ 8. If a patient receiving an anticoagulant is begun on diphenylhydantoin sodium for arrhythmias, what adjustment should be made in the dosage of the anticoagulant? (a) it should be reduced (b) it should be increased (c) it should be discontinued (d) no change is necessary

_b_ 9. Why is digitalis not considered a true antiarrhythmic drug? (a) it does not act directly on the heart muscle (b) it does not convert the atria to a normal sinus rhythm (c) it cannot be used to treat dangerous ventricular arrhythmias (d) it slows the heart rate excessively

_c_ 10. What is the drug of choice for treating tachyarrhythmias due to digitalis intoxication? (a) quinidine sulfate (b) procainamide hydrochloride (c) diphenylhydantoin sodium (d) epinephrine

_c_ 11. What effect might propranolol have on a diabetic patient? (a) it might require that insulin dosage be increased (b) it might require that insulin dosage be decreased (c) it might mask the symptoms of hypoglycemia (d) it might mask the symptoms of diabetic acidosis

_d_ 12. Which of the following antiarrhythmic drugs is a beta adrenergic blocking agent? (a) quinidine sulfate (b) procainamide hydrochloride (c) lidocaine hydrochloride (d) propranolol hydrochloride

_a_ 13. What is the action of a beta adrenergic blocking agent? (a) it inhibits the sympathetic nervous system (b) it inhibits the parasympathetic nervous system (c) it depresses the adrenal cortex (d) it depresses a portion of the central nervous system

_b_ 14. Which of the following may be a side effect of propranolol hydrochloride? (a) hyperglycemia (b) respiratory distress from bronchospasm (c) urinary retention from decreased bladder tone (d) hypertension

III. *Calculation*

_____ 1. Dilantin 250 mg. I.V. push is ordered. The medication vial is labeled 50 mg./2cc. How many cc. will you give?

19

Diuretics

Diuretics are drugs that increase the amount of urine produced by the kidneys. Although diuretics are occasionally used in nonedematous conditions, their principal use is to relieve the excessive sodium and water retained in body tissues in the condition called edema. With the exception of the newer potent diuretics, these drugs should be used only when renal function is good.

A patient with severe edema may be maintained on daily administration of a diuretic until his "dry weight" is reached. "Dry weight" is normal body weight without the presence of excess fluid. Once the patient has reached his dry weight, he may be maintained by taking the same diuretic every other day or by daily administration of a less potent diuretic to prevent recurrence of the edema.

NURSING RESPONSIBILITIES

When a patient is receiving a diuretic, the nurse must be very alert to his safety and comfort. Accurate records of intake and output must be maintained, along with daily records of weight. Body weight provides the best data for judging whether a patient is losing fluid too fast or is beginning to gain fluid again. Weighing should be done at the same time every day, preferably on the same scale. It is important to note any changes in the patient's food intake or activity level, because these could alter the body weight without indicating a change in fluid balance.

The nurse should also consider the patient's comfort when establishing the time for administration of the diuretic. For example, if a rapid acting diuretic is to be given once a day, the patient would be more comfortable receiving the drug during the morning, so it would not disturb his sleep at night. The patient should be told beforehand about the urgency and frequency of urination that will occur, to prevent him from becoming alarmed when diuresis begins. Be certain that a bedpan or urinal as well as the call bell is within easy reach of the patient. The patient with edema may be weak and have difficulty moving about. If the nurse does not respond at once to the patient's signal light, he may attempt to get up and go into the bathroom without assistance, risking injury from falling rather than the embarrassment of voiding in the bed.

CLASSIFICATION OF DIURETICS

There are eight broad classes of diuretics: (1) oral sulfonamides; (2) newer high-potency diuretics; (3) organic mercurials; (4) carbonic anhydrase inhibitors; (5) osmotic diuretics; (6) potassium-sparing diuretics; (7) acidifying salts; and (8) xanthine compounds.

All the most effective diuretics act by interfering with tubular reabsorption of sodium. When sodium is not reabsorbed, water as well as ions such as potassium, chloride, hydrogen, and bicarbonate, may also be kept from reabsorption. The water loss is desirable, if not too rapid or excessive, but the loss of ions can lead to severe and dangerous side effects. The most common side effect of diuretics is *hypokalemia*, or potassium loss. This can lead to irregularities in the heartbeat, especially if the patient is also taking digitalis, which is often the case in the treatment of edema associated with congestive heart failure. Hypokalemia can also lead to muscle weakness and pain, drowsiness, dizziness, confusion, and other neuromuscular symptoms. Hypokalemia may cause a patient with cirrhosis to lapse into hepatic coma.

Also possible as a side effect is *hyperkalemia*, which occurs only with the potassium-sparing diuretics; this may lead to cardiac arrest.

When sodium, potassium, hydrogen, and chloride ions are lost and bicarbonate is allowed to accumulate, *alkalosis* may occur. Diuretic therapy with the sulfonamides, the newer potent drugs, or the mercurials may lead to alkalosis. On the other hand, when chloride ions are allowed to accumulate and bicarbonate is removed, *acidosis* may occur. Diuretics such as the carbonic anhydrase inhibitors and the acidifying salts may lead to acidosis.

Overdosage of a diuretic that removes both sodium and chloride ions can lead to "low salt syndrome," or hyponatremia. The sulfonamides, mercurials, and newer potent diuretics are the most likely to cause this syndrome. Low salt syndrome is the condition that occurs when fluid losses are replaced by large quantities of plain water; the symptoms and treatment are the same as those for heat prostration.

Diuretic therapy can, of course, lead to severe dehydration. This is a severe threat with the new potent diuretics. Dehydration in turn can lead to poor skin turgor and to skin breakdown in immobilized patients.

Sulfonamides

This class of drugs is related chemically to the antibacterial sulfonamides. Although not all sulfonamides are thiazides, most of the commonly used sulfonamide diuretics are thiazides: sodium chlorothiazide (Diuril); benzthiazide (Aquatag); and methyclothiazide (Enduron). The thiazides are still widely used because they are less likely than other diuretics to cause excessive diuresis and electrolyte imbalance. In addition, they are convenient for administration, as they are given orally. They are not as potent or as effective as the newer diuretics, and therefore are not used in emergency situations.

Thiazides can lead to hypokalemia; patients maintained on these drugs should therefore be instructed to include foods high in potassium in their daily diet. Oranges, bananas, and raw mushrooms are not only high in potassium, but also low in sodium. Thus they are good foods to recommend to patients who must restrict their sodium intake while on diuretic therapy. A thiazide diuretic may be given in combination with a potassium-sparing diuretic to correct the potassium imbalance.

Patients with diabetes mellitus or gout should be observed closely while taking thiazide diuretics, because the drugs cause an increase in uric acid and glucose levels in the blood. The insulin requirement of the diabetic patient may increase, and the patient with gout may need his gout medication increased as well.

Potent Diuretics

These new diuretics, furosemide (Lasix) and ethacrynic acid (Edecrin) are very potent. They are particularly useful in emergency situations because they can be given intravenously and have a rapid onset of action. They are potent enough that they can be given to patients with renal failure to force some kidney function if necessary. Although these drugs are useful in severe and emergency situations, they are also more likely than other diuretics to cause severe dehydration and electrolyte imbalances. In therapy with these drugs, it is important to avoid too rapid or too much fluid loss, which might lead to cardiovascular collapse or clot formation.

Mercurials

These are the oldest potent diuretics but the least used today. They are rapid acting but must be given by injection. The mercurials can cause direct tissue toxicity and, although less likely to cause hypokalemia than drugs of the two classes discussed above, can lead to hypochloremic alkalosis. Patients can become unresponsive to mercurials if they are given too frequently. An acidifying salt may be given in conjunction with one of the mercurials to counteract the alkalosis and restore responsiveness to the mercurial drug.

Potassium-Sparing Diuretics

These drugs remove edema fluid and sodium from the body without removing potassium; they can, in fact, cause hyperkalemia. Spironolactone (Aldactone), the most commonly used potassium-sparing diuretic, blocks the action of aldosterone. This drug can be used to combat the symptoms of hyperaldosteronism, but is also used frequently in combination with one of the thiazide or mercurial diuretics to decrease the possibility of hypokalemia. Drugs are available which combine a potassium-sparing and a potassium-depleting diuretic in one preparation. An example is Aldactazide, a drug preparation that contains both spironolactone and hydrochlorothiazide. The other potassium-sparing diuretic is triamterene (Dyrenium).

Carbonic Anhydrase Inhibitors

These weak but safe diuretics are useful when mild diuresis is needed, in such instances as premenstrual edema, pregnancy edema, and retention of fluid accompanying corticosteroid therapy. Because drugs of this class, such as acetazolamide sodium (Diamox), may cause excretion of bicarbonate, the patient must be watched for signs of metabolic acidosis. The carbonic anhydrase inhibitor drugs are useful in nonedematous conditions, as for reducing intraocular pressure in glaucoma and as adjunct therapy with anticonvulsants in the treatment of epilepsy.

Table 19–1. Diuretics.

Generic Name	Trade Name	How Supplied	Routes	Usual Dose	Comments
mercaptomerin sodium	Thiomerin	ampuls 1 cc., 2 cc. / vials 10 ml., 30 ml. 125 mg./ml.	Sc / I.M. (deep) I.V.	0.2–2 ml. daily	I.M. injections are painful; massage of the site often helps to relieve the pain.
spironolactone	Aldactone	tablets 25 mg.	P.O.	25 mg. q.i.d.	Children's daily dose is 1.5 mg./lb. of body weight.
acetazolamide *Used for Glaucoma, save eyesight*	Diamox	tablets 125 mg., 250 mg. capsules 500 mg. (sustained release) vials 500 mg.	P.O. / I.V.	250 mg. q.d. or q.o.d.	
urea	Ureaphil	vials 150 cc. 40 Gm./vial	I.V.	1 Gm./kg. of body weight or 8–20 Gm. several times a day. Not to exceed 1.5 Gm./kg.	Given in 30% solution; rate not to exceed 60 gtts/minute. Dose should not exceed 120 Gm. daily. Should be freshly prepared each dose.
benzthiazide	Aquatag	tablets 25 mg., 50 mg.	P.O.	50 mg. b.i.d.	Larger doses may be necessary until "dry weight" is obtained.
furosemide	Lasix	tablets 20 mg., 40 mg. ampuls 2 cc. 10 mg./cc. 10 cc. 10 mg./cc.	P.O. I.M. I.V.	40–80 mg. P.O. q.d. 20–40 mg. I.M. or I.V.	Exposure of the drug to light may cause discoloration, which does not alter its potency. This drug is contraindicated in women of childbearing potential. I.V. doses should be given slowly.
ethacrynic acid	Edecrin	tablets 25 mg., 50 mg.	P.O.	50–200 mg. P.O. q.d.	Edecrin should not be given intramuscularly or subcutaneously. When some 5% dextrose solutions are used to reconstitute the dry material, the solution may appear hazy. I.V. use of these solutions is not recommended. Discard unused solution after 24 hours. Edecrin is not recommended for pregnant women or nursing mothers.
sodium ethacrynate	Sodium Edecrin	vials 50 cc. 1 mg./cc.	I.V.	50 mg. I.V., or 0.5–1 mg. per kg. of body weight	

fast acting. Dose response continues to climb.

toxic, causes deafness

Osmotic Diuretics

These drugs, urea (Urevert) and mannitol (Osmitrol) increase the fluid volume through the kidney. They are used to continue urine formation in situations that could lead to kidney shutdown, such as following massive burns or trauma and following open heart surgery. They are useful for reducing intracranial pressure caused by cerebral edema. They may also be used to relieve pressure within the eye.

Acidifying Salts

Drugs of this class, such as ammonium chloride, are weak diuretics which may be used as adjuncts to the mercurial diuretics discussed above.

Xanthines

These drugs are very weak diuretics such as caffeine, theobromine, and theophylline. They are no longer widely used as diuretics. Theophylline may be used for its dual actions of diuresis and bronchodilation in the treatment of pulmonary edema. The xanthines and the acidifying salt diuretics are those usually found in medications sold without a prescription for such conditions as premenstrual edema.

REFERENCES

Kee, Joyce L. "Fluid and Electrolyte Imbalances." *Nursing 72* 2:22, January 1972.

Lee, Carla A., "Extracellular Volume Imbalance." *American Journal of Nursing* 74:888, May 1974.

Reed, Gretchen Mayo. "Confused about Potassium? Here's a Clear, Concise Guide." *Nursing 74* 3:20, March 1974.

Rodman, Morton J. "Drugs Used in Cardiovascular Disease: Part III, Treating Edema." *RN 36*:55, May 1973.

Schneider, William, Boyce, B. A. "Complications of Diuretic Therapy." *American Journal of Nursing 68*:1903, September 1968.

APPLICATION QUESTIONS

I. *True-False*

For each statement below, write **a** if the statement is true or **b** if it is false.

_a_ 1. Overdosage of one of the potent diuretics can lead to the low salt syndrome.

_b_ 2. Spironolactone (Aldactone) is likely to cause hypokalemia.

_b_ 3. Thiazide diuretics are given intravenously in emergency situations.

_a_ 4. Combining spironolactone (Aldactone) with a thiazide diuretic aids in preventing potassium imbalance.

_a_ 5. The pain and irritation experienced when mercurials are given parenterally may be minimized by massaging the injection site.

___ 6. Most diuretics act by interfering with tubular reabsorption of sodium.

_b_ 7. Hyperchloremia is another name for alkalosis.

_a_ 8. Hyperkalemia can cause cardiac arrest.

_a_ 9. When a diabetic is begun on a thiazide diuretic, his insulin requirement may be increased.

_a_ 10. Furosemide (Lasix) may be used in the presence of renal failure.

_b_ 11. When a patient is receiving spironolactone (Aldactone) in combination with a mercurial diuretic, he must be taught to include foods high in potassium in his daily diet.

II. *Multiple Choice*

For each of the following questions, indicate the letter providing the *best* answer.

_a_ 1. Acidosis is most likely to develop when a patient is taking which of the following drugs? (a) Diamox (b) Diuril (c) Edecrin (d) Thiomerin

_b_ 2. For which of the following reasons would a mercurial diuretic be used instead of a thiazide? (a) convenience in administration (b) higher degree of potency (c) fewer toxic reactions

_d_ 3. Which of the following drugs would be most effective when given intravenously in the emergency treatment of acute pulmonary edema? (a) ammonium chloride (b) benzthiazide (Aquatag) (c) hydrochlorothiazide (Hydrodiuril) (d) furosemide (Lasix)

_a_ 4. Fluid and electrolyte imbalance would be of the most concern in which of the following patients? (a) a 75-year-old atherosclerotic man receiving Lasix (b) a 90-year-old lady with a history of pulmonary edema being maintained on chlorothiazide (Diuril) every other day (c) a 30-year-old woman with premenstrual tension on acetazolamide (Diamox) (d) a 50-year-old alcoholic being maintained on hydrochlorothiazide (Hydrodiuril)

_c_ 5. Resistance to the mercurial diuretics can be controlled by adding to the regimen a diuretic of which of the following types? (a) osmotic (b) carbonic anhydrase inhibitor (c) acidifying salts (d) xanthine

d 6. Alkalosis occurs when which of the following ions is not excreted and is allowed to accumulate? (a) potassium (b) hydrogen (c) chloride (d) bicarbonate

c 7. What is the most common electrolyte imbalance resulting from excessive diuretic activity? (a) hyperkalemia (b) hypochloremia (c) hypokalemia (d) hyperchloremia

d 8. If a patient's diuretic dose is being adjusted according to daily weights, which of the following related activities would be important to record on the chart? (1) a large holiday meal brought in by the family (2) an exercise program started in physical therapy (3) the refusal of his prescribed hospital diet (4) the N.P.O. period prior to a GI series
(a) 3 (b) 2, 4 (c) 1, 2, 4 (d) 1, 2, 3, 4

b 9. Which of the following is *not* a symptom of hypokalemia? (a) muscle weakness and pain (b) wakefulness (c) confusion (d) dizziness

a 10. What is the major function of diuretic drugs? (a) to increase the amount of urine produced by the kidneys (b) to decrease the amount of sodium excreted by the kidneys (c) to maintain volume and composition of urine within normal limits (d) to regulate blood plasma production

b 11. Which of the following is the best muscle in which to inject an organic mercurial? (a) lateral thigh (b) gluteus maximus (c) deltoid (d) ventrogluteal

a 12. In consideration of the comfort of a patient, what time of day would be best to administer a mercurial diuretic? (a) 8 A.M. (b) noon (c) 6 P.M. (d) 10 P.M.

a 13. What happens to sodium when it is not reabsorbed by the kidney tubules? (a) it is excreted in the urine (b) it returns to the blood (c) it leaks into interstitial spaces (d) it is excreted by the skin

b 14. Which of the following statements best describes "dry weight"? (a) the patient's weight before diuretics are administered (b) the patient's weight before edema occurred (c) the patient's weight immediately following the morning bath (d) the patient's weight after two weeks of diuretic therapy

b 15. If a patient is begun on a diuretic drug, which of the following actions could the nurse institute without a doctor's order? (1) daily weight (2) intake and output (3) 200 mg. sodium diet (4) daily chemistry tests
(a) 2 (b) 1, 2 (c) 2, 4 (d) 1, 2, 3, 4

c 16. When a patient is receiving furosemide (Lasix) or ethacrynic acid (Edecrin) the nurse should be alert to which of the following complications? (1) cardiac irregularities (2) decubitus ulcers (3) acidosis (4) low salt syndrome
(a) 1, 3 (b) 3, 4 (c) 1, 2, 4 (d) 1, 2, 3, 4

b 17. A diuretic of which of the following types would be used to combat cerebral edema? (a) thiazide (b) osmotic (c) xanthine (d) sulfonamide

c 18. Which of the following types of diuretics act by increasing the fluid volume through the kidney? (a) potent diuretics (b) mercurials (c) osmotics (d) potassium-sparing

III. *Calculations*

A child weighing 35 pounds is to receive a total daily dose of Aldactone on the basis of 1.5 mg/lb.

_____ 1. How many mg. should the child receive daily?

_____ 2. Since Aldactone is supplied only in scored tablets containing 25 mg. each, what quantity of tablets would this child receive at any one time, if the total daily dose is divided into four equal doses through the day?

20

Antihypertensive Agents

A patient whose diastolic pressure is consistently higher than 90 mm. of Hg is considered to have hypertension. The height of the diastolic pressure is directly proportional to the severity of the hypertension as well as to the likelihood of organ damage.

PRIMARY AND SECONDARY HYPERTENSION

Hypertension is usually discussed in terms of primary hypertension (essential hypertension) and secondary hypertension. Secondary hypertension refers to high blood pressure with a known underlying cause, such as renal disease or the adrenal medullary tumor called *pheochromocytoma*. Primary hypertension refers to high blood pressure occurring with no known underlying cause. If a patient has secondary hypertension, treatment is directed at the underlying cause; if he has primary hypertension, treatment is directed solely at lowering blood pressure and preventing complications of the condition. This chapter deals mainly with drug treatment of primary hypertension.

Prolonged hypertension can lead to damage in the blood vessels and tissues of the brain, heart, and kidneys. It can also lead to retinal damage, cardiac muscle hypertrophy, abnormal electrocardiogram, proteinuria, and elevated blood levels of urea nitrogen and serum creatinine. In addition, the patient with hypertension is susceptible to myocardial infarction, cerebral vascular accident, aortic aneurysm, and other cardiovascular and kidney complications.

The treatment regimen for primary hypertension includes rest, modified diet, and drug therapy. *Mild hypertension*, with a diastolic pressure between 90 and 105 mm. of Hg, may require no drug therapy other than a minor tranquilizer. If the diastolic pressure is between 105 and 115 mm. of Hg, the treatment regimen

may include weight reduction, restricted sodium intake, more rest, and a diuretic drug. If he feels it is necessary, the physician may add one of the rauwolfia antihypertensive drugs to the regimen of a patient with mild hypertension. *Moderate hypertension*, with a diastolic pressure between 115 and 130 mm. of Hg, and with no evidence of organ damage, may be treated with a diuretic, a rauwolfia drug, and another antihypertensive agent such as hydralazine hydrochloride (Apresoline). *Severe hypertension*, with diastolic pressure over 130 mm. of Hg and with evidence of organ damage, would be treated with the same regimen as moderate hypertension, but one of the antihypertensive agents would be replaced with a more potent drug such as methyldopa (Aldomet). If a patient demonstrates *malignant hypertension*, in which organ damage occurs rapidly and leads to kidney and other organ failure, he may be treated with guanethidine sulfate (Ismelin).

DIURETICS

The diuretic drugs are discussed in Chapter 19. The thiazide diuretics are those most commonly used for treating hypertension. Diuretics not only reduce the volume of circulating blood, but they also increase the effectiveness of antihypertensive agents such as methyldopa and guanethidine.

When treating malignant hypertension or hypertensive crisis (an acute medical emergency), intravenous administration of one of the more potent diuretics such as furosemide or sodium ethacrynate would be used.

SYMPATHOLYTIC AGENTS

Since the sympathetic nervous system is responsible for constricting most of the peripheral vessels, sympatholytic drugs (sympathetic blocking agents) would cause dilation of these vessels. Almost all the sympathetic blocking agents cause arterial vasodilation, dilation of the veins, and slowing and weakening of the heart beat. These actions respectively result in reduced peripheral resistance, reduced amount of blood returning to the heart, and reduced cardiac output. All these actions lead to a reduction in blood pressure. Because of the potency of sympatholytic drugs, however, even a slight overdosage can result in excessive and dangerous lowering of the blood pressure. If blood pressure falls too greatly, poor kidney perfusion can occur, leading to kidney failure as well as heart failure. Remember that both digitalis and the sympathetic blocking agents slow the heart; when given in combination, they can lead to excessive bradycardia.

Patients receiving antihypertensive medications, particularly elderly patients with arteriosclerosis, are particularly subject to *postural hypotension*. Because the medication interferes with the autonomic nervous system, when a patient stands up too quickly from a recumbent position, the vessels do not constrict fast enough in response, and blood pools toward the gravitational force, depriving the brain of blood and resulting in dizziness and fainting. Of course, patients should be told to avoid sudden changes in posture to avoid postural hypotension.

Because the sympathetic nervous system has many actions, sympathetic blocking agents may cause a variety of side effects. For example, patients with gastric ulcers or colitis may experience an exaggeration of symptoms due to the increase in gastric secretions and motility caused by the drug. The increase in gastrointestinal tract activity can cause abdominal cramping and diarrhea in any patient taking these drugs.

Sympatholytic agents can be classified according to where in the sympathetic pathway they act. *Ganglionic blocking agents* inhibit impulses at the sympathetic ganglia. *Adrenergic neuron blocking agents* reduce the amount of neurohormone at the nerve ending. *Adrenergic blocking agents* keep the receptor sites in the body organs and vessels from responding to the impulses.

Adrenergic Neuron Blocking Agents

These drugs are the most commonly used sympathetic blocking agents in the treatment of hypertension. They act specifically on the sympathetic pathways, without interfering with parasympathetic pathways. Drugs in this classification include the rauwolfia alkaloids, methyldopa, and guanethidine sulfate.

Rauwolfia Alkaloids. Reserpine (Serpasil) is the most widely used rauwolfia alkaloid. It is an old drug that has been used for centuries. It was once used as a

tranquilizer because of its calming influence on the central nervous system.

Reserpine is most often administered with a thiazide diuretic. The heart-slowing activity of reserpine may add to the effectiveness of digitalis, but it could lead to excessive bradycardia. This drug can be injected intramuscularly or intravenously in emergency situations. Although it may be slower acting than other drugs and may make the patient excessively sleepy, reserpine is used because of its relative safety. Even if an overdose is given, the use of reserpine rarely leads to a rapid or excessive drop in blood pressure.

Methyldopa (Aldomet). One major advantage of this drug is that it does not reduce cardiac output or blood flow through the kidneys. It is therefore a drug of choice for patients with poor kidney function. Methyldopa is less likely to cause postural hypotension, but it is similar to reserpine in that it can cause drowsiness. Administering methyldopa with a diuretic can increase the antihypertensive effect.

Although methyldopa is relatively safe, it has on rare occasions caused liver damage and hemolytic anemia. It is therefore not administered to patients with existing disorders of these types.

Note: methyldopa should never be confused with the antiparkinsonism drug *levodopa* (see Chapter 10), although their names are quite similar.

Guanethidine Sulfate (Ismelin). This drug is a very effective antihypertensive agent. Combining guanethidine sulfate with a diuretic increases its effectiveness, so a smaller dose of guanethidine may be used. Because this drug is long acting, the nurse may need to teach the patient or a member of his family how to take the blood pressure each morning to determine if the daily dose is necessary.

Guanethidine is never used in the treatment of pheochromocytoma or given by injection in hypertensive crisis, because it could cause an *increase* in blood pressure in those instances.

Ganglionic Blocking Agents

Drugs in this classification are not commonly used in the treatment of hypertension because they block both sympathetic and parasympathetic fibers. This action can lead to a wide variety of discomforting side effects, such as constipation, urinary retention, blurring of vision from mydriasis, sexual impotence in men, and dry skin and mouth. These drugs are contraindicated for patients with glaucoma.

Drugs in this classification include trimethaphan camsylate (Arfonad) and mecamylamine hydrochloride (Inversine). Arfonad, when given by intravenous drip, usually produces an immediate drop in blood pressure and can rapidly lead to dangerous shock levels.

Adrenergic Blocking Agents

Drugs of this classification include phentolamine (Regitine) and phenoxybenzamine hydrochloride (Dibenzyline); they are generally reserved for the treatment of pheochromocytoma. They block the sympathetic effects on the arterioles but do not affect the heart.

MISCELLANEOUS ANTIHYPERTENSIVE AGENTS

Hydralazine Hydrochloride (Apresoline).   This drug has a direct vasodilating action. It is usually used in less serious stages of hypertension and is considered useful for patients with poor kidney function. Hydralazine hydrochloride is most often given in combination with reserpine and a diuretic drug. Because hydralazine hydrochloride may cause an increase in heart rate, it is desirable to combine it with reserpine, which has a heart-slowing effect.

Other side effects of hydralazine may include headache, dizziness, and an increase in anginal pain. This drug is contraindicated in the presence of hypertensive heart disease.

Pargyline Hydrochloride (Eutonyl).   This drug is a monoamine oxidase inhibiting drug. It is of the same classification as the MAO inhibitor antidepressant drugs (see Chapter 7). It is effective in lowering blood pressure, but because it is subject to all the side effects, cautions, and contraindications of any MAO inhibitor drug, its use is reserved for those patients who do not respond to other antihypertensive drugs.

Table 20–1. Antihypertensive agents.

Generic Name	Trade Name	How Supplied	Routes	Usual Dose	Comments
methyldopa	Aldomet	tablets 125 mg., 250 mg., 500 mg.	P.O.	500 mg.–2.0 Gm.	Not recommended for use in pregnant patients. Parenteral form is used to control acute hypertensive crisis.
methyldopate hydrochloride		ampuls 5 cc. 250 mg./5 cc.	I.V.	250–500 mg. q. 6h.	
hydralazine hydrochloride	Apresoline	tablets 10 mg., 25 mg., 50 mg., 100 mg.	P.O.	50 mg. P.O. q.i.d.	Initial doses are small, then dosage is increased until desired effect is reached.
		ampuls 1 cc. 20 mg./cc.	I.V. I.M.	20–40 mg. repeat p.r.n.	
reserpine	Serpasil	tablets 1 mg., 0.25 mg., 0.1 mg.	P.O.	maintenance dose 0.1 mg.–0.25 mg. q.d. Initial dose 0.5 mg. to 1 mg. I.M., followed by 2–4 mg. at three-hour intervals until blood pressure reaches the desired levels.	Should be given after meals to lessen gastro-intestinal discomfort.
		elixir 0.2 mg./tsp. (4 cc.)			
		multiple dose vials 10 cc., 2.5 mg./cc. ampuls 2 cc. 2.5 mg./cc.	I.M.		
phentolamine	Regitine	tablets 50 mg.	P.O.	50 mg. P.O. q.i.d.	Regitine blocking test may be used for diagnosis of pheochromocytoma. Also used to prevent dermal necrosis following I.V. administration or extravasation of norepinephrine.
		ampuls 1 cc. 5 mg./cc.	I.V. I.M.	5 mg. I.V.	

Handwritten annotations: "Symptoms - depression" (next to reserpine row); "Guanethitidine" (below reserpine row)

REFERENCES

AAGAARD, GEORGE N. "Treatment of Hypertension." *American Journal of Nursing* 73:621, April 1973.

COLEMAN, VERNON. "The Top Drugs—Aldomet." *Nursing Times* 69:531, April 1973.

RODMAN, MORTON J. "Drugs Used in Cardiovascular Disease: part 2, Treating Hypertension." *RN* 36:41, April 1973.

APPLICATION QUESTIONS

I. *True-False*

For each statement below, write **a** if the statement is true or **b** if it is false.

_a_ 1. Varied adverse drug interactions limit the use of pargyline hydrochloride (Eutonyl).

_a_ 2. Primary hypertension and essential hypertension are the same disease.

_b_ 3. The treatment of essential hypertension is aimed toward relieving the underlying cause.

_a_ 4. The thiazide type diuretics increase the effectiveness of antihypertensive drugs when administered in combination.

_a_ 5. Ganglionic blocking drugs may have an adverse effect on male sexual functioning.

_a_ 6. The higher the diastolic pressure, the greater the degree of severity of hypertension.

II. *Multiple Choice*

For each of the following questions, indicate the letter providing the *best* answer.

_d_ 1. Ganglionic blocking agents would be contraindicated for patients with which of the following? (a) peptic ulcer (b) athlete's foot (c) hypertensive crisis (d) glaucoma

_c_ 2. Which of the following statements describes the effect on the cardiac rate when hydralazine and reserpine are given together? (a) the tachycardia effects of both drugs increase the cardiac rate (b) bradycardia results from the vagal stimulation effects of the two drugs (c) the drugs have an antagonist reaction, and the cardiac rate remains the same (d) neither drug affects the cardiac rate

_b_ 3. Which of the following would be the antihypertensive drug of choice for a patient with poor kidney function? (a) reserpine (Serpasil) (b) methyldopa (Aldomet) (c) pargyline hydrochloride (Eutonyl) (d) guanethidine sulfate (Ismelin)

_a_ 4. Guanethidine sulfate (Ismelin) is contraindicated in the treatment of hypertension caused by pheochromocytoma for which of the following reasons? (a) it may cause a rise in blood pressure (b) it may cause a rapid drop in blood pressure (c) it may cause blindness (d) its action is too slow

_b_ 5. The general action of sympathetic blocking agents is described by which of the following statements? (1) reducing tone of smooth muscle in blood vessels (2) pooling peripheral venous blood (3) strengthening the heart contractions (4) slowing the heartbeat (a) 1 (b) 1, 2, 4 (c) 2, 3, 4 (d) 1, 3, 4

_c_ 6. Which of the following blood study reports would be seen in advanced cases of hypertension? (a) decreased BUN, increased creatine, increased urine protein (b) increased BUN, increased creatine, decreased urine protein (c) increased BUN, increased creatine, increased urine protein (d) decreased BUN, decreased creatine, decreased urine protein.

_a_ 7. What is the drug of choice for patients whose high blood pressure is caused by pheochromocytoma? (a) phentolamine (Regitine) (b) methyldopa (Aldomet) (c) pargyline hydrochloride (Eutonyl) (d) rauwolfia serpentina (Raudixin)

_c_ 8. All drugs used for treating hypertension affect the circulation in what ways? (a) they reduce peripheral resistance and increase cardiac output (b) they increase peripheral resistance and increase cardiac output (c) they decrease peripheral resistance and decrease cardiac output (d) they increase peripheral resistance and decrease cardiac output

III. *Matching*

Identify the drug classification acting at each point in the sympathetic pathway.

_a_ 1. Stops impulses at sympathetic ganglia

_c_ 2. Keeps the receptors in the heart and vessels from responding to neurohormone

_b_ 3. Decreases the amount of neurohormone at the nerve ending

(a) ganglionic blocker
(b) adrenergic neuron blocker
(c) adrenergic blocker.

IV. *Discussion*

For each patient statement given below, write **a** if teaching is needed or **b** if no teaching is indicated. If you answer that teaching is needed, outline the content you would teach.

_____ 1. "Well, actually my high blood pressure never did bother me much, not anything like the pills I'm supposed to take to cure it."

_____ 2. "The nurse in the hospital taught my mother how to take her blood pressure before she takes her medicine, but her eyes are so bad I don't know how she does it."

_____ 3. "The doctor has me on a pill for my hypertension and a diuretic pill, too. I think I'll stop that diuretic one, though; it's just too inconvenient to have to go to the bathroom that much."

_____ 4. "Mother sure gets sleepy and naps a lot since she started those blood pressure pills. I try to call her frequently though so that she will have to get up and go to the kitchen to answer the phone."

_____ 5. "Ever since the doctor brought Herman's blood pressure down with those pills, he's had diarrhea. I guess the lower blood pressure makes him susceptible to intestinal viruses."

V. *Calculation*

_____ 1. A patient is to receive 375 mg. of Aldomet I.V. The ampul indicates that there are 250 mg./5 cc. How many cc. will you administer?

Beater Blocker.
1) Propranolog - hypertension > violinest
tremor, migraine

Vasodilators

Vessel diseases are predominantly ischemic diseases. Ischemia results from a temporary decrease in blood supply to an area. Although permanent damage does not usually result from this temporary anemia and hypoxia, pain and decreased capacity of the part may occur. Ischemic diseases are usually classified as coronary, peripheral, or cerebral vascular diseases. Although many drugs, such as anticoagulants, thrombolytic agents, analgesic and anti-inflammatory agents, and anti-infective drugs, may be used in treating vascular disease, this chapter deals strictly with the use of vasodilating drugs.

Vasodilating drugs fall into three broad categories: (1) the nitrates and nitrites; (2) drugs that alter autonomic nervous system vasomotor control; and (3) drugs that act directly on the muscles of the blood vessels. Drugs in the first category are used primarily in the treatment of coronary vascular disease (angina pectoris), whereas drugs in the last two categories are used primarily for peripheral vascular disease and occasionally for cerebral vascular disease.

DRUGS USED FOR CORONARY ISCHEMIA

Angina pectoris is an ischemic disease caused by spasms of the coronary vessels. The main symptom of the disease is sudden, severe chest pain, usually preceded by emotional stress or physical exertion. There is usually no permanent damage from an anginal attack, but angina could be a warning that the patient is likely to suffer an acute myocardial infarction. Drugs relieve anginal pain by dilating coronary vessels to increase blood flow, and also by dilating peripheral veins to pool blood in the extremities, decrease the blood returning to the heart, and thereby reduce the workload of the heart.

Nitrates and Nitrites

Nitrates and nitrites are the most widely used antianginal drugs; they may be used to treat an attack or to prevent an attack.

Amyl nitrite and octyl nitrate are the two most rapid acting vasodilators. They could be used for treating an acute anginal attack, but are not often used because of the inconvenience of administration. These drugs can only be administered by inhalation. Nitrates taken sublingually are more convenient and are therefore more often used. Nitrates administered sublingually include nitroglycerin, erythrityl tetranitrate (Cardilate), and isosorbide dinitrate (Isordil). These drugs may also be taken in large oral doses or in sustained release oral preparations for long-term prophylaxis. Nitroglycerin is the most commonly used drug for treating the pain of an acute angina attack. Nitroglycerin is usually effective within two minutes after a small tablet is placed under the tongue.

Side Effects of Nitrates. Patients may complain of headache when taking nitrates. As the headache decreases, the effectiveness of the nitrates usually decreases. Tolerance to these drugs develops quickly, and it is important to stress to the patient that he should not be taking the drug unless it is definitely indicated. Poor response to the drug may also be due to deterioration of the chemical. These pills must be stored in tightly sealed *glass* containers—*not* in plastic because the plastic and exposure to air will hasten deterioration. Nitrates may also cause a drop in blood pressure because of peripheral vasodilation. Patients should be instructed always to lie down, or at least to sit down, when taking the drugs to avoid dizziness, faintness, and injury from falling. Postural hypotension may also set off a reflex racing of the heartbeat, leading to an undesirable increase in the workload of the heart. Nitrates should be used with caution by patients with glaucoma, since the vasodilation will aggravate the increased intraocular pressure.

Nursing Care. Since most patients learn to recognize their need for nitroglycerin and thus require the drug immediately, hospitalized patients are very often allowed to keep this medication at their bedside. The nurse must still be aware of and record the number of pills taken each day, the frequency, the activity of the patient prior to his need for the drug, and the patient's response to the medication. The nurse must also observe for mental confusion or any other situation that might contraindicate allowing the patient to medicate himself.

Long-Term Prophylaxis. The effectiveness of nitrates for prophylaxis against an anticipated attack or for long-term, around-the-clock therapy is questioned. The exception to this would be if a patient knew of impending exposure to cold, exercise, or excitement. In such situations, sublingual nitroglycerin may provide protection for about half a hour; isosorbide dinitrate may provide a longer effect; and erythrityl tetranitrate may provide even longer lasting protection, but it is delayed in its onset. If a nitrate drug does not prove effective in preventing attacks when taken frequently for prophylaxis, but tolerance to the drug still develops, its use must be questioned. As the patient becomes tolerant, it becomes more difficult to relieve the pain of an acute attack.

The patient with angina may lessen the number of attacks by adjusting his lifestyle so as to avoid cold, to avoid stressful situations, and to follow his prescribed regimen. It may be effective to maintain the patient on an antianxiety agent such as chlordiazepoxide, to reduce his response to stress and thereby reduce anginal attacks.

DRUGS USED TO TREAT PERIPHERAL VASCULAR DISEASE

Peripheral ischemia usually results either from vasospasm as in Raynaud's disease, or from organic damage to the walls of the blood vessels, as in Buerger's disease, atherosclerosis, and arteriosclerosis. Poor peripheral circulation can lead to pain, numbness, pallor, cyanosis, and eventually to necrosis and gangrene.

Vasodilating drugs are most beneficial when the etiology of the disease is vasospasm. When vessels are damaged and their walls are rigid from lipid plaque deposits, they do not respond well because they have lost their elasticity.

Administering vasodilating drugs to a patient with organic damage to the vessel walls may dilate the collateral vessels. Some physicians believe this aids in perfusing the ischemic area, while others feel it shunts blood away from the area.

Whether the patient is maintained on drug therapy or not, he should be taught to keep the body warm at all times; to avoid chilling; to avoid applying heat directly to the affected part; not to use commercial chemicals for removing corns and calluses from the feet; not to cut corns or calluses on the feet; to check the temperature of bath water with a part of the body not affected before submerging the ischemic part; to do light exercise, such as walking; to keep weight within recommended limits; to rest in positions that aid blood flow (if there is venous difficulty in the legs, the patient should rest with the legs elevated; if there is arterial disease in the legs, he should rest with the head elevated); to avoid clothing that constricts or causes pooling of blood; to avoid smoking; and not to take drugs which could cause vasoconstriction, such as ephedrine, amphetamines, and headache remedies containing ergotamine.

Drugs That Alter Autonomic Nervous System Vasomotor Control

The sympathetic response normally acts to dilate the vessels of the skeletal muscles and to constrict the cutaneous and superficial vessels. Since the adrenergic receptors in skeletal muscle vessels are basically beta type, and the receptors in the vessels of the skin are alpha type, alpha adrenergic *blocking* agents would be most effective in treating superficial vasospasm disease, such as Raynaud's disease, frostbite, and acrocyanosis. On the other hand, beta adrenergic *stimulating* agents would be most effective in treating vessel diseases of the skeletal muscle, such as intermittent claudication.

Alpha Adrenergic Blocking Agents. Phenoxybenzamine hydrochloride (Dibenzyline) is one of the most effective alpha adrenergic blocking agents. It tends to produce a relatively prolonged peripheral vasodilating effect when taken orally. The drug must be given in gradually increasing doses until its full effect is obtained. If large doses are given immediately, generalized vasodilation and hypotension may occur. This drug is used more for treating hypertension than for treating peripheral vascular diseases.

Because of the relationship between the sympathetic nervous system and blood pressure, patients should be watched carefully while on sympathetic blocking agents. A rapid drop in blood pressure might precipitate tachycardia or even congestive heart failure, especially in elderly patients.

Tolazoline hydrochloride (Priscoline) has adrenergic blocking properties and may be used in treating Raynaud's disease. It is very short acting but is available in sustained release form to prolong action. This drug stimulates gastric acid secretion and can cause epigastric distress, nausea, and vomiting. It may also cause tachycardia, and is therefore contraindicated for patients with coronary disease. Tolazoline hydrochloride may be given parenterally into a vein, muscle, subcutaneous tissue, or even directly into an artery; it may also be given orally.

Phentolamine (Regitine) is an alpha adrenergic blocking drug used primarily for treating pheochromocytoma (see Chapter 20). However, its vasodilating effect is useful when the drug is infiltrated into an area where intravenous infusion of levarterenol bitartrate (Levophed) has leaked into surrounding tissue. Levarterenol bitartrate can cause drastic local vasoconstriction, leading to tissue necrosis and ulceration if not quickly counteracted.

Beta Adrenergic Stimulating Drugs. Nylidrin hydrochloride (Arlidin) and isoxsuprine hydrochloride (Vasodilan) are the two beta adrenergic stimulating agents most commonly used for treating intermittent claudication and other occlusive vascular diseases of the skeletal muscle vessels. These drugs have also been used for increasing cerebral blood flow in the presence of arteriosclerosis, and for increasing labyrinth arterial blood flow when treating arterial spasms of the inner ear. Side effects are rare with these drugs, but heart palpitations, hypotension, and nervousness may occur.

Parasympathomimetic (Cholinergic) Drugs. These drugs increase blood flow in vessels that dilate in response to acetylcholine. They may be given to dilate cutaneous vessels in treating Raynaud's disease. Because such drugs as methacholine chloride (Mecholyl) also stimulate other acetylcholine receptor sites, they may produce some undesirable side effects, such as diarrhea.

Direct Acting Vasodilating Drugs

Some drugs act directly on the smooth muscles of the vessels to cause dilation. The principal drug of this class is papaverine hydrochloride (Vasal), a nonaddicting opium alkaloid. Cyclandelate (Cyclospasmol), and drugs such as nicotinyl alcohol (Roniacol) that are derivatives of the B-complex vitamins, are also in this group.

These drugs do not seem very effective when given orally, but they do cause facial flushing, so the patient may feel that they are doing some good. The patient may be discouraged and want to stop taking the drug when facial flushing stops, but the nurse must en-

Table 21-1. Vasodilators.

Generic Name	Trade Name	How Supplied	Routes	Usual Dose	Comments
nitroglycerin		tablets 0.2, 0.3, 0.4, 0.6 mg.	sublingually	0.3–0.6 mg.	If pain does not stop, sublingual tablets may be repeated in 15 minutes. If drug does not relieve pain in 30 minutes, the physician should be called.
	Nitro-Bid Nitrospan	sustained release tablets 2.5, 6.5 mg.	P.O.	1 tablet q. 12h.	
tolazoline hydrochloride	Priscoline	tablets 25 mg.	P.O.	25–50 mg. P.O. q.i.d.	Start with low doses and increase as necessary. Intra-arterial approach should be used only in carefully selected cases, after maximum benefits have been reached with other methods.
		sustained release tablets 80 mg.	P.O.		
		multiple dose vials 10 cc. 25 mg./cc.	I.M. I.V. S.C.	10–50 mg. q.i.d. for parenteral.	
			intra-arterial	25 mg. initially, then 50–75 mg. 2 or 3 times per week for intra-arterial	
nylidrin hydrochloride	Arlidin	tablets 6 mg.–12 mg.	P.O.	3–12 mg. P.O. t.i.d. or q.i.d.	
papaverine hydrochloride	Vasal	sustained release capsule 150 mg.	P.O.	150 mg. q. 8–12h.	Should be used wit caution in patients with glaucoma

courage him to continue, as short-term therapy is of no value. Parenteral administration of papaverine hydrochloride may be used for arteriolar dilation; however, large doses given in this manner may lead to cardiac arrhythmias. Remember that vasodilators must be used with caution in patients with glaucoma, because the drugs may aggravate the glaucoma.

CEREBRAL VASODILATING DRUGS

In addition to the beta adrenergic stimulating drugs already mentioned, all the direct acting vasodilating drugs are claimed to be useful for cerebral vasodilation. There is little evidence that any of these drugs can dilate blood vessels beyond the degree of dilation brought about naturally as a body reaction to poor circulation and hypoxia caused by the organic vessel damage. These drugs are occasionally prescribed and are claimed to assist in improving memory, mood, and behavior, especially in elderly patients suffering cerebral arteriosclerosis. One of the most commonly used preparations for this purpose is sustained release papaverine hydrochloride (Pavabid, Vasal).

REFERENCES

ALLENDORF, ELAINE, and KEEGAN, M. HONOR. "Teaching Patients About Nitroglycerin." *American Journal of Nursing* 75:1168, July 1975.

KRATZ, ALLEN M., and KRATZ, JUDITH L. "Vasodilators." *Nursing 73* 3:33, May 1973.

RODMAN, MORTON J. "Drug Management in Peripheral Vascular Disease." *RN* 29:61, August 1966.

APPLICATION QUESTIONS

I. *True-False*

For each statement below, write **a** if the statement is true or **b** if it is false.

_b_ 1. Amyl nitrate is given sublingually for relief of angina.

_a_ 2. Nitroglycerin is one drug which is often self-administered by hospitalized patients.

_b_ 3. Patients who faithfully follow a medicinal regimen, including the long-lasting nitrates, will not suffer angina.

_b_ 4. All vasodilator drugs are useful in preventing angina attacks.

_a_ 5. Angina may be considered a warning that more serious heart conditions may be imminent.

_b_ 6. If angina pain is not relieved by nitroglycerin in five minutes, the doctor should be called.

_a_ 7. Patients should continue to take direct acting vasodilator drugs even though flushing no longer takes place.

_a_ 8. Pain usually accompanies hypoxia and ischemia.

_b_ 9. Tolazoline hydrochloride (Priscoline) is a drug safely used to relax vascular spasm in angina pectoris.

_a_ 10. Normal vessels respond more readily to sympathetic blocking agents than do vessels with organic disease.

II. *Multiple Choice*

For each of the following questions, indicate the letter providing the *best* answer.

_c_ 1. Symptoms commonly associated with peripheral vascular disease include which of the following? (1) pain (2) tingling (3) pallor or cyanosis (4) ecchymosis
(a) 1, 3 (b) 2, 4 (c) 1, 2, 3 (d) 2, 3, 4

_e_ 2. Drugs that dilate constricted blood vessels are most effective in the treatment of which of the following? (1) Buerger's disease (2) Raynaud's disease (3) frostbite (4) acrocyanosis
(a) 1 (b) 2, 3 (c) 2, 3, 4 (d) 1, 2, 3

_a_ 3. Which of the following vasodilating drugs, when administered as indicated, would be considered the safest with the fewest serious side effects? (a) isoxsuprine hydrochloride (Vasodilan) orally (b) methacholine chloride (Mecholyl) orally (c) papaverine hydrochloride parenterally (d) phenoxybenzamine hydrochloride (Dibenzyline) orally

_b_ 4. Which of the following is the dosage pattern usually used with the drug phenoxybenzamine hydrochloride (Dibenzyline)? (a) large doses gradually reduced (b) small doses gradually increased (c) alternating large and small doses (d) doses every other day

_c_ 5. Drugs that act as sympathetic blocking agents may produce which of the following serious complications? (a) rectal bleeding (b) bradycardia (c) hypotension (d) laryngeal edema

_d_ 6. Tolazoline hydrochloride (Priscoline) may be administered through which of the following routes? (1) intravenously (2) intra-arterially (3) orally (4) subcutaneously
(a) 1, 3 (b) 1, 2, 4 (c) 2, 3, 4 (d) 1, 2, 3, 4

_a_ 7. Which of the following drugs is used to counteract the vasoconstricting effects of levarterenol bitartrate (Levophed) if it has infiltrated into tissue? (a) phentolamine (Regitine) (b) isoxsuprine hydrochloride (Vasodilan) (c) tolazoline hydro-chloride (Priscoline) (d) nicotinic acid

_C_ 8. Adverse effects of the nitrates include: (1) flushing (2) increased intraocular pressure (3) syncope (4) peripheral vasoconstriction
(a) 2, 3, 4 (b) 1, 3, 4 (c) 1, 2, 3 (d) 1, 2, 3, 4

_b_ 9. Pharmacological actions of the nitrates include which of the following? (1) dilatation of coronary vessels (2) pooling of peripheral blood (3) constriction of peripheral vessels (4) reduction of venous return
(a) 2, 3 (b) 1, 2, 4 (c) 1, 3, 4 (d) 1, 2, 3, 4

_b_ 10. What advice should the nurse give to a patient regarding the relationship of activity to taking nitroglycerin for pain? (a) continue with mild activity (b) sit or lie down immediately (c) remain active for ten minutes, then lie down (d) wait to take the drug until it is possible to be prone.

III. *Matching*

Match each classification of vasodilators with its action.

_c_ 1. beta adrenergic stimulants

_d_ 2. alpha adrenergic blockers

_a_ 3. cholinergics

_b_ 4. direct acting vasodilators

(a) mimic action of the neurohormone acetylcholine

(b) reduce the tone of smooth muscle surrounding vessels

(c) stimulate vasodilator receptors in skeletal muscles

(d) block transmission of vasoconstrictive impulses in superficial vessels

IV. *Discussion*

For each patient statement given below, write **a** if teaching is needed or **b** if teaching is not indicated. If you answer that teaching is needed, outline the content you would include.

_____ 1. "My nitroglycerin doesn't seem to stop the pain like it used to, but at least my head doesn't ache for hours like it used to when I took them."

_____ 2. "Winters are hard for me, but I find I can take one of my nitroglycerin tablets before I go out in the cold morning and I have less difficulty."

_____ 3. "Oh! I want you to see my fancy new plastic pill case my daughter brought me to carry my nitroglycerin in."

_____ 4. "Maybe if I took nitroglycerin like my neighbor does, my chest wouldn't hurt so bad, but my eyes are so bad from my glaucoma that I can't see those tiny pills."

_____ 5. "One thing about nitroglycerin is that you don't have to buy it very often. I guess I've had these pills for five years at least."

_____ 6. "Ever since I've been taking that timed-out medicine for my heart, I don't seem to get such a red face when I take my nitroglycerin for pain."

22

Antilipemic Drugs

Lipids are fats or fatlike substances that are insoluble in water. Certain lipids are carried in the blood in combination with plasma proteins; these are called *lipoproteins*. People whose plasma shows consistently elevated levels of lipoproteins tend to develop lipid deposits in various body tissues. An example of such deposits is xanthoma, a yellow-orange growth that erupts like a rash or as a nodule on elbows, eyelids, and elsewhere.

Some authorities suggest that hyperlipoproteinemia also causes the atherosclerotic plaques within artery walls that lead to ischemic vascular disease.

The two lipids most commonly studied and discussed are cholesterol and triglycerides.

TREATMENT OF HYPERLIPOPROTEINEMIA

Hyperlipoproteinemia is classified into five types, all of which may be treated with diet therapy. Any current textbook dealing with therapeutic nutrition should provide a complete explanation of the diet therapy. Types III, IV, V, and sometimes type II may be treated with drug therapy in combination with diet. Type I is a rare disease for which no drug is effective.

There are several antilipemic drugs available today, although their usefulness in preventing the complications of atherosclerosis has not yet been firmly established.

Because these drugs do not relieve any symptoms and, in fact, may cause some uncomfortable side effects initially, patients may want to discontinue drug therapy.

Drug therapy should be initiated only for patients who demonstrate lipid disorders on laboratory testing and who are considered "high risk" for myocardial infarction, stroke, or other complications of atherosclerosis. Drug therapy should be instituted in combination with diet therapy, a prescribed exercise regimen and no smoking.

Clofibrate

Clofibrate (Atromid-S) is the most widely used antilipemic drug. It is most effective when hypertriglyceridemia is the predominant lipid abnormality, as in types III and IV hyperlipoproteinemia. It may be given in combination with other drugs for treating hypercholesterolemia, as in types II and V hyperlipoproteinemia.

Clofibrate also seems to counteract the tendency of blood to form clots. This, of course, indicates a need to reduce the dosage of anticoagulant drugs and to increase the frequency of prothrombin time testing if these drugs are given in combination. Anticoagulant dosage may be reduced by as much as one-third to one-half when clofibrate treatment is begun.

Xanthomas have disappeared after beginning treatment with clofibrate, and regression of exudative retinopathy has occurred in diabetic patients.

Side effects of clofibrate include nausea, abdominal distress, loose stools, and headache. These effects seem to decrease as treatment is continued, but the patient may need much encouragement to continue therapy until the distress subsides. Liver toxicity, muscle aches, cramps, and weakness have also been reported on occasion.

Nicotinic Acid

Nicotinic acid (Niacin), a vitamin of the B-complex group, reduces plasma levels of both cholesterol and triglycerides when administered in relatively large doses. It is useful in types II, III, and IV hyperlipoproteinemia. Side effects of the large daily doses may include heartburn, flatulence, and other gastrointestinal symptoms. Aluminum nicotinate (Nicalex) is a derivative of nicotinic acid which is claimed to reduce the gastrointestinal distress. Any nicotinic acid product may initially cause skin flushing and itching. The nurse should remind patients taking these drugs that the discomforting side effects are likely to disappear in time, and should suggest that they take the drugs after a meal to decrease the irritation.

Sodium Dextrothyroxine

Sodium dextrothyroxine (Choloxin) is a form of thyroid hormone. It is most effective for reducing pure hypercholesterolemia (type II hyperlipoproteinemia). Sodium dextrothyroxine is less likely than other thyroid hormones to stimulate general body metabolism and thus increase the needs of body tissues for oxygen—an undesirable effect for patients with heart disease. Because only a slight overdose of this drug could set off an attack of angina pectoris or precipitate cardiac arrhythmias or congestive heart failure, it is generally reserved for patients who have both hypothyroidism and hypercholesterolemia. The patient must be observed closely for heart palpitations, nervousness, or tremors. Dosages of anticoagulants must be reduced if they are taken with sodium dextrothyroxine. Diabetics may need increased amounts of insulin if treated with this drug.

Cholestyramine resin

Cholestyramine resin (Questran) is a drug used mainly for relief of pruritus in patients with primary biliary cirrhosis and cholestatic jaundice. It relieves itching by removing bile salts that have accumulated in the patient's skin. Taken orally, this drug binds bile salts in the intestines; they are excreted in the feces instead of being reabsorbed. In response to this, the body breaks down liver cholesterol to replace the missing bile salts. This process can lead to a reduction of blood cholesterol by about 20 percent in the average person.

Side effects of cholestyramine resin may include heartburn, nausea, and either constipation or diarrhea. The drug is very unpalatable, and its bad taste, along with the initial side effects, may be very discouraging to the patient. The nurse should encourage the patient to continue taking the drug, because the initial side effects usually decrease. Patients should not swallow the dry powder as it may irritate or block the esophagus. The drug may be mixed with pulpy foods or juices such as orange or apricot juice. Because cholestyramine resin can prevent acidic drugs and fat-soluble vitamins from being absorbed, the patient may require fat-soluble vitamin supplements, and drugs such as anticoagulants, antiarthritic drugs, phenobarbital, and thyroxine should be given at the longest possible interval before or after the dose of cholestyramine resin.

Estrogens

Estrogens were the first drugs used for reducing cholesterol. However, if these drugs are administered to male patients in doses large enough to be effective, gynecomastia and other feminizing effects may occur. Recent reports indicate that when estrogens are used to reduce cholesterol, they increase triglycerides; this

Table 22–1. Antilipemic drugs.

Generic Name	Trade Name	How Supplied	Routes	Usual Dose	Comments
cholestyramine	Questran	powder packets 4 Gm.	P.O.	1 packet t.i.d. (a.c.)	Dose not to exceed six packets daily. Place powder in 4–6 oz. of fluid and allow it to stand approximately one minute before stirring. Since cholestyramine may bind other drugs given concurrently, other drugs should be administered at least one hour before or 4–6 hours after cholestyramine dose.
clofibrate	Atromid-S	capsules 500 mg.	P.O.	1 capsule q.i.d.	For adults only. Caution should be exercised when administered to pregnant women or when anticoagulants are administered concurrently.

may account for the increased incidence of thrombophlebitis and other clot disorders. Today, estrogens are used as antilipemic drugs only in postmenopausal women.

REFERENCES

DI PALMA, JOSEPH R. "Drugs for Hyperlipidemia." *RN* 37:55, March 1974.

"Drug Update: Cholestyramine." *Nursing 74* 4:70, April 1974.

RODMAN, MORTON J. "Drugs That Reduce Blood Cholesterol." *RN 32:77*, February 1969.

APPLICATION QUESTIONS

I. *True-False*

For each statement below, write **a** if the statement is true or **b** if it is false.

_a_ 1. Discomforting side effects of the antilipemic drugs may decrease in severity with continued drug use.

_a_ 2. Xanthomas are a form of lipid deposits.

_b_ 3. It has been proven that atherosclerosis results from high levels of circulating cholesterol.

_a_ 4. Nicotinic acid lowers plasma levels of both cholesterol and triglycerides.

_b_ 5. Sodium dextrothyroxine decreases the need for insulin in the diabetic.

_b_ 6. Estrogens are used as antilipemic agents only in male patients.

II. *Multiple Choice*

For each of the following questions, indicate the letter providing the *best* answer.

_a_ 1. Cholestyramine powder is best administered in which of the following manners? (a) mixed with applesauce (b) as powder to be followed with milk (c) mixed to paste form and eaten (d) mixed in cool water

_b_ 2. Which of the following drugs is also used for relief of pruritus in biliary obstruction? (a) clofibrate (Atromid-S) (b) cholestyramine (Questran) (c) estrogen (d) nicotinic acid (Niacin)

_a_ 3. Which of the following nutritional supplements would be given to a patient receiving cholestyramine? (a) fat-soluble vitamins (b) water-soluble vitamins (c) minerals (d) powdered egg whites

_d_ 4. Side effects of clofibrate may include which of the following? (1) nausea and vomiting (2) loose stools (3) xanthomas (4) headache (a) 1, 3 (b) 1, 2 (c) 3, 4 (d) 1, 2, 4

_c_ 5. What adjustment should be made in the dosage of an anticoagulant when it is added to a clofibrate treatment regimen? (a) no adjustment (b) increased (c) decreased

_b_ 6. Which of the following antilipemic drugs is a form of thyroid hormone? (a) cholestyramine (Questran) (b) sodium dextrothyroxine (Choloxin) (c) nicotinic acid (Niacin) (d) sitosterols (Cytellin)

_c_ 7. Which of the following properties of clofibrate is an added benefit to patients in reducing heart attacks? (a) dilates the coronary vessels (b) lowers blood pressure (c) counteracts clotting (d) functions as an antidepressant

III. Matching

Indicate which of the following side effects occurs with each of the following drugs.

_a_ 1. Interferes with absorption of acidic drugs

_d_ 2. Produces a feminizing effect in males

_c_ 3. Precipitates angina attacks

_b_ 4. Causes skin flushing and itching

(a) cholestyramine
(b) nicotinic acid
(c) sodium dextrothyroxine
(d) estrogens

23

Drugs That Affect Blood Coagulation

Coagulation of blood is a very complex interaction of many factors. It is not the intention of this chapter to explain this process; rather, the process will be greatly simplified with the intent of offering a basic understanding of the action and therapeutic implications of anticoagulant, thrombolytic, and hemostatic drugs.

Blood has the ability to remain fluid most of the time, and yet when injury occurs, it clots to prevent excessive loss. Blood clotting occurs in three stages. Table 23–1 presents a very simplified diagram of that process, obviously not including many of the clotting factors listed in Table 23–2.

Blood clotting factors and anticlotting factors are normally in a delicate state of balance within the body. If their equilibrium shifts, disorders of bleeding and clotting may occur. Disorders will occur if any of the factors are missing or deficient, or if other substances such as vitamin K, which is necessary for the synthesis of prothrombin in the liver, are inhibited from action. The two types of drugs used to treat disorders involving excessive clot formation are anticoagulants and thrombolytic agents. Drugs used to control excessive bleeding are called hemostatic agents.

NEED FOR ANTICOAGULANTS

It is important that the nurse be mindful that many clotting disorders can be prevented by avoiding stasis of blood during periods of immobility. Leg exercises, ambulation, proper positioning to prevent pressure, and proper hydration are important measures for preventing clot formation. When clotting does occur, however, the patient's regimen changes, because ambulation and exercise could cause a portion of a clot to break loose and travel through the circulation until it becomes lodged in a vessel small enough to com-

Table 23–1. The three stages of clot formation

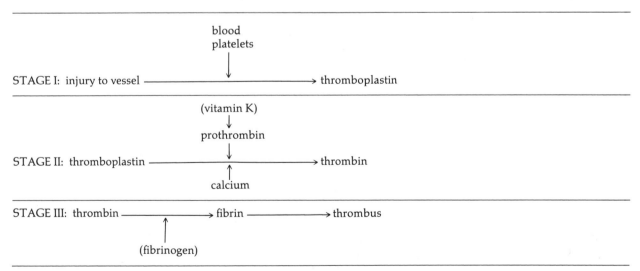

Table 23–2. Blood clotting factors

I	Fibrinogen
II	Prothrombin
III	Thromboplastin
IV	Calcium
V	Proaccelerin
VII	Proconvertin
VIII	Antihemophilic factor
IX	Christmas factor
X	Stuart-Prower factor
XI	Plasma thromboplastin antecedent
XII	Hageman factor
XIII	Fibrin stabilizing factor

pletely impede its progress. There it will completely occlude the vessel. Clots usually form in veins, where stasis can occur. If an embolus breaks off from a thrombus in a vein, it travels in vessels that become larger and larger as the venous blood returns to the heart. The first smaller vessels the embolus encounters, then, are the vessels in the lungs as the blood is pumped through the lungs for oxygenation. It is not difficult to see why pulmonary embolism is one of the more common (and more dangerous) complications of immobility. Since emboli usually lodge in arteries or arterioles, complete occlusion leads to lack of perfusion, severe pain, and tissue death. Clots formed in veins create serious conditions requiring treatment to prevent them from becoming emboli. Clots lodged in the arteriolar system are emergency conditions requiring immediate treatment before extensive tissue destruction occurs.

Anticoagulant Drugs

Only the two major anticoagulant drugs, sodium heparin and sodium warfarin (a coumarin derivative) will be discussed in this chapter. Sodium heparin acts on circulating clotting factors to prevent immediately the extension of clots already formed. Sodium warfarin acts in the liver by inhibiting vitamin K in the synthesis of prothrombin and other blood clotting factors; thus it reduces the amount of circulating clotting factors.

Sodium Heparin. This drug is injected intravenously in emergency situations. It prevents the formation of thrombin and permits fibrinogen to stay in a liquid state. Sodium heparin is used for immediate treatment of conditions such as thrombophlebitis,

pulmonary embolism, and acute myocardial infarction. Remember that anticoagulants do not break up formed clots; they prevent extension of the clot and allow the body's natural defenses to dispose of the clot.

When a patient is receiving sodium heparin, clotting time must be tested frequently. Normal clotting time is 5 to 10 minutes. Patients on anticoagulant therapy are maintained at between 20 and 30 minutes. If clotting time is allowed to increase further, serious spontaneous bleeding may occur. If overdose or bleeding occurs while a patient is receiving sodium heparin, the antidote *protamine sulfate* is used as its chemical antagonist. Since sodium heparin can only be given parenterally, and requires frequent injections, it is not often used for long-term therapy or for patients who are not hospitalized.

Sodium Warfarin (Coumadin). The coumarin derivatives are oral anticoagulants. Oral anticoagulants might take several days to reduce the clotting ability of the blood effectively, as they work in the liver to reduce the amount of circulating clotting factors. They do not act on already-formed clotting factors to prevent extension of clots, as sodium heparin does. A patient with a clotting disorder is often begun on both sodium heparin and sodium warfarin (Coumadin) at the same time. When laboratory tests reveal that sodium warfarin is having effect, the sodium heparin, which was used for the immediate emergency, is discontinued. The sodium warfarin is then continued for long-term and even outpatient therapy.

When a patient is receiving sodium warfarin in the hospital, his prothrombin time must be tested before every dose. The nurse must never give a dose of the drug before the doctor is aware of the daily prothrombin time and acknowledges that the patient should receive the next dose. Results of prothrombin time may be given both in seconds and in percent of the control. Normal prothrombin time is 10 to 15 seconds, or 100 percent. During anticoagulation therapy, the patient's prothrombin time is kept between 20 and 30 percent of the control, or 3 to 5 seconds. If overdose or bleeding occurs, fat soluble vitamin K (Phytonadione) is the antidote for the oral anticoagulants.

When a patient is discharged from the hospital but must continue taking sodium warfarin, prothrombin time testing may only be done once a week, or even once or twice a month. The patient must be made to understand how important these tests are and that he should always keep his appointments for prothrombin time testing.

NURSING RESPONSIBILITIES WHEN A PATIENT IS ON ANTICOAGULANT THERAPY

The nurse must become familiar with normal dosage ranges and with the significance of laboratory test results in order to guard against overdosage as well as to insure effectiveness of anticoagulant therapy. Not all patients respond to anticoagulants in the same manner. Patients with poor nutritional status may be more responsive to the drugs and require lower dosages. On the other hand, patients with diarrhea, which inhibits absorption of the drug, or those who simply metabolize the drug quickly, may require higher doses.

The effectiveness of an anticoagulant drug is frequently affected by other drugs taken simultaneously. If the patient is receiving a drug that potentiates the action of the anticoagulant, such as chloral hydrate, cholestyramine, clofibrate, sodium dextrothyroxine, phenylbutazone, quinidine, salicylates, anabolic steroids, or some of the broad-spectrum antibiotics such as the sulfonamides, the dosage of the anticoagulant may need to be reduced to prevent uncontrolled bleeding. Drugs such as antacids, barbiturates, estrogens, griseofulvin, meprobamate, corticosteroids, and thiazide diuretics may antagonize anticoagulants and necessitate an increase in dosage to insure effectiveness.

Patient Teaching

When a patient is sent home on anticoagulants, the nurse must explain to him that he must not medicate himself with *any* medications without checking first with the physician. Many over-the-counter drug items contain chemicals which interfere with the anticoagulants. Patients should also be encouraged to keep their weight within recommended limits, avoid drastic changes in their dietary intake, and avoid excessive intake of alcohol in order to prevent changes in their response to the anticoagulants.

The nurse must observe for signs of bleeding and explain to the patient, without unduly alarming him, the significance of such observations. Since mucous membranes are some of the most delicate tissues in the body, bleeding may be detected there first. Observe contents of emesis basins and bedpans for traces of blood. Tarry stools may indicate bleeding high in the intestinal tract. "Coffee ground" emesis could indicate partially digested blood. A patient with an indwelling urinary catheter could be more susceptible to bleeding because of the constant irritation of

the mucous membranes of the urethra. Nosebleeds should be reported promptly, as should excessive bruising. The patient should be cautioned against contact sports, since he is likely to bruise.

The nurse must explain to the patient taking oral anticoagulants the importance of carrying vitamin K tablets and of carrying an identification card explaining that he is taking the medication. In the hospital, the nurse should be sure that injectable vitamin K is available if patients are receiving oral anticoagulants, and should also be sure there is a supply of injectable protamine sulfate if patients are receiving heparin.

THROMBOLYTIC AGENTS

Anticoagulants do not break up clots, but merely prevent extension of existing clots and permit the body to dispose of the formed clots. This normal process in the body, called *fibrinolysis*, occurs by the action of an enzyme called plasmin or fibrinolysin. This enzyme is formed within the clot by the action of certain activators upon a precursor substance called profibrinolysin or plasminogen.

Currently, two partially purified plasminogen activators are being used experimentally to speed up the rate at which formed clots are broken down. These two substances are called *streptokinase* and *urokinase*. Injected streptokinase has shown some effectiveness but tends to cause allergy reactions and fever. Urokinase, when injected intravenously with heparin, has accelerated clot breakdown with little toxic effect except to increase the incidence of bleeding.

HEMOSTATIC AGENTS

The second major difficulty a patient can experience with regard to the clotting mechanism is the tendency to bleed excessively and *not* to form clots. When excessive bleeding occurs, the patient may require the use of hemostatic agents.

Local pressure or sutures usually supply any aid necessary for normal clotting to occur after a break in a vessel. A patient may require a hemostatic agent if massive capillary damage makes it difficult to tie off all the bleeding vessels, or if he lacks one or more of the clotting factors. Hemostatic agents may act locally or systemically.

Locally Acting Hemostatic Agents

Thrombin, when applied directly as a powder, reacts with the fibrinogen in the blood and quickly forms a clot. Thrombin may also be taken in solution by

Table 23–3. Drugs that affect blood coagulation

Generic Name	Trade Name	How Supplied	Routes	Usual Dose	Comments
sodium warfarin	Coumadin	tablets: 2 mg., 2-1/2 mg., 5 mg., 7-1/2 mg., 10 mg., 25 mg.	P.O.	2–10 mg. q.d.	The dosage of this drug must be individualized for each patient, as indicated by the prothrombin time.
		vials: 50 mg., 75 mg., to be reconstituted	I.V. I.M.		
sodium heparin	Panheprin	multiple dose vials 10 cc. 1000 U./cc. 5000 U./cc. multiple dose vials 5 cc. 10,000 U./cc. 20,000 U./cc. multiple dose vials 4 cc. 10,000 U./cc. multiple dose vials 2 cc. 40,000 U./cc. ampuls 1 cc. 10,000 U./cc. 20,000 U./cc.	I.V. I.M. S.C.	dosage is individualized according to periodic blood coagulation time determinations	Protamine sulfate 1% solution, by slow infusion, will neutralize heparin. Usual aim of therapy is to maintain the clotting time approximately 2-1/2 to 3 times the control value. Safety for use in pregnancy has not been established. I.M. injection is not usually used because of the danger of hematoma formation.
aminocaproic acid	Amicar	vials 20 cc. 250 mg./cc. syrup 250 mg./cc. in 16 fl. oz. bottles tablets 500 mg.	I.V. P.O. P.O.	initial dose 5 Gm. followed by 1 to 1-1/4 Gm. hourly thereafter until plasma levels of 0.130 mg./cc. of the drug is reached	Rapid I.V. injection of undiluted Amicar is not recommended. Administration of more than 30 Gm. in 24 hours is not recommended. Safety for use in pregnancy has not been established.
antihemophilic factor (human)	Hemofil Humafac	bottles	I.V.	4–40 U./kg. body wt.	Dosage must be individualized according to the weight of the patient, the severity of the bleeding, the severity of the blood condition, the source of the bleeding, the presence of inhibitors, and other factors as determined by the physician.
streptokinase-streptodornase	Varidase	tablets 10,000 U. vials 25,000 U. vials 125,000 U.	P.O. I.M. Topical	one tablet q.i.d. 5,000 U. b.i.d. p.r.n.	I.M. dose should be accompanied by systemic administration of broad spectrum antibiotic.

mouth or through a nasogastric tube to control bleeding ulcers in the stomach. It would be very dangerous ever to inject thrombin, as it could lead to diffuse clotting in the circulatory system

There are many types of specially treated absorbable surgical cotton and sponges (oxidized cellulose, absorbable gelatin) that can be applied and left in place in a surgical wound to control bleeding.

Systemically Acting Hemostatic Agents

Defects in the clotting mechanism may occur from drug reactions or from genetic defects in clotting factors, as in the disease *hemophilia*. Until recently, transfusions of whole blood or plasma were the only treatments available to help replace a missing clotting factor. Today, concentrates of various clotting factors are available. For example, there is a factor VIII concentrate (Hemofil) for treating classic hemophilia (type A). Type B hemophilia (Christmas disease) can be treated with a concentrate of factor IX (Konyne).

Vitamin K may be used to treat *hypoprothrombinemia*. Vitamin K, although a fat-soluble vitamin, is available in both water-soluble and fat-soluble forms for drug therapy. The water-soluble salts of menadione (Synkayvite, Hykinone) are preferred for oral administration in the presence of biliary tract disease. Phytonadione, the fat-soluble vitamin K (Aqua Mephyton, Konakion) is considered more effective in other situations.

Hypofibrinogenemia, a deficiency in fibrinogen, can be treated with transfusions of whole fresh blood or plasma. Aminocaproic acid (Amicar) is a synthetic antifibrinolytic substance available today for treating this disease, which results from the excessive breakdown of circulating fibrinogen and fibrin deposits.

Ascorbic acid (vitamin C) may control capillary fragility and oozing if there is a deficiency of the vitamin; estrogen can control uterine bleeding caused by hormonal imbalance. There is no conclusive evidence that these substances can be used as hemostatic agents in situations other than those mentioned.

REFERENCES

DiPALMA, JOSEPH R. "Precautions with the Anticoagulants." *RN* 34:57, October 1971.

HUSSAR, DANIEL A. "Anticoagulants." *Nursing 73* 3:11, April 1973.

KOPROWICZ, DIANNE C. "Drug Interactions with Coumarin Derivatives." *American Journal of Nursing* 73:1042, June 1973.

MAYER, GLORIA GILBERT. "Disseminated Intravascular Coagulation." *American Journal of Nursing* 73:2067, December 1973.

SHAPIRO, RUTH MAYER. "Anticoagulant Therapy." *American Journal of Nursing* 74:439, March 1974.

APPLICATION QUESTIONS

I. *True-False*

For each statement below, write **a** if the statement is true or **b** if it is false.

_b_ 1. Coumarin derivatives act directly on clotting factors in the circulating blood.

_b_ 2. Sodium heparin and coumarin derivatives are never given simultaneously.

_b_ 3. Sodium heparin dissolves clots which are fully formed.

_a_ 4. Oral anticoagulants may take several days to attain their clinical effectiveness.

_a_ 5. Fever is a toxic side effect seen with the use of the drug streptokinase.

_a_ 6. Sodium heparin is generally not used for outpatient therapy.

_a_ 7. Hemofil is used in the management of classical hemophilia.

II. *Multiple Choice*

For each of the following questions, indicate the letter providing the *best* answer.

_a_ 1. Which of the following patients would probably be *most* susceptible to the effects of anticoagulant drugs? (a) a skid row alcoholic, 56 years of age (b) an 80-year-old retired bank president (c) a teenage football player (d) a 30-year-old housewife

_a_ 2. The action of the coumarin derivatives is best described by which of the following statements? (a) they prevent vitamin K from carrying out its metabolic function (b) they dissolve clots (c) they inhibit production of the Christmas factor (d) they inhibit production of thrombocytes.

_c_ 3. Oral anticoagulant therapy should reduce the circulating prothrombin activity to what percent of normal? (a) 70–80 percent (b) 60–70 percent (c) 20–30 percent (d) 10–15 percent

_c_ 4. How does sodium heparin interfere with the normal clotting process? (a) it inhibits the production of prothrombin (b) it prevents the combining of thromboplastin and fibrinogen (c) it maintains fibrinogen in a liquid state (d) it reduces the effectiveness of platelets _b_ 5. A dislodged blood clot in the femoral vein might be likely to cause which of the following complications? (a) myocardial infarction (b) pulmonary embolism (c) stroke (d) gangrene of the leg

_b_ 6. What is the specific antidote for sodium warfarin (Coumadin)? (a) water-soluble vitamin K (b) fat-soluble vitamin K (c) protamine sulfate (d) thrombin

_c_ 7. Which of the following are clotting factors? (1) prothrombin (2) thromboplastin (3) calcium (4) vitamin K
(a) 1, 2 (b) 2, 3 (c) 1, 2, 3 (d) 1, 2, 3, 4

_b_ 8. Thrombin may _not_ be used in which of the following ways? (a) in powder form on a wound (b) in slow intravenous infusion (c) in solution through Levine tube (d) in a tooth socket with gauze

_c_ 9. Nursing measures used to prevent venous stasis during inactivity would include which of the following? (1) passive or active exercises (2) elevation of the knee gatch of the bed (3) turning frequently (4) keeping the head of the bed elevated
(a) 4 (b) 2, 4 (c) 1, 3 (d) 1, 2, 3

_d_ 10. The effectiveness of sodium heparin is determined by which of the following laboratory tests? (a) platelet count (b) prothrombin time (c) CBC (d) clotting time

_b_ 11. The specific antagonist of sodium heparin is which of the following drugs? (a) warfarin (b) protamine sulfate (c) vitamin K (d) thrombin

_b_ 12. Normal clotting time falls within which of the following ranges? (a) 20–30 seconds (b) 5–10 minutes (c) 20–30 minutes (d) 1–2 hours

_d_ 13. Oxidized cellulose (Hemopak) is used in which of the following clinical situations? (1) ruptured liver (2) gallbladder surgery (3) to approximate a fracture (4) intestinal resection
(a) 1, 2, 3 (b) 1, 3, 4 (c) 2, 3, 4 (d) 1, 2, 4

III. _Matching A_

The following drugs interact with anticoagulants and require an adjustment in the dosage of the drug. Indicate for each whether the anticoagulant dosage should be increased or decreased.

_a_ 1. Sodium phenobarbital
_b_ 2. Phenylbutazone
_a_ 3. Thiazide diuretics
_b_ 4. Clofibrate

(a) increase the dose of anticoagulant
(b) decrease the dose of anticoagulant

_b_ 5. Broad-spectrum antibiotics
_b_ 6. Aspirin
_a_ 7. Birth control pills
_a_ 8. Meprobamate

IV. _Matching B_

Indicate whether anticoagulants are indicated or contraindicated in each clinical condition.

_a_ 1. Thrombophlebitis
_a_ 2. Pulmonary embolism
_b_ 3. Cerebral hemorrhage
_b_ 4. Colitis

(a) indicated
(b) contraindicated

V. _Matching C_

Match each drug with its classification.

_a_ 1. Streptokinase
_b_ 2. Aminocaproic acid
_c_ 3. Warfarin sodium
_a_ 4. Urokinase
_b_ 5. Phytonadione

(a) thrombolytic
(b) hemostatic
(c) anticoagulant

VI. _Nursing Action_

Of the following nursing activities, select the five that relate _specifically_ to anticoagulant therapy.

_c_ 1.
_d_ 2.
_f_ 3.
_h_ 4.
_i_ 5.

(a) force fluids
(b) bedtime feeding
(c) check color of urine
(d) report amount and color of emesis
(e) daily weight
(f) observe old I.V. sites carefully
(g) keep padded tongue blade at bedside
(h) observe number and character of stools
(i) perineal pad count
(j) weekly shampoo

VII. *Discussion*

For each patient statement given below, write **a** if teaching is needed, or **b** if no teaching is indicated. If you answer that teaching is needed, outline the content you would include.

_____ 1. "I sure am glad the doctor took me off my Coumadin today. Back to normal at last! My hockey team has been hurtin', and I can make it to practice tonight."

_____ 2. "Mama's phlebitis really hurts her. That blood-thinning medicine the doctor has her on may be good, but we've found that aspirin helps her feel better."

_____ 3. "Well, I guess this anticoagulant medicine means no more heavy drinking for awhile. Guess I'll stay sober this New Year's Eve."

_____ 4. "Even with that blood-thinning medicine, I haven't been feeling as spry as I should. But I've gotten some real high-power vitamins from the drug store, and those should help."

_____ 5. "The new drug to keep my blood from clotting seems to upset my stomach—or it may be nerves—but either way, Alka-Seltzer helps."

VIII. *Calculations*

_____ 1. A patient is to receive heparin 1200U. S.C. The vial on hand is labeled 5000 U./cc. Using a T.B. syringe, how many cc. would you administer?

_____ 2. There is an order for heparin 18,000U. S.C. There are three strengths of heparin available for use: 1000U./cc.; 10,000U./cc.; and 40,000U./cc.

(a) Which strength would be best to use, considering the dose and route of the medication?

(b) How many cc. would you administer?

Acute Myocardial Infarction

A survey of drug therapy for patients with acute myocardial infarction is actually a summary of most drugs already discussed in this section, as well as some drugs discussed in other sections. Since acute myocardial infarction is fairly common in the United States, we shall discuss the drug therapy commonly used in treating myocardial infarction and its complications.

TREATMENT OF COMPLICATIONS

Arrhythmias

Cardiac arrhythmias are the most common cause of death in the first few days following acute myocardial infarction. The abnormal rhythm may be fast or slow. The most common arrhythmia is premature ventricular contraction (PVCs or extrasystoles). The nurse observes the cardiac monitor for PVC patterns and becomes aware of patterns that may lead to dangerous ventricular tachycardia or even the fatal arrhythmia of ventricular fibrillation. In these potentially dangerous situations, lidocaine may be administered intravenously; it usually suppresses the rapid run of PVCs within less than a minute. The dose may be repeated in about five minutes if the rhythm persists. Some patients may respond better to a slow intravenous drip of procainamide hydrochloride (Pronestyl) over a prolonged period of time. When either drug is used, the nurse must carefully observe the cardiac monitor as well as the patient's blood pressure. The drugs may cause too rapid a drop in blood pressure or may depress cardiac impulse conduction. When an intravenous solution of an antiarrhythmic drug is discontinued, it must be done very gradually and never stopped abruptly. Following initial control of the arrhythmia with intravenous medication, the patient may be maintained on an oral antiarrhythmic drug such as quinidine or procainamide hydrochloride.

If the arrhythmia is a slow one (bradycardia), an adrenergic drug such as atropine sulfate or isoproterenol hydrochloride (Isuprel) is used. These drugs, when given intravenously, depress the vagal impulses on the heart and thus speed up the heart rate. When these drugs are given, the nurse must observe the pulse and the cardiac monitor and adjust the infusion rate to prevent drug-induced tachyarrhythmias.

Cardiac Arrest

When the ventricles begin to fibrillate or stop beating altogether, the patient is in cardiac arrest. Keeping oxygen supplied to the brain is necessary if the patient is to live. The nurse must immediately begin cardiopulmonary resuscitation and prepare for cardioversion. In this situation, the physician may choose to inject a drug such as epinephrine (Adrenalin) or isoproterenol hydrochloride (Isuprel) directly into the heart chambers. Since the patient is in acidosis from the corresponding respiratory arrest, a systemic alkalinizing drug such as sodium bicarbonate should be given before the adrenergics to increase their effectiveness.

Cardiogenic Shock (Dopamine, Intropin)

If a patient goes into cardiogenic shock following acute myocardial infarction, death will quite probably follow. However, careful observation and careful administration of drug therapy may sustain the patient through this complication. A vasopressor such as levarterenol bitartrate (Levophed) or metaraminol bitartrate (Aramine) is given by infusion to keep the patient's systolic pressure at about 90 to 100 mm. of Hg. Levarterenol bitartrate must not be allowed to leak out of the vein into surrounding tissue, as vast tissue destruction will occur. Close monitoring of the blood pressure is essential when a patient is receiving intravenous vasopressor drugs, because slight changes in the drip rate can result in wide fluctuations of the blood pressure. Central venous pressure monitoring should also be done to prevent overloading of the circulation, specifically the left ventricle.

Heart Failure

To prevent pulmonary edema resulting from failure of the left ventricle, a rapid acting digitalis glycoside such as digoxin (Lanoxin) or deslanoside (Cedilanid-D) is given in combination with a rapid acting diuretic such as furosemide (Lasix) or ethacrynate sodium (Edecrin). Care must be taken when using these drugs to prevent digitalis intoxication or excessive diuresis. Apical and radial pulses, intake and output, and daily weights must be carefully observed and recorded.

GENERAL DRUG THERAPY

Use of Anticoagulant Drugs

Most patients are treated with anticoagulant drugs immediately following the attack. Sodium heparin is injected for immediate results, and the patient is begun on oral warfarin sodium (Coumadin) as soon as possible for long-term therapy. After about a week, the sodium heparin is discontinued and the oral anticoagulant continued. The patient's prothrombin time is usually kept between 20 and 30 percent of normal.

Use of Vasodilating Drugs

Some physicians advocate the long-term use of long acting nitrates after recovery from an acute myocardial infarction. The administration of rapid acting nitrates, papaverine, and other vasodilators could have an adverse effect on the patient's circulation if given immediately following an attack. The use of coronary vasodilating drugs following acute myocardial infarction is a current controversy.

Use of Analgesics and Sedatives

Narcotic analgesics such as morphine or meperidine hydrochloride (Demerol) are usually administered to relieve the severe chest pain accompanying an acute myocardial infarction. The nurse understands that narcotics can decrease respiration and may consider this when morphine is ordered for a patient who is quite dyspneic following an attack. However, the nurse should not hesitate to give the narcotic as ordered, since the response to pain as well as the response to the stress and anxiety of this situation will increase the patient's oxygen requirements and cardiac workload. Morphine has a calming effect which

will ultimately reduce the oxygen needs and the cardiac workload. After a few days, the patient may not need morphine and may be maintained on meperidine hydrochloride in combination with promethazine hydrochloride (Phenergan) or with only an antianxiety agent such as chlordiazepoxide (Librium).

REFERENCES

BIDDLE, THEODORE, and YU, PAUL. "Understanding and Treating Arrhythmias Accompanying Myocardial Infarction." *Nursing Clinics of North America* 7:481, September 1972.

JENKINS, ADELINE C., ed. "Drugs Used in the Care of the Cardiac Patient." *Nursing Clinics of North America* 4:645, December 1969.

LAWSON, BETTY. "Clinical Assessment of Cardiac Patients in Acute Care Facilities." *Nursing Clinics of North America* 7:431, September 1972.

RODMAN, MORTON J. "Drugs Used in C.C.U." *RN 32*:53, December 1969.

RODMAN, MORTON J. "Drugs Used in Cardiovascular Disease: Part 1, Managing Cardiac Emergencies." *RN 36*:71, March 1973.

SHINN, ARTHUR, et al. "Drug Interactions of Common C. C. U. Medication." *American Journal of Nursing* 74:1432, August 1974.

APPLICATION QUESTIONS

I. *True-False*

For each statement below, write **a** if the statement is true or **b** if it is false.

_b_   1. Dysrhythmias occur only in the first few hours following an infarction.

_a_   2. Isoproterenol (Isuprel) is an adrenergic drug.

_b_   3. When infusing an adrenergic vasopressor drug in treating cardiogenic shock, it is desirable to keep the diastolic blood pressure reading between 90 and 100 mm. of Hg.

____   4. The anticoagulant drug used for its immediate action following an acute myocardial infarction is warfarin sodium (Coumadin).

_b_   5. Rapid acting nitrates and papaverine are used in the period immediately following an acute myocardial infarction.

II. *Multiple Choice*

For each of the following questions, indicate the letter providing the *best* answer.

_a_ 1. Which drug would be given first if a patient develops ventricular fibrillation? (a) I.V. lidocaine (Xylocaine) (b) I.V. epinephrine (Adrenalin) (c) I.V. levarterenol bitartrate (Levophed)

_c_ 2. The drug of choice for *initial* treatment of bradycardia is: (a) quinidine (b) lidocaine (c) atropine (d) papaverine

_d_ 3. Adrenergic drugs are most likely to prove effective in the treatment of cardiac arrest when preceded by the infusion of which of the following? (a) vitamin K (b) sodium heparin (c) meperidine hydrochloride (d) sodium bicarbonate

_a_ 4. An increase in the CVP reading should be an impetus for which of the following nursing actions? (a) adjusting the rate of the I.V. (b) securing the defibrillator (c) increasing the oxygen liter rate (d) elevating the foot of the bed

_b_ 5. Which of the following combinations is most likely in the treatment of heart failure following an acute myocardial infarction? (a) digoxin (Lanoxin) and isoproterenol hydrochloride (b) deslanoside (Cedilanid-D) and ethacrynate sodium (Edecrin) (c) furosemide (Lasix) and ethacrynate sodium (Edecrin) (d) Ouabain and digoxin (Lanoxin)

_d_ 6. Careful monitoring of the vital signs is important in the care of patients receiving which of the following drugs? (1) atropine sulfate (2) lidocaine (3) levarterenol bitartrate (4) digoxin (Lanoxin) (a) 3 (b) 1, 2 (c) 3, 4 (d) 1, 2, 3, 4

_a_ 7. Arrange the following drugs in the order in which they would be given to a patient with a myocardial infarction, beginning with his acute illness and continuing through convalescence. (1) morphine sulfate (2) meperidine hydrochloride and promethazine hydrochloride (3) sodium phenobarbital (a) 1—2—3 (b) 3—2—1 (c) 2—1—3 (d) 3—1—2

III. *Matching*

Match each drug with its use following an acute myocardial infarction.

_____ 1. levarterenol bitartrate (Levophed)

_____ 2. isoproterenol hydrochloride (Isuprel)

_____ 3. sodium bicarbonate

(a) counteract acidosis

(b) regulate heartbeat

(c) elevate blood pressure

III. *Matching*

1. c	2. b	3. a

CHAPTER 25

I. *True-False*

1. a	2. b	3. a
4. b	5. b	6. a
7. a	8. b	9. a
10. b	11. a	12. b

II. *Multiple Choice*

1. d	2. b	3. b
4. c	5. a	6. b
7. a	8. b	9. b
10. d	11. c	12. b

III. *Matching*

1. b	2. a	3. b
4. a	5. b	

IV. *Discussion*

1. a	2. b	3. a
4. a	5. a	

CHAPTER 26

I. *True-False*

1. b	2. b	3. a
4. b	5. b	6. b
7. b	8. a	

II. *Multiple Choice*

1. b	2. c	3. c
4. b	5. c	6. d
7. a		

III. *Matching*

1. a	2. b	3. b
4. a	5. c	6. a
7. c	8. a	9. c
10. a		

CHAPTER 27

I. *True-False*

1. b	2. a	3. a
4. a	5. a	6. b
7. b	8. a	9. b
10. a	11. a	12. b
13. b	14. a	15. a
16. a	17. a	18. b
19. b	20. b	21. a
22. a		

II. *Multiple Choice*

1. b	2. b	3. b
4. b	5. b	6. c
7. a	8. b	9. a
10. b	11. c	12. b
13. a	14. a	15. b
16. c	17. c	18. b

III. *Matching*

1. a	2. a	3. b
4. a	5. b	6. b

IV. *Discussion*

1. a	2. a	3. a
4. a		

CHAPTER 28

I. *True-False*

1. b	2. b	3. a
4. b	5. a	6. a
7. b	8. b	9. a
10. b		

II. *Multiple Choice*

1. c	2. b	3. c
4. c	5. a	6. a
7. b	8. b	9. c
10. b	11. d	

III. *Matching*

1. b	2. b	3. a
4. b	5. a	6. a
7. a		

CHAPTER 29

I. *True-False*

1. a	2. b	3. b
4. b	5. b	6. a
7. a	8. b	

II. *Multiple Choice*

1. c	2. d	3. b
4. b	5. b	6. a
7. b	8. c	9. a
10. d	11. c	12. d
13. b	14. b	

III. *Symptom–Cause A*

1. d	2. a	3. c

IV. *Symptom–Cause B*

1. b	2. c	3. a

III. *Calculation*

1. 52.5 mg. 2. ½ tablet

CHAPTER 20

I. *True-False*

1. a 2. a 3. b
4. a 5. a 6. a

II. *Multiple Choice*

1. d 2. c 3. b
4. a 5. b 6. c
7. a 8. c

III. *Matching*

1. a 2. c 3. b

IV. *Discussion*

1. a 2. a 3. a
4. a 5. a

V. *Calculation*

1. 7.5 cc.

CHAPTER 21

I. *True-False*

1. b 2. a 3. b
4. b 5. a 6. b
7. a 8. a 9. b
10. a

II. *Multiple Choice*

1. c 2. c 3. a
4. b 5. c 6. d
7. a 8. c 9. b
10. b

III. *Matching*

1. c 2. d 3. a
4. b

IV. *Discussion*

1. a 2. b 3. a
4. a 5. a 6. a

CHAPTER 22

I. *True-False*

1. a 2. a 3. b
4. a 5. b 6. b

II. *Multiple Choice*

1. a 2. b 3. a

4. d 5. c 6. b
7. c

III. *Matching*

1. a 2. d 3. c
4. b

CHAPTER 23

I. *True-False*

1. b 2. b 3. b
4. a 5. a 6. a
7. a

II. *Multiple Choice*

1. a 2. a 3. c
4. c 5. b 6. b
7. c 8. b 9. c
10. d 11. b 12. b
13. d

III. *Matching A*

1. a 2. b 3. a
4. b 5. b 6. b
7. a 8. a

IV. *Matching B*

1. a 2. a 3. b
4. b

V. *Matching C*

1. a 2. b 3. c
4. a 5. b

VI. *Nursing Action*

1. c 2. d 3. f
4. h 5. i

VII. *Discussion*

1. a 2. a 3. b
4. a 5. a

VIII. *Calculations*

1. 0.24 cc. 2(a). 40,000 U./cc. 2(b). 0.45 cc.

CHAPTER 24

I. *True-False*

1. b 2. a 3. b
4. b 5. b

II. *Multiple Choice*

1. a 2. c 3. d
4. a 5. b 6. d
7. a

III. *Matching A*

1. a   2. b   3. b

IV. *Matching B*

1. a   2. b   3. b
4. b   5. a

CHAPTER 15

I. *True-False*

1. b	2. b	3. a
4. a	5. b	6. a
7. a	8. a	9. a
10. a	11. a	12. b

II. *Multiple Choice*

1. b	2. c	3. b
4. b	5. d	6. c
7. a	8. d	9. a
10. b	11. b	12. b
13. c	14. d	

III. *Matching*

1. c   2. a   3. b

IV. *Drug Use—Drug Action*

1. a   2. d   3. b
4. c   5. b

V. *Calculation*

1. 0.7 cc.

CHAPTER 16

I. *True-False*

1. b	2. a	3. b
4. b	5. a	6. b
7. a	8. b	9. a
10. a	11. b	12. b
13. a	14. b	15. a
16. a	17. b	18. a
19. b		

II. *Multiple Choice*

1. a	2. a	3. a
4. d	5. a	6. b
7. a	8. c	9. b
10. a	11. a	12. b
13. b	14. a	15. b
16. b	17. c	18. b

III. *Calculation*

1. 0.5 cc.

CHAPTER 17

I. *True-False*

1. a	2. a	3. b
4. a	5. a	6. a

II. *Multiple Choice*

1. b	2. a	3. c
4. b	5. b	6. d
7. b	8. a	9. c
10. d	11. c	12. d

III. *Matching A*

1. b   2. a   3. b

IV. *Matching B*

1. b   2. c   3. a

V. *Discussion*

1. a   2. a   3. b

VI. *Calculation*

1. 0.25 cc.

CHAPTER 18

I. *True-False*

1. b	2. a	3. a
4. b	5. b	6. a

II. *Multiple Choice*

1. c	2. b	3. a
4. a	5. c	6. d
7. a	8. a	9. b
10. c	11. c	12. d
13. a	14. b	

III. *Calculation*

1. 10 cc.

CHAPTER 19

I. *True-False*

1. a	2. b	3. b
4. a	5. a	6. a
7. b	8. a	9. a
10. a	11. b	

II. *Multiple Choice*

1. a	2. b	3. d
4. a	5. c	6. d
7. c	8. d	9. b
10. a	11. b	12. a
13. a	14. b	15. b
16. c	17. b	18. c

III. *Situation A*

1. a	2. b	3. a
4. b		

IV. *Situation B*

1. b	2. a	3. a
4. b	5. b	6. a

V. *Calculations*

1. 7.5 cc.; 1½ teaspoons	2. 5 tablets of 0.5 Gm strength and 1 tablet of 0.1 Gm strength

CHAPTER 11

I. *True-False*

1. b	2. a	3. b
4. b	5. b	6. b

II. *Multiple Choice*

1. c	2. a	3. a
4. d	5. c	6. a
7. b	8. b	9. d
10. c	11. a	

III. *Calculations*

1. 200 mg./day; 2 cc.	2. 1.4 cc.

CHAPTER 12

I. *True-False*

1. b	2. b	3. a
4. a	5. b	6. a
7. b	8. b	9. b
10. b	11. b	12. b
13. a	14. b	15. b

II. *Multiple Choice*

1. b	2. b	3. c
4. d	5. c	6. c
7. a	8. b	9. c
10. b	11. a	12. a

III. *Matching A*

1. b	2. b	3. a
4. b	5. a	6. a
7. b		

IV. *Matching B*

1. c	2. a	3. c
4. c	5. b	6. a
7. a	8. a	

V. *Matching C*

1. a	2. a	3. b
4. a	5. a	6. a
7. b		

VI. *Matching D*

1. b	2. c

VII. *Calculations*

1. 0.7 cc.	2. 0.75 cc.	3. 0.63 cc.

CHAPTER 13

I. *True-False*

1. a	2. b	3. b
4. b	5. a	6. a
7. b	8. b	9. a
10. b	11. a	12. a
13. b	14. a	

II. *Multiple Choice*

1. d	2. c	3. b
4. d	5. a	6. a
7. d	8. d	9. a
10. b	11. a	12. c
13. c	14. c	15. c
16. d	17. d	

III. *Matching A*

1. a	2. b	3. a

IV. *Matching B*

1. b	2. a	3. c

V. *Matching C*

1. c	2. b	3. a
4. d		

CHAPTER 14

I. *True-False*

1. b	2. a	3. b
4. a	5. b	6. a
7. b	8. b	9. a
10. a	11. b	12. b
13. b		

II. *Multiple Choice*

1. a	2. c	3. d
4. b	5. a	6. a
7. b		

Answers

CHAPTER 1

I. True-False
1. b   2. b

II. Multiple Choice
1. a   2. d   3. b
4. c   5. d

III. Matching A
1. b   2. a   3. c

IV. Matching B
1. b   2. e   3. d
4. c   5. a

V. Matching C
1. c   2. d   3. a
4. b

V. Matching C
1. e   2. c   3. d
4. a   5. b

VI. Drug Interactions
1. a   2. b   3. a
4. b   5. a   6. c
7. a   8. a

VII. Nursing Action
1. a   2. a   3. b
4. b   5. a   6. a
7. a   8. a   9. a

VIII. Discussion
1. b   2. a   3. a
4. a   5. a   6. a
7. a   8. b

CHAPTER 2

I. True-False
1. b   2. a   3. b
4. b   5. b   6. b
7. a   8. b   9. a
10. b   11. a   12. a
13. b

II. Multiple Choice
1. a   2. b   3. c
4. d   5. b   6. c
7. c   8. c   9. e
10. a

III. Matching A
1. e   2. a   3. d
4. b   5. c

IV. Matching B
1. c   2. a   3. b
4. d   5. e

CHAPTER 3

I. True-False
1. a   2. b   3. a
4. b   5. b   6. a
7. a

II. Multiple Choice
1. b   2. a   3. c
4. a   5. b

III. Situation A
1. c   2. a   3. d
4. b   5. e   6. b
7. a

IV. Situation B
1. b   2. a   3. a
4. b   5. a   6. a

V. Calculation Problems
1. 1.5 Gm.   2. 100 mg.

CHAPTER 4

I. *True-False*

1. b	2. a	3. a
4. b	5. b	6. b
7. b	8. a	9. a
10. a	11. b	12. a
13. a	14. a	15. b
16. b	17. a	18. a
19. a	20. b	21. b
22. a		

II. *Multiple Choice*

1. a	2. b	3. d

III. *Matching*

1. a	2. c	3. b

CHAPTER 5

I. *True-False*

1. b	2. b	3. a
4. a	5. a	6. b
7. b	8. a	9. a
10. a	11. b	12. a
13. b	14. a	

II. *Multiple Choice*

1. b	2. a	3. d
4. b	5. c	6. a
7. b	8. a	9. b
10. d		

III. *Matching*

1. b	2. a	3. d
4. c		

CHAPTER 6

I. *True-False*

1. a	2. a	3. b
4. a	5. b	6. b
7. a	8. b	

II. *Multiple Choice*

1. b	2. d	3. d
4. d	5. b	6. a
7. c		

III. *Calculations*

1. 1 tablet of 16 mg.	2. 0.4 cc.	3. 15 cc.

CHAPTER 7

I. *Multiple Choice*

1. a	2. d	3. b
4. c	5. d	6. b
7. b	8. a	9. b
10. d	11. d	12. a
13. d	14. d	15. d
16. a	17. a	

II. *Calculation*

1. 13 cc.

CHAPTER 8

I. *True-False*

1. b	2. a	3. a
4. b	5. b	6. b

II. *Multiple Choice*

1. d	2. b	3. d
4. a	5. b	6. c
7. d	8. a	

III. *Matching A*

1. b	2. a	3. c

IV. *Matching B*

1. b	2. b	3. b
4. c		

CHAPTER 9

I. *True-False*

1. a	2. b	3. a
4. a	5. a	6. a
7. a	8. b	9. a
10. a		

II. *Multiple Choice*

1. c	2. d	3. b
4. b	5. c	

CHAPTER 10

I. *True-False*

1. a	2. b	3. a
4. b	5. b	

II. *Multiple Choice*

1. d	2. d	3. b
4. c	5. b	6. c
7. a	8. d	

Antianemic Drugs

Red blood cells (erythrocytes) are used in the body to transport oxygen from the lungs to the tissues. Erythrocytes are composed of hemoglobin, the pigment that combines with oxygen for transport, and stroma, the supporting structure of the hemoglobin. An abnormality in the size or shape of erythrocytes or a decrease in their number creates the condition called anemia, which may be of many types. Many nutrients are required for the manufacture of red cells, but the most important are iron, required for hemoglobin, and vitamin B_{12} and folic acid, needed for stroma.

TYPES OF ANEMIA

Anemias requiring therapy with hematinics are classified as either iron deficiency anemia or megaloblastic anemia. The former is referred to as hypochromic microcytic anemia, and the latter is referred to as hyperchromic macrocytic anemia.

Iron Deficiency Anemia

This condition occurs when an individual loses more iron per day than his dietary intake supplies. Symptoms of iron deficiency anemia are vague and may include fatigue, irritability, headache, dizziness, and loss of appetite.

Since the patient has been receiving less than adequate iron through his diet for a period of time, he has used iron from his body storage sites and has often depleted these reserves by the time he seeks medical attention for treatment. Iron therapy is aimed at relieving the patient's symptoms, increasing the red cell and hemoglobin levels to normal, and restoring the iron reserves in the body storage sites. Although the patient may begin to feel better very quickly, he should realize that it may take several months before the iron reserves are back to normal.

Simple inorganic iron salts provide the necessary iron for treating iron deficiency anemia. Iron is also supplied in complex compounds, enteric coated tablets, and sustained release capsules. The latter products usually cost more and can cause an unnecessary expense to a patient on long-term therapy.

Treatment. Iron may be administered orally, intramuscularly, or even intravenously if necessary. Oral iron preparations are better absorbed if taken when there is no food in the stomach. Iron can be quite irritating to the gastrointestinal system, however, and often must be given with food to minimize the irritation. Liquid preparations or concentrated drops may stain the teeth, so they should be placed on the back of the tongue or given through a straw to prevent this. The patient receiving oral iron therapy should be told that his stools may appear dark red or black, and that this is normal. He should also be asked about any bowel difficulties in order that the constipation or diarrhea that may accompany therapy can be corrected. Intramuscular iron injections should be given deep in a large muscle; local reaction may occur at the injection site, consisting of swelling, tenderness, and discoloration of the skin. An intravenous iron injection may be painful and cause phlebitis. Systemic reactions to parenteral iron may include headache, nausea, flushing, joint pain and swelling, and hypotension.

Iron Toxicity. There are three types of iron toxicity: (1) acute iron poisoning caused by the ingestion of an overdose of iron; (2) acute toxicity or allergic reaction to injected iron; and (3) chronic toxicity from long-term parenteral overdosage.

Acute iron poisoning is usually accidental, occurring when a young child swallows several pills. Because of the corrosive effect of iron, hemorrhaging may occur in the gastrointestinal tract. Acute iron poisoning may lead to shock and death. The toxicity is treated symptomatically as well as by administering the antidote, deferoxamine mesylate (Desferal). Deferoxamine mesylate is a chelating agent that binds iron and converts it into a harmless complex to be excreted by the kidney.

An acute allergic reaction to injected iron is usually a hypotensive or an anaphylactic shock reaction. It is treated as an allergic response, according to the severity of the shock.

Chronic toxicity, or long-term parenteral overdosage, results in the depositing of iron in vital organs, skin, and bone marrow (hemosiderosis). Eventually damage to these tissues occurs (hemochromatosis). Deferoxamine has been found to be effective in converting some of this stored iron for excretion by the kidney, but of course it is best to avoid the situation by calculating parenteral doses carefully.

Megaloblastic Anemia

The megaloblastic anemias cause symptoms similar to iron deficiency anemia, with the addition of glossitis and gastrointestinal disturbances. Megaloblastic anemia may be caused by the lack of vitamin B_{12} or by the lack of folic acid. It is important to determine which of these substances is deficient and treat the disease accordingly.

Vitamin B_{12} Deficiency. This may occur in two ways—through inadequate intake of the vitamin, or through failure to absorb it. The American diet usually contains more than adequate amounts of vitamin B_{12}, which is found in abundance in animal

Table 25–1. Hematinics and hematinic antidotes.

Generic Name	Trade Name	How Supplied	Routes	Usual Dose	Comments
ferrous sulfate	Feosol	elixir equivalent to 220 mg./5 cc. in 12 fl. oz. bottles capsules 250 mg. tablets 325 mg.	P.O.	Adults: 1–2 tsp. t.i.d. 1 capsule q.d. 1 tablet t.i.d. or q.i.d.	Children's dose individualized; mix elixir with water only.
folic acid	Folvite	tablets 0.25 mg., 1 mg. vials 10 cc., 5 mg./cc.	P.O. I.M. S.C.	1 mg. daily	Doses of 1 mg. daily are effective for treatment and prophylaxis of folate deficiency; however, daily doses may range from 1 to 20 mg.
iron dextran	Imferon	ampuls 2 cc., 5 cc. 50 mg./cc. vials 10 cc. 50 mg./cc.	I.V. I.M.	Daily dose not to exceed: 0.5 cc. infants under 10 lbs.; 1.0 cc. under 20 lbs.; 2.0 cc. under 110 lbs.; 5.0 cc. others	Use Z-track technique for intramuscular injections. Inject deep and only into upper outer quadrant of the buttock for adults.
deferoxamine mesylate	Desferal	ampuls 500 mg. powder for reconstitution with sterile water.	I.V. I.M.	I.M.: 1 Gm. initially, 0.5 Gm. q. 4h. for 2 doses, then 0.5 Gm. q. 4–12h. Not to exceed 6 Gm./24h. I.V.: Not to exceed 15 mg./kg. body wt./h.	I.M. preferred route unless patient is in shock.
cyanocobalamin; vitamin B_{12}	Rubramin	vials 10 cc., 100 μg./cc., 1 cc., 10 cc., 1000 μg./cc. disposable syringe 1 cc., 100 μg./cc. 1 cc., 1000 μg./cc.	I.M.	Monthly maintenance dose of 100 micrograms for pernicious anemia.	μg. = mcg.

protein foods. However, some individuals do develop megaloblastic anemia from inadequate intake of vitamin B_{12}; a strict vegetarian who does not consume beans, milk, eggs, or other foods with moderate amounts of B_{12} might become anemic. However, the more common vitamin B_{12} deficiency anemia is *pernicious anemia*. This condition is characterized by the lack of a substance, called *intrinsic factor*, normally secreted by the mucosa of the stomach. Intrinsic factor is necessary for the absorption of vitamin B_{12} from the digestive system.

Since a patient with pernicious anemia lacks intrinsic factor, administering large doses of vitamin B_{12} by mouth would not relieve the deficiency. Pernicious anemia is treated with monthly injections of cyanocobalamin. It is very important to stress to the patient that he needs to receive the injections every month, even if he is feeling better. He will need to do this for the rest of his life.

Folic Acid Deficiency.   Folic acid is found in abundance in leafy green vegetables. Because the requirements for this vitamin are so small, foods other than green vegetables that contain small amounts of folic acid may adequately meet the daily requirements. Folic acid deficiency megaloblastic anemia occurs in deficiency states such as malabsorption syndromes, alcoholism, or in poor and elderly patients. It may also occur when folic acid demands in the body are great, as in a woman with successive pregnancies. Folic acid deficiency may easily be reversed by oral ingestion or intramuscular injections of the vitamin.

Both cyanocobalamin and folic acid are nontoxic substances. The body readily excretes any excess of these vitamins. There are no side effects or toxic effects known for either vitamin, even in very high doses.

REFERENCES

RODMAN, MORTON J. "Drugs for Treating Nutritional Anemias." *RN* 35:61, June 1972.

WILSON, PATIENCE. "Iron-Deficiency Anemia." *American Journal of Nursing* 72:502, March 1972.

APPLICATION QUESTIONS

I. *True-False*

For each statement below, write **a** if the statement is true or **b** if it is false.

_____ 1. Adequate amounts of substances essential for building hemoglobin are present in the normal well balanced diet.

_____ 2. Macrocytic anemia is caused by a smaller intake of iron than the amount lost each day.

_____ 3. Individuals vary in the amount of iron needed to maintain normal body reserves.

_____ 4. Usually, a person with iron deficiency anemia is also suffering from megaloblastic anemia.

_____ 5. Folic acid is given immediately to patients suffering from megaloblastic anemia to relieve symptoms while diagnostic procedures are being done.

_____ 6. Simple iron salts, properly administered, effectively treat simple deficiency anemias.

_____ 7. Vitamin B_{12} causes little or no local or systemic toxicity, even when given in large doses.

_____ 8. When a patient being treated with an iron preparation begins to feel better, it is an indication that iron storage sites have been replenished.

_____ 9. Intramuscular administration of iron can cause skin discoloration at the injection site.

_____ 10. Pernicious anemia is best treated with oral doses of vitamin B_{12}.

_____ 11. Less expensive iron preparations are often as therapeutic as the expensive ones.

_____ 12. Iron preparations cannot be given I.V.

II. *Multiple Choice*

For each of the following questions, indicate the letter providing the *best* answer.

_____ 1. Deficiency anemia results from which of the following? (1) insufficient dietary intake (2) poorly absorbed nutrients (3) loss of nutrients (4) removal of the liver
(a) 1 (b) 2, 4 (c) 1, 3, 4 (d) 1, 2, 3

_____ 2. Which of the following symptoms is seen in megaloblastic anemia but *not* in iron deficiency anemia? (a) fatigue (b) glossitis (c) loss of appetite (d) headache

_____ 3. Which of the following statements correctly expresses the relationship between the ingestion and the absorption of dietary iron? (a) absorption capacity remains stable despite ingestion or body need (b) absorption varies with intake in accordance with body need (c) all that is ingested is absorbed (d) absorption capacity is a fixed proportion of iron intake

_____ 4. What is the most appropriate way of administering liquid oral iron preparations to avoid discoloration of the teeth? (a) place concentrated drops on the tip of the tongue (b) mix the solution with a teaspoon of baking soda (c) draw through a straw placed to the back of the mouth (d) brush teeth immediately after taking solution

_____ 5. In which of the following conditions are oral iron preparations contraindicated? (a) ulcerative colitis (b) pulmonary emphysema (c) postpartum anemia (d) menopause

_____ 6. Systemic complications which may occur in parenteral administration of iron salts include which of the following? (1) headache (2) joint pain (3) flushing (4) hypertension
(a) 1, 3 (b) 1, 2, 3 (c) 3, 4 (d) 2, 4 (e) 1, 2, 3, 4

_____ 7. What is hemosiderosis? (a) a chronic toxic response to iron injections characterized by a build-up of the metal in vital organs (b) an anemic condition marked by inadequate utilization of iron (c) an acute systemic allergic response to injected iron preparations (d) a change in the shape of erythrocytes caused by an excess of iron

_____ 8. What is the principal danger of accidentally ingesting large quantities of iron preparations? (a) staining and erosion of tooth enamel (b) corrosion of the mucosa of the gastrointestinal tract (c) excessive, irreversible deposition of iron around vital organs (d) anaphylactic shock

_____ 9. What is the action of deferoxamine mesylate (Desferal)? (a) it speeds the excretion of iron by the bowel (b) it converts iron to a harmless complex for excretion by the kidney (c) it neutralizes iron salts (d) it blocks the receptor sites of iron salts

_____ 10. Which of the following foods would be the best source of vitamin B_{12}? (a) potatoes (b) green peas (c) whole wheat bread (d) roast beef

_____ 11. Folic acid deficiency may develop in which of the following conditions? (1) pregnancy (2) alcoholism (3) gastrectomy (4) celiac disease
(a) 1, 4 (b) 2, 3 (c) 1, 2, 4 (d) 1, 2, 3, 4

_____ 12. Which of the following foods would be the best source of folic acid? (a) chicken (b) asparagus (c) eggs (d) rye bread

III. _Matching_

Match each red blood cell abnormality with the anemia in which it is seen.

_____ 1. Large cells

_____ 2. Small cells

_____ 3. Immature cells

_____ 4. Pale cells

_____ 5. Highly pigmented cells

(a) iron deficiency anemia

(b) megaloblastic anemia

IV. _Discussion_

For each patient statement given below, write **a** if teaching is indicated, or **b** if it is not. If you answer that teaching is needed, outline the content you would include.

_____ 1. "I've just adopted a new belief about meats—the Lord didn't intend us to eat meat of any kind; I'm through eating it, myself."

_____ 2. "Mary loves her iron syrup; I have to keep it out of her reach, and Tom knows it must be kept up there too."

_____ 3. "The doctor said I had pernicious anemia, but _I'm cured_. One shot and I feel so much better I don't think I'll need to go back."

_____ 4. "I haven't been feeling very peppy lately, so I'm taking these fancy multiple vitamins I can buy at the drug store. They haven't helped much, so I guess I'm just suffering from old age."

_____ 5. "I think I'm going to have to stop taking those iron pills the doctor gave me. I've been constipated, and when I do have a bowel movement, it looks like there's blood in it."

Drugs for Treating Endocrine Disorders

SECTION SEVEN

Introduction to Endocrine Disorders and Pituitary Hormones

Endocrine disorders result from alteration or absence of those hormones secreted by the endocrine glands. These are hormones secreted by the pituitary gland and the pituitary target glands, as well as by the parathyroid glands, the pancreas, and the adrenal medulla. Since the actions of the neurohormone epinephrine, secreted by the adrenal medulla, are similar to those of the neurohormone norepinephrine of the sympathetic nervous system, those two hormones are discussed together in Chapter 16. The major hormonal disorder of the pancreas is diabetes mellitus. That disease is discussed separately in Chapter 29.

POSTERIOR PITUITARY

The posterior lobe of the pituitary gland is called the *neurohypophysis*. The two hormones released from this gland are oxytocic hormone (oxytocin) and vasopressin (antidiuretic hormone, ADH). The oxytocic hormone exerts its main effect on the smooth muscle of the uterus and the breast; it has its major pharmacological use in obstetrics. This hormone is discussed in Chapter 27.

The antidiuretic hormone, vasopressin, influences the smooth muscles of the body and acts on renal tubules to increase their ability to reabsorb water. It thereby has an "antidiuretic" action. Lack of this hormone leads to a condition called diabetes insipidus, characterized by excessive diuresis and loss of large volumes of very dilute urine.

Extracts of posterior pituitary glands of animals are used to prevent dehydration in patients with diabetes insipidus. Milder forms of the disease may be treated by inhalation of a powdered form of the extract. More severe cases may require the more potent posterior pituitary injection (Pituitrin), the purer form of vasopressin injection (Pitressin), or the longer acting vasopressin tannate injection (Pitressin Tannate).

Overdosage of these drugs can lead to water intoxication, characterized by fluid retention and a decrease in sodium (hyponatremia). If signs of drowsiness, mental confusion, and decreased urine production occur, indicating impending water intoxication, the drug should be withheld. Determination of urine specific gravity may be ordered frequently while the patient is hospitalized and being regulated on the drug, as a means of determining need and dosage of the hormone.

Other adverse effects of posterior pituitary drugs result from contraction of the smooth muscles of the intestines and blood vessels. Gastrointestinal side effects may include abdominal cramps and diarrhea; the vasoconstriction may lead to an elevation in blood pressure and constriction of the coronary vessels. This drug must be used with extreme caution in patients with previous cardiovascular disease, as it could precipitate an anginal attack or even an acute coronary attack.

Patients may become allergic to the foreign protein present in even the purified extracts of animal glands. A synthetic product called lypressin (Diapid) is now available with antidiuretic activity. It is applied to nasal mucosa as a liquid nasal spray, and is less irritating than the dry posterior pituitary powder. Lypressin helps to avoid the sneezing, asthmatic wheezing, and dyspnea sometimes seen with the dry powder. It may, however, cause some running of the nose, nasal itching, congestion, and, rarely, ulceration of the mucosa. Symptoms of overdosage and the cautions for patients with coronary artery disease are the same as for the posterior pituitary preparations.

ANTERIOR PITUITARY

The anterior pituitary, also called the adenohypophysis, is considered to be the master gland of the endocrine system. The names of most hormones secreted by the adenohypophysis have the suffix *-tropic*.

This suffix indicates that the hormone has a stimulating effect on something else. The names also indicate the target organ or substance stimulated by the hormone.

The secretion of most anterior pituitary hormones is regulated by a negative feedback mechanism with the hormones secreted by the target organ. For example, the pituitary gland secretes adrenocortico*tropic* hormone, which stimulates the adrenal cortex to secrete cortical hormones. When these cortical hormones reach a sufficiently high level in the blood, they suppress the pituitary secretion of the "-tropic" hormone. Low blood levels of cortical hormones, on the other hand, stimulate the release of the pituitary adrenocorticotropic hormone.

Melanocyte-Stimulating Hormone (MSH)

This pituitary hormone controls pigmentation of the skin. It has no pharmacological significance. Treatment of disorders of pigmentation is discussed in Chapter 33.

Somatotropin (STH), or Human Growth Hormone (HGH)

Somatotropin stimulates growth. Without this hormone a child may suffer hypopituitary dwarfism. Recently, this hormone has been made available in small quantities by extracting it as HGH, from the pituitary glands of corpses. Injections of this hormone three times each week for several years have helped dwarfed adolescents develop to the height of small, but normal, adults. The major drawback of the hormone injections is their insulin-antagonizing effect, which may precipitate diabetes mellitus in susceptible people. Glucose tolerance testing must be done frequently when this drug is being administered.

Luteotropin (LTH), Lactogenic Hormone, or Prolactin

The main action of this hormone is control of the secretion of milk during lactation. It has no pharmacological significance, although other hormones may be administered to *suppress* this hormone during the postpartum period.

The Gonadotropic Hormones

The follicle stimulating hormone (FSH) and the luteinizing hormone (LH) are the gonadotropic hormones. Because of the many therapeutic and diagnostic uses of these hormones and the hormones secreted by the gonads, they are discussed in a separate chapter in this section (Chapter 27).

Thyrotropin or Thyroid Stimulating Hormone (TSH)

Because this hormone and the hormones of its target gland, the thyroid, have therapeutic and diagnostic uses, they are discussed in a separate chapter in this section (Chapter 28).

Adrenocorticotropin or Adrenocorticotropic Hormone (ACTH)

This pituitary hormone influences the secretion of cortical hormones by the cortex of the adrenal gland. These hormones are frequently used as anti-inflammatory agents as well as for treating hormonal deficiencies. They are discussed in Chapter 30.

Hormone Replacement Following Hypophysectomy

The hormone replacement regimen necessary after removal of the pituitary gland (hypophysectomy) may vary somewhat according to the physician involved. The nurse should have some idea of the complexity of this situation. When the pituitary gland, or "master gland," is removed, many other endocrine functions are inhibited.

Immediately following surgery, the patient will most likely receive cortocosteroid drugs because the absence of ACTH will prevent the patient's own adrenal glands from functioning. Since these hormones are especially vital in coping with stress situations, failure to replace them after such a serious stress as surgery could lead to a very grave situation.

During the postoperative period, the patient's urinary output and urine specific gravity must be observed carefully to determine if there is a need to replace vasopressin. Replacement of sex steroids will be instituted as the physician perceives the need; in the interim, however, the patient is no longer secreting the gonadotropic hormones and thus cannot secrete sex hormones.

The patient needs to understand the importance of follow-up visits with the physician in order to insure proper regulation of replacement hormones. The need for some hormones, such as those secreted by the thyroid gland, may not become evident until a later visit to the physician. This is because the thyroid gland stores its hormone, and the patient may not show signs of hypothyroidism until the stored hormone has been depleted.

Table 26-1. Miscellaneous endocrine drugs

Generic Name	Trade Name	How Supplied	Routes	Usual Dose	Comments
vasopressin tannate	Pitressin in oil	ampuls 1 cc. 5 U./cc.	I.M.	0.3–1 cc. as required	This drug is also given by subcutaneous injection. It should never be given I.V. Nose drops and powder forms are snuffed onto the nasal mucosa.
	Pitressin Aqueous Solution				Aqueous solution may be given I.V.
dihydrotachysterol	Hytakerol	capsules 0.125 mg. bottles 15 cc. 0.25 mg./cc.	P.O.	Strictly individualized maintenance dose 1–7 cc. or 2–14 capsules weekly.	Careful control of the calcium level of the blood and urine must be maintained.
		ampuls 1 cc. 0.25 mg./cc.	I.M.	Weekly injections; dosage individualized.	

PARATHYROID

The parathyroids are endocrine glands, but they are not under the influence of the pituitary gland. The parathyroids secrete the hormone parathormone, which influences the concentrations of calcium and phosphorus in the blood, and the migration of these elements between the blood and the bones. The hormone acts by preventing reabsorption and thereby promoting urinary excretion of phosphorus. The secretion of the hormone is regulated by the blood levels of calcium and phosphorus. Hyperparathyroidism, in which blood phosphorus levels become abnormally high, can be treated by surgical removal of the glands. Hypoparathyroidism is characterized by a low blood calcium level, and results in tetany.

Tetany

Because of the need for calcium by the nervous system, tetany results in such neuromuscular symptoms as muscular hypertonia, tremor, and spasmodic contractions. The aim of treatment is to raise the blood calcium to a normal level. This is done with the oral or parenteral administration of calcium salts and vitamin D.

Acute hypocalcemic tetany is treated with intravenous calcium lactate and simultaneous parenteral administration of parathormone solution and vitamin D. Dihydrotachysterol (Hytakerol) can be given orally as a substitute for vitamin D, both during the crisis and for maintenance therapy. This drug should be used with caution for pregnant women and patients with kidney stones. Dosage should be controlled by frequent determinations of blood calcium levels. Overdosage would be characterized by symptoms of hypercalcemia: weakness, headache, nausea, anorexia, vomiting, and vertigo.

REFERENCES

DiPalma, Joseph. "The Pituitary Hormones: Potential Wonder Workers." *RN 29*:65, January 1966.

Kahn, Edgar, et al. *Correlative Neurosurgery*. Second edition. Springfield, Ill.: C. C. Thomas, 1969.

Pryor, J. P. "Hyperparathyroidism." *Nursing Times 69*:1558, November 1973.

Rodman, Morton J. "The Pituitary Hormones." *RN 31*:55, June 1968.

APPLICATION QUESTIONS

I. *True-False*

For each statement below, write **a** if the statement is true or **b** if it is false.

_____ 1. Vasopressin is used in the treatment of diabetes mellitus.

_____ 2. Thyroid hormones must be replaced immediately following hypophysectomy.

_____ 3. Vasopressin is another name for the antidiuretic hormone.

_____ 4. MSH extracts are given to promote growth.

_____ 5. Dihydrotachysterol (Hytakerol) is a synthetic preparation of parathormone.

_____ 6. Overdose of dihydrotachysterol (Hytakerol) can lead to hypocalcemia.

_____ 7. Secretion of parathormone is controlled by a hormone from the anterior pituitary gland.

_____ 8. Sex steroids usually need to be replaced following hypophysectomy.

II. *Multiple Choice*

For each of the following questions, indicate the letter providing the *best* answer.

_____ 1. An overdose of an antidiuretic hormone can lead to which of the following? (a) polyuria (b) hyponatremia (c) hypotension (d) constipation

_____ 2. Posterior pituitary extract should be used with caution if which of the following conditions exist? (a) megacolon (b) hypotension (c) angina pectoris (d) tuberculosis

_____ 3. A patient with diabetes insipidus who has developed an allergy to his medication would best be switched to treatment with which of the following drugs? (a) oxytocin (Pitocin) (b) thyrotropin (Thytopar) (c) lypressin (Diapid) (d) vasopressin tannate (Pitressin)

_____ 4. The administration of high doses of adrenocortical steroids has what effect on the pituitary production of corticotropin? (a) increases production (b) decreases production (c) has no effect on production

_____ 5. What is the function of vasopressin? (a) it acts on the adrenal cortex to aid in the production of cortisone (b) it acts on the islet cells of the pancreas to stimulate the production of insulin (c) it acts on the renal tubules to increase their reabsorption ability (d) it acts on the smooth muscle of the intestine to decrease motility

_____ 6. Urine specific gravity is often used to determine the need for which of the following hormones? (a) thyrotropin (b) adrenocorticotropin (c) somatotropin (d) vasopressin

_____ 7. Which of the following tests must be done frequently for a patient receiving human growth hormone? (a) glucose tolerance test (b) white cell count (c) liver function tests (d) urinalysis (e) glomerular filtration rate

III. *Matching*

For each hormone listed, indicate whether it is secreted by the anterior pituitary, the posterior pituitary, or whether it is not secreted by the pituitary.

_____ 1. adrenocorticotropin

_____ 2. vasopressin

_____ 3. oxytocin

_____ 4. melanocyte-stimulating hormone

_____ 5. parathormone

_____ 6. luteotropin

_____ 7. progesterone

_____ 8. prolactin

_____ 9. thyroxine

_____ 10. luteinizing hormone

(a) anterior pituitary

(b) posterior pituitary

(c) not secreted by the pituitary

Hormones Influencing or Secreted by the Gonads

Two pituitary gonadotropic hormones influence the gonads of both males and females. The follicle stimulating hormone (FSH) stimulates growth of the ovarian follicle in females, as well as influencing the secretion of the female sex hormone, estrogen. In males, FSH stimulates the production of spermatozoa. The second pituitary gonadotropic hormone is the luteinizing hormone (LH); in males this hormone may be called interstitial cell stimulating hormone (ICSH), because it stimulates the testicular secretion of the male sex hormone, testosterone.

Following ovulation in females, LH is responsible for converting the ruptured sac of the ovarian follicle into the corpus luteum and stimulating the corpus luteum to secrete the second female sex hormone, progesterone. If the ovum becomes fertilized and pregnancy occurs, the corpus luteum continues to secrete progesterone, but *not* under the influence of LH. Rather, secretion is then stimulated by human chorionic gonadotropin (HCG) which is secreted first by the trophoblasts, and then eventually by the placenta. Detection of human chorionic gonadotropin in a woman's urine is the basis of some pregnancy tests.

PITUITARY AND GONAD FEEDBACK MECHANISMS

In females, the secretion of FSH and the female sex hormones is controlled by a negative feedback mechanism: high blood levels of estrogen or progesterone suppress FSH, whereas low blood levels stimulate the pituitary to release FSH. LH is not controlled in this manner. Although high levels of progesterone *suppress* LH, high blood levels of estrogen *stimulate* its production. This is necessary because FSH is secreted at the beginning of the menstrual cycle, causing growth of the ovarian follicle and production of estrogen. Estrogen then serves as the stimulus for the release of LH from the pituitary, since LH is needed for the ripening and rupture of the ova.

In the male, the pituitary gonadotropins and the sex hormone testosterone are controlled by negative feedback. High blood levels of testosterone suppress the pituitary secretion of both FSH and LH (or ICSH). High doses of testosterone lead eventually to a decrease in spermatogenesis and possible sterility because of the suppression of FSH.

MALE SEX HORMONES

The male sex hormone, testosterone, has both androgenic (sexual) and anabolic (tissue building) activities. Testicular secretions, then, not only stimulate the development of secondary sex characteristics and growth of the sex organs in boys at puberty, but also influence the growth of skeletal muscle, bone, hair, and skin, and stimulate protein metabolism in general so that dietary nitrogen is retained in the tissues. The greater growth and size of the male's skeletal structure in comparison to that of the female is attributable to testosterone. When testosterone is first secreted at puberty, there is a sudden growth spurt in which the bones become thicker and longer. But testosterone then ends bone growth by converting cartilaginous tissues at the ends of the long bones into bone.

Eunuchism and Eunuchoidism

Pharmacologically, testosterone and its derivatives are used mainly as replacement therapy in males who lack the hormone. Eunuchism is the complete absence of the hormone, usually as a result of castration. Eunuchoidism is a result of testicular hypofunction, which may be primary (caused by disease of the testicles) or secondary (caused by dysfunction of the pituitary). Differentiation between primary and secondary eunuchoidism may be done by injecting human chorionic gonadotropin, which will stimulate testicular function if the disorder is secondary to pituitary dysfunction. Secondary eunuchoidism can be treated with HCG, but it is more often treated with a long-lasting male hormone preparation. Other conditions of hormone deficiency are also treated in this way, because the hormone is much less expensive for long-term maintenance therapy.

Treatment may be instituted with testosterone injections of one of the longer acting esters such as testosterone cypionate (Depo-Testosterone Cypionate). Oral preparations are also available, such as methyltestosterone (Metandren) or its synthetic derivative fluoxymesterone (Halotestin). Fluoxymesterone is claimed to be more potent and less likely to cause the jaundice that sometimes occurs with methyltestosterone. The natural hormone, testosterone, cannot be taken orally because it is rapidly destroyed in the liver.

Treatment of Sterility

Oligospermia. Lack of viable, motile sperm, or oligospermia, cannot usually be corrected by testosterone alone, because high dosage of the hormone suppresses FSH. Occasionally, however, after testosterone is given and then withdrawn, the temporarily suppressed pituitary may respond with a rebound secretion of a greater amount of FSH.

Cryptorchism. Undescended testicle, or cryptorchism, may be caused by an obstruction of the inguinal canal or by a lack of testosterone. This condition may cause sterility if the testicle is not brought down into the scrotum. If the condition results from lack of hormone, it may be treated with HCG. Dosage must be carefully regulated, however, to avoid precipitating premature puberty in young boys.

Male Climacteric

The male climacteric is a condition analogous to menopause in women, but relatively rare. The symptoms are similar to those of the menopause, including hot flashes, heart palpitations, nervous irritability, fretting over minor matters, failure of concentration and memory, and insomnia. A true hormone deficiency responds readily to replacement therapy, and cardiovascular and mental symptoms will disappear. The patient will gain in physical vigor, sense of well-being, and restoration of lost libido and potency.

Before proceeding with long-term treatment of men in their middle or late years, prostate gland growths must be ruled out as the cause of the symptoms. If such growths are present, male hormone may stimulate their activity. Prostatic carcinoma is dependent on testosterone, and stimulating this tumor could lead to rapid growth and metastasis. Since prostatic hypertrophy is not uncommon in men over forty years of age, periodic examinations *must* be done if a patient is maintained on hormone replacement therapy.

Side Effects of
Testosterone Therapy

Adverse effects of male sex hormone replacement therapy may include steroid-induced sodium and fluid retention which could lead to hypertension or precipitate congestive heart failure in patients with previous cardiovascular difficulties. Testosterone therapy may also lead to chronic priapism and increased libido, which could be embarrassing socially and personally for the patient. Remember that testosterone suppresses FSH and can therefore cause a reduction in spermatogenesis. Remember also that the hormone can stimulate prostate gland growths, and so periodic prostate examinations are necessary.

If testosterone is given to a prepubertal boy, care must be taken to avoid premature puberty and to prevent premature closure of the epiphyses, which would prevent the boy from attaining his adult height.

Androgen Therapy for Women

In women, male hormones antagonize the effects of excessive estrogen and suppress secretion of pituitary gonadotropic hormones. They can be used, then, for treatment of gynecological conditions such as uterine bleeding, dysmenorrhea, premenstrual tension, and postpartum breast engorgement. Since oral estrogen-progesterone preparations are now available, they are obviously preferable to the androgens because the androgens cause masculinization.

Cancer of the breast which has spread beyond the reach of surgery or radiation treatment may be treated with androgen therapy. Although these drugs have masculinizing effects, the patient may be willing to endure the virilization and possible development of acne for the feeling of well-being and the relief of pain brought about by the treatment. The nurse must help the patient understand the changes in her body and the increased libido she is experiencing. When cancer patients are treated with male hormones, they must also be observed for hypercalcemia. If this occurs, the drug must be discontinued and fluids forced to avoid the formation of kidney stones.

Use of Male Hormones as Anabolic Agents

Because of its anabolic activity, testosterone can produce a positive nitrogen balance in patients who are in negative nitrogen balance. It has thus been used for stimulating the appetite and reversing the processes responsible for protein wastage and subsequent weight loss in debilitated patients. Although the hormone brings about a return of appetite and feeling of well-being, its sexual effects have limited its usefulness for women and children, and have even presented some undesirable effects in men.

Complete separation of the anabolic and androgenic effects of testosterone has not yet been achieved, but some synthetic anabolic steroids are available that stimulate muscle growth and strength with fewer androgenic effects. These drugs include nandrolone phenpropionate (Durabolin), methylandrostenediol dipropionate (Anabolin), and stanozolol (Winstrol).

Patients treated with corticosteroids, especially those who are inactive or confined to bed, will sometimes receive anabolic steroids to counteract the catabolic effects of the corticosteroids and prevent the development of osteoporosis. Convalescent patients and patients who have suffered severe trauma or stress may be in negative nitrogen balance, which may be helped with the administration of anabolic agents. Aplastic amenia in men, women, and children has also responded to the anabolic activity of these drugs.

FEMALE SEX HORMONES

The ovaries synthesize two types of hormones: the estrogens and the progestins. Estrogens cause the secondary sex characteristics and changes in the sex organs in girls at puberty; together with the progestins, they set the stage for pregnancy and childbearing. Estrogens influence growth in the myometrium and the endometrium of the uterus. They rebuild the endometrial epithelium during the first half of the ovulatory cycle, stimulate the endocervical glands to secrete a thin watery fluid, and keep the mucosa of the vaginal tract thick—all activities which foster conception. Estrogens also affect the mammary gland ducts at puberty, during pregnancy, and during each ovulatory cycle.

Estrogens have an anabolic action, but it is less potent than that of the androgens. Estrogens affect the elasticity of the skin, the mineral deposits in the bones, and the fat distribution in the body. In addition, they help retain nitrogen and turn it into protein. At puberty, estrogen converts the cartilage at the ends of the long bones into bone to halt growth.

Whereas the actions of estrogen foster conception, the actions of progesterone foster survival of the fertilized ovum, the embryo, and the fetus. Progesterone prepares the uterine mucosa for reception and implantation of the zygote and decreases uterine muscle contraction to prevent the embryo from becoming dislodged. Throughout pregnancy, progesterone counteracts uterine spasms that could cause spontaneous abortion. The decrease in progesterone production late in pregnancy apparently allows the myometrium to become sensitive to the contractile effects of oxytocin in order to begin labor and delivery of the baby.

During pregnancy, progesterone causes mammary gland secretory sacs to grow and fill with milk; however, postpartum lactation is controlled by the pituitary hormone prolactin, and administration of progesterone at that time actually suppresses lactation.

Estrogen Therapy

Menopause and Postmenopause. Reduction of ovarian function at the time of the female climacteric or "change of life" is accompanied by menstrual irregularities, hot flashes, heart palpitations, sweating, headache, dizziness, insomnia, crying spells, and anxiety. These symptoms can be relieved by properly individualized doses of estrogen preparations such as conjugated estrogens (Premarin). A tranquilizer or antidepressant may be added for relief of some of the mental and emotional disturbances.

Physicians sometimes recommend that women continue taking estrogens following the menopause for their effects on nonsexual metabolism. Postmenopausally, estrogens are used to aid in keeping the breasts firm and the skin supple, and to help avoid osteoporosis and coronary atherosclerosis.

Osteoporosis. Osteoporosis can occur in men or women and can be treated with estrogens, androgens, or a combination of the two. Drug therapy is usually accompanied by a high protein and milk diet with supplementary calcium salts, vitamin D, and fluorides. Prophylactic therapy for osteoporosis is considered especially desirable for patients under treatment with corticosteroids.

Coronary Atherosclerosis. There is actually little evidence that estrogens lower plasma lipid levels or delay the development of atherosclerosis in coronary vessels. But since premenopausal women are relatively free of coronary artery disease, and postmenopausal women have the same incidence of the disorder as men, the use of estrogens for preventing heart attack in both men and women has been advocated recently. Although estrogens employed for this purpose appear to be harmless for women, they can cause some disturbing effects when employed for male patients. The physical changes accompanying these hormones, such as gynecomastia, and the mental effects, such as depression and loss of libido, may cause great concern to male patients.

Senile Vaginitis. The reduction of estrogenic effects on the vaginal mucosa leads to atrophic changes and an increased tendency toward vaginitis after the menopause. This condition can be corrected by estrogens administered orally as well as by topical vaginal creams and suppositories.

The nurse must never assume that because a woman is about fifty years old (or because the patient may be a nurse herself) that she understands gynecological disorders and treatments. It is because these assumptions are sometimes made that some women are too embarrassed to ask questions. The nurse must help the patient understand the changes occurring in her body. Explain to the patient that she may wear a sanitary napkin to prevent soiling her clothing when topical medications are used. The physician may also approve wearing a tampon for this purpose. Explain how to apply topical creams and how to use the applicators that come with the medications. The patient should be told to keep suppositories in the refrigerator and to peel off the foil before inserting them. Suppositories must be placed high in the vagina to prevent expulsion before they have melted.

Hypogonadism. Estrogens may be used to treat women with hypogonadism. This occurs when the ovaries are removed surgically before the menopause, or when a girl fails to develop sexually because of congenital absence of the ovaries, failure of the ovaries to respond to the pituitary gonadotropins, or pituitary dysfunction.

Postpartum. Estrogens are often used to prevent postpartum breast engorgement in women who do not wish to breast feed. After the breasts have been emptied of milk following delivery, either by using a breast pump or through a dose of oxytocin, estrogen suppresses production of the pituitary hormone prolactin and thus inhibits lactation.

Halting Growth. Since estrogen production at puberty halts growth by its action on the cartilage of the long bones, a girl whose puberty is delayed or who does not produce estrogen will continue to grow. In such instances, estrogens may be administered to avoid excessive height.

On the other hand, use of estrogens in young children, as in the case of juvenile vaginitis, may prevent the child from achieving her adult height by causing premature closure of the epiphises. For this reason, it is best to use topical estrogens if at all possible.

Cancer. Although estrogens have not been known to *cause* cancer, their use is not recommended if cancer of the breast or genital cancer is already present. Since these neoplasms may be estrogen-dependent, administration of estrogen would nourish the cancer and lead to more rapid metastasis.

Women who are at least five years past the menopause with cancer of the breast may be treated with estrogens for symptomatic relief, because in such cases the cancer is most likely *not* estrogen-dependent. Men with cancer of the prostate may also be treated with estrogens to antagonize the androgens required by this androgen-dependent neoplasm (see Chapter 39).

"Morning-After Pill." The synthetic estrogen diethylstilbestrol (DES) has been referred to as the "morning-after pill" for preventing implantation of a fertilized ovum after intercourse. Although this drug is not routinely used for this purpose because of its discomforting side effects and the lack of substantial data concerning its use, it is sometimes utilized to prevent pregnancy after rape. When a rape victim comes to a clinic, physician's office, or emergency room following the initial trauma, the psychological effect of the incident may cause her to exhibit any of a number of emotional responses. After the emotional responses have subsided somewhat, the woman may then begin to formulate questions concerning the effects of the rape and the medications she has been given. It is of utmost importance that the nurse be sure the patient has a *written* phone number of the clinic, nurse's office, or physician's office where she can call if she needs some questions answered. The side effects of DES, such as nausea, vomiting, abdominal cramping, vaginal spotting, and others, may be very distressful to the patient; she may not realize that the symptoms are from the drug. If prophylactic antibiotics have also been prescribed to prevent venereal disease and other vaginal infections, the woman may have additional side effects (see Chapter 35). The patient may also be concerned about publications citing the relationship of DES to cancer in children. The nurse can explain that this correlation has been found

only in children of women treated with DES *during* pregnancy.

Progesterone Therapy

Progesterone is useful in treating some menstrual disorders and in selected cases of endocrine infertility and habitual abortion. The massive oral doses or frequent painful injections necessary to treat these conditions limits the use of the natural hormone. The synthetic progestins, however, may be used with fewer drawbacks to treat conditions such as menorrhagia, metrorrhagia, amenorrhea, and dysmenorrhea. Synthetic progestins have also been used to control endometriosis and premenstrual tension.

Uterine Bleeding. Excessive uterine bleeding sometimes responds to "medical curettage," thus averting the need for surgical dilation and curettage. This is done by oral administration of a progestogen such as norethindrone (Norlutin) several times a day for a week or two, followed by withdrawal of the drug. This leads to shedding of the endometrium.

If bleeding is the result of the ovary's failure to produce enough progesterone, as in an anovulatory cycle in which there is no corpus luteum, bleeding may be irregular, prolonged, and excessive. Administration and withdrawal of a progestin can be used to bring this condition under control.

Dysmenorrhea and Premenstrual Tension. Oral administration of synthetic progestins early in the menstrual month has been reported to bring about painless menstruation in cases of dysmenorrhea. Estrogens and combinations of estrogens and progestins have also been used for treating this condition.

There is a theory that the symptoms of premenstrual tension are caused by inadequate production of progesterone by the corpus luteum. Oral progestins, administered during the latter half of the menstrual month, either alone or in combination with diuretics and sedatives, have been effective in relieving symptoms of premenstrual tension.

Habitual Abortion. Progesterone and the synthetic progestins have been used for treatment of habitual aborters—those women who have had three or more consecutive miscarriages. Use of progestins is based on the assumption that some abortions result from failure of the placenta to secrete enough hormone to counteract the contractile effects of estrogens. Daily oral doses of medroxyprogesterone acetate (Provera) have been used for maintaining a pregnancy. Injections of the long acting ester derivative hydroxyprogesterone acetate (Prodox) may also be used.

Diagnostic Use of Progestational Steroids Progestational steroids may be used to determine whether the ovaries of a patient with amenorrhea are capable of producing estrogen. Since bleeding following the administration and withdrawal of the drug indicates the presence of estrogen, absence of bleeding indicates the absence of estrogen.

This same procedure can be used as a pregnancy test. The absence of bleeding following withdrawal of the oral progestin could indicate that the corpus luteum is still producing progesterone, which indicates pregnancy.

Estrogen-Progestin Therapy

Treatment of Amenorrhea. Cyclic administration of the two types of female hormones can be used to treat primary amenorrhea (when menstruation has never occurred) or secondary amenorrhea (when menstruation has previously occurred but is no longer occurring). Several cycles of drug therapy may induce the resumption of normal cyclic function in patients with secondary amenorrhea.

Oral Contraceptives. Administration of the sex steroids inhibits pituitary gonadotropic hormones and thereby suppresses ovulation. Progestin has an added contraceptive value in that it stimulates the endocervical glands to produce a thick secretion that prevents the passage of sperm into the uterus. Most oral contraceptive products contain a potent estrogen and one of the progestins. They were administered in either the combination method or the sequential method. Although both methods provide almost completely effective contraception, the effectiveness of the sequential products appears to be somewhat less than that of the combination products and they have been taken off the market.

The *combination* products contain both steroids in a single tablet which is taken for twenty-one consecutive days, beginning on the fifth day of the menstrual cycle. The first day of menstruation is considered as the first day of the cycle. No tablets are taken for the final seven days of the cycle. Some oral contraceptive products, such as Norinyl 28 Day, include seven tablets with inert ingredients so that the woman maintains the habit of taking one tablet every day.

Women today are likely to discuss contraceptives with the nurse. It is very important that the patient understand her course of treatment, and whether she takes a pill *every* day or only for twenty-one days and does not take any pills for seven days. The patient must understand the importance of telling the physician about spotting or breakthrough bleeding. This is not usually a cause for alarm, but a phone call to the doctor can set the woman's mind at ease, and the physician may arrange to increase the dosage to prevent further bleeding. The woman must also understand the importance of consulting the physician if a menstrual period does not occur when the hormones are withdrawn. Absence of menstruation could indicate that pregnancy has occurred.

The nurse must understand that these drugs may have undesirable side effects resembling those in early pregnancy, such as nausea, vomiting, headache, dizziness, weight gain, breast fullness, and occasionally acne, chloasma, and melasma. The nurse may reassure the patient that these discomforts often subside after several cycles of taking the drug. Nausea may be decreased by taking the pill at bedtime with a glass of milk.

The use of prostaglandins for birth control is under investigation and may provide an alternative means of contraception. These drugs are discussed in Chapter 38.

Adverse Effects of Female Sex Hormones

Women are still confused as to the use of female sex hormones, especially estrogen, and worry about the possibility that they cause cancer. The nurse can offer reassurance that side effects of estrogens are relatively few, minor, and controllable.

Although no truly toxic effects have been traced to the steroid combinations used for cyclic therapy and oral contraception, long-term studies are still being done. Some studies suggest that oral contraceptives, especially those with relatively high doses of estrogen, increase the risk of developing thromboembolic disease. The risk seems small for most women, but women with a history of thromboembolism should not take these drugs. If any clotting disorder occurs while the patient is taking these drugs, they should be discontinued promptly.

Small doses of estrogens and oral contraceptives often produce symptoms similar to those occurring at the beginning of pregnancy. Breakthrough bleeding or spotting may occur but is often relieved by raising the dosage of estrogen.

Postmenopausal women placed on cyclic estrogen therapy should understand that they will have a menstrual period when the hormones are withdrawn. They should be told that this is actually pseudomenstruation; they have not become fertile again and are not likely to become pregnant.

Adverse effects may occur with large doses of estrogens. Gastrointestinal symptoms are the most common, including anorexia, nausea, vomiting, and diarrhea. Other side effects may include headache and

dizziness. Large doses of estrogens administered for long intervals can also cause irregular uterine bleeding. This can be avoided by withdrawing the medication for a week or so after several weeks of treatment—this results in a normal menstrual period. Predictable cyclic bleeding is best assured by taking a progestational hormone together with the estrogen for the last few days before withdrawal of both medications.

Caution is required when administering estrogens or oral contraceptives to patients with a history of liver disease, mental depression, or conditions that might be influenced by steroid-induced fluid retention, such as epilepsy, migraine headaches, asthma, or cardiovascular disease. Patients with thyroid disease, diabetes, or other endocrine disorders should be watched for signs of change in their conditions while taking these drugs. Since the presence of estrogen tends to favor the growth of uterine fibroids, estrogen therapy and oral contraceptives are contraindicated if fibroids are present.

Treatment of Infertility

The administration of small daily oral doses of synthetic progestins combined with estrogens has been claimed to help some infertile women conceive and bear children. This therapy is based on the assumption that these cases of infertility are due to inadequate secretion of progesterone by the corpus luteum to maintain an adequate secretory endometrium.

Infertility stemming from failure to ovulate may be treated with progestins. Although the progestins suppress ovulation, withdrawal of progestin therapy may cause a reflex increase in production of FSH and LH which stimulates production of ova.

Treatment of anovulatory infertility has also been successful with products such as menotropins (Pergonal), which is a product rich in gonadotropin. After these injections stimulate ovarian follicles to mature, injections of human chorionic gonadotropin cause rupture of the ripened follicle and release of the ovum.

The orally effective drug clomiphene citrate (Clomid) is also used to treat anovulatory infertility, although it is neither a female sex hormone nor a gonadotropin. It is thought to act by stimulating the patient's own pituitary gland to produce gonadotropins.

The undesirable effects of the drugs used to treat anovulatory infertility result from overstimulation of the ovaries. Use of these drugs has resulted in the development of painfully enlarged ovaries and ovarian cysts. Development of ovarian cysts warrants discontinuation of the drug to prevent cystic rupture.

REVIEW AND APPLICATION OF CLINICAL PHARMACOLOGY

154

Table 27-1. Hormones influencing and secreted by the gonads.

Generic Name	Trade Name	How Supplied	Routes	Usual Dose	Comments
testosterone cypionate	Depo-Testosterone	vials 1 cc. 100 mg./cc., 200 mg./cc. vials 10 cc. 50 mg./cc., 100 mg./cc. 200 mg./cc.	I.M.	200–400 mg. every 3–4 weeks	Given for the drug's anabolic effect. Dose varies according to the condition being treated. When given with coumarin, dosage of coumarin may be lowered.
nandrolone phenpropionate	Durabolin	vials 5 cc. 25 mg./cc. vials 2 cc. 50 mg./cc. ampuls 1 cc. 25 mg./cc.	I.M.	25–50 mg. weekly	
conjugated estrogens	Premarin	tablets 2.5 mg., 1.25 mg., 0.625 mg., 0.3 mg. ampuls 25 mg. (for reconstitution)	P.O. I.V. I.M.	1.25 mg. q.d. cyclically (3 weeks on, 1 week off) 25 mg. to be repeated in 6–12 hours p.r.n.	Dosage is adjusted upward or down-ward according to the response of the patient.
medroxyproges-terone acetate	Provera	tablets 2.5 mg., 10 mg.	P.O.	5–10 mg. q.d. cyclically	
norethindrone	Norlutin	tablets 5 mg.	P.O.	5–20 mg. P.O. q.d. cyclically	
clomiphene citrate	Clomid	tablets 50 mg.	P.O.	50–100 mg. P.O. q.o.d. 5 days	Three courses of 5 days each may be given.

Prospective parents should also be made aware of the high incidence of multiple births occurring when these drugs are employed.

Prostaglandins may also be found useful for treating certain types of infertility. These drugs are discussed in Chapter 38.

McEwan, J. A. "Menopause, Myths and Medicine." *Nursing Times* 69:1483, November 1973.

Rodman, Morton J. "The Male Sex Hormone and Anabolic Steroids." *RN* 30:41, May 1967.

Soika, Cynthia. "Combatting Osteoporosis." *American Journal of Nursing* 73:1193, July 1973.

REFERENCES

Benjamin, Harry, and Ihlenfeld, Charles L. "Transsexualism." *American Journal of Nursing* 73:457, March 1973.

Benton, Barbara D. A. "Stilbestrol and Vaginal Cancer." *American Journal of Nursing* 74:900, May 1974.

Burgess, Ann W., and Holmstrom, Lynda L. "The Rape Victim in the Emergency Ward." *American Journal of Nursing* 73:1740, October 1973.

DiPalma, Joseph R. "The Pill, Pro and Con." *RN* 34:61, January 1971.

Kistner, Robert. "The Infertile Woman." *American Journal of Nursing* 73:1937, November 1973.

APPLICATION QUESTIONS

I. *True-False*

For each statement below, write **a** if the statement is true or **b** if it is false.

_____ 1. The pituitary hormone FSH stimulates testicular secretion.

_____ 2. Testosterone has anabolic action.

_____ 3. Eunuchism can be treated with testosterone.

_____ 4. The symptoms of the male climacteric are similar to those of the menopause.

_____ 5. Anabolic agents may be given to counteract the catabolic effects of corticosteroids.

_____ 6. Secretion of testosterone is influenced by the pituitary hormone FSH.

_____ 7. The follicle stimulating hormone is referred to as ICSH in males.

_____ 8. High blood levels of estrogen stimulate the secretion of LH.

_____ 9. Estrogen counteracts the contractile effects of progesterone on the myometrium.

_____ 10. Progestins convert the proliferative endometrium to the secretory endometrium.

_____ 11. Ovarian sex steroids suppress ovulation.

_____ 12. Male patients receiving estrogens may experience increased libido.

_____ 13. Taking estrogens causes cancer.

_____ 14. Progesterone is an ovarian hormone.

_____ 15. Some clinical conditions respond to progestins and estrogens given in combination.

_____ 16. Estrogens may be given to control excessive height in prepubertal girls.

_____ 17. Female sex hormones have proved effective for treatment of dysmenorrhea and premenstrual tension.

_____ 18. Progesterone is given to prevent pregnancy after rape.

_____ 19. Chorionic gonadotropin is secreted by the corpus luteum.

_____ 20. Progesterone may be given during lactation to increase milk production.

_____ 21. There is an increased incidence of multiple births when fertility drugs are used.

_____ 22. Fertility drugs may cause development of ovarian cysts.

II. *Multiple Choice*

For each of the following questions, indicate the letter providing the *best* answer.

_____ 1. Why are anabolic agents given to convalescing patients? (a) to decrease the clotting time (b) to correct negative nitrogen balance (c) to facilitate use of oxygen (d) to aid in elimination of protein wastes

_____ 2. Which of the following statements is true regarding the rationale for using testosterone in treating oligospermia? (a) large doses will decrease production of LH (b) discontinuing the drug may result in rebound increase in sperm production

(c) administering the drug stimulates FSH (d) small doses stimulate spermatogenesis directly

_____ 3. When testosterone is being used for treatment of undescended testicles in prepubertal boys, be sure to observe the reports of which of the following diagnostic procedures? (a) CBC (b) X-ray of bones (c) lung scan (d) urinalysis

_____ 4. When testosterone is added to the medicinal regimen of a patient already receiving coumarin, what adjustment should be made in the coumarin dosage? (a) raise the dosage (b) lower the dosage (c) omit the drug (d) make no change

_____ 5. Which of the following drugs is used to maintain the fetus in women who abort habitually? (a) menotropins (b) medroxyprogesterone acetate (c) glucocorticoids (d) testosterone

_____ 6. Infertility due to failure to ovulate may be treated with which of the following drugs? (1) menotropins (Pergonal) (2) female sex steroids (3) testosterone (4) clomiphene citrate (Clomid) (a) 2 (b) 1, 4 (c) 1, 2, 4 (d) 1, 2, 3, 4

_____ 7. Sex steroids produce their contraceptive effects by which of the following? (1) suppressing ovulation (2) stimulating secretion by the endocervical glands (3) stimulating pituitary gonadotropins (4) inhibiting estrogen production (a) 1, 2 (b) 3, 4 (c) 2, 4 (d) 1, 2, 3

_____ 8. What is the drug of choice for controlling excessive uterine bleeding? (a) estrogens (b) progestins (c) testosterone (d) gonadotropin

_____ 9. To determine whether the ovaries of a patient with amenorrhea are capable of producing estrogens, which of the following drugs may be administered? (a) progesterone (b) gonadotropin (c) estrogen (d) thyroid extract

_____ 10. What conditions may exist if a patient fails to menstruate after being given progestational steroids? (1) the pituitary gland is not functioning (2) the ovaries are not producing enough natural estrogen (3) the corpus luteum is secreting progesterone (4) the ovaries are secreting an excess of estrogen (a) 1 (b) 2, 3 (c) 1, 4 (d) 3, 4

_____ 11. Why are estrogens used after menopause? (1) to prevent osteoporosis (2) to decrease the chance of atherosclerosis (3) to keep the vaginal mucosa thick (4) to increase libido (a) 4 (b) 1, 3 (c) 1, 2, 3 (d) 1, 2, 3, 4

_____ 12. When might estrogens be used for treating cancer of the breast? (a) in premenopausal patients (b) in postmenopausal patients (c) at any time (d) never

_____ 13. Which of the following types of cancer respond to treatment with estrogens? (1) advanced cancer of

the prostate (2) premenopausal genital cancer (3) cancer of the uterus (4) cancer of the ovary
(a) 1 (b) 1, 2 (c) 3, 4 (d) 2, 4

_____ 14. The nausea which sometimes accompanies oral contraceptives may be diminished by taking the tablet in which of the following ways? (a) with milk at bedtime (b) after breakfast (c) at the same time each day (d) after some physical exercise

_____ 15. Breakthrough bleeding, a possible adverse reaction to oral contraceptives, may be overcome by which of the following? (a) refraining from coitus during ovulation periods (b) increasing the dosage of the drug (c) reducing emotional stress (d) taking the pill at bedtime

_____ 16. Oral contraceptives have been proven to have which of the following effects? (1) stimulate fibroid growths of the uterus (2) increase possibility of thrombolytic disorders (3) cause cancer of cervix (4) decrease libido
(a) 2 (b) 2, 4 (c) 1, 2 (d) 3, 4

_____ 17. Estrogens should be used cautiously for patients with which of the following conditions? (1) diabetes (2) epilepsy (3) tuberculosis (4) migraine headaches
(a) 1, 2 (b) 3, 4 (c) 1, 2, 4 (d) 2, 3, 4

_____ 18. The presence of chorionic gonadotropin in a woman's urine would indicate which of the following? (a) pituitary dysfunction (b) pregnancy (c) ovulation (d) excessive estrogen production

III. Matching

Indicate whether *androgens* (or anabolic agents) may be used therapeutically in the following conditions, or whether they would be contraindicated if the condition is present.

_____ 1. Breast cancer

_____ 2. Cryptorchism

_____ 3. Prostate cancer

_____ 4. Aplastic anemia

_____ 5. Benign prostatic hypertrophy

_____ 6. Hypertension

(a) may be used therapeutically

(b) contraindicated

IV. Discussion

For each patient statement given below, write **a** if teaching is needed, or **b** if no teaching is needed. If teaching is needed, outline the content you would include.

_____ 1. "I know it just must be my imagination, but it seems like practically overnight since I went through the change—my skin is wrinkled, my hair is thinner, and I need glasses for the first time in my life."

_____ 2. "I do need to see the doctor again, another vaginal infection—how many is that now since I started this menopause bit?"

_____ 3. "I've been taking Premarin since the menopause, and you know, when I stop taking the pills for a few days, I have a period. Do you think I can still get pregnant?"

_____ 4. "I hate the pill. I feel so miserable when I'm taking them, but from what all my friends say, that's just part of it and nothing can be done. They're all the same."

Drug Treatment of Thyroid Disorders

The pituitary hormone thyrotropin (thyroid stimulating hormone, TSH) increases the thyroid's ability to take up iodine from the blood, and can actually cause the thyroid to increase in size. In addition, thyrotropin stimulates the thyroid to utilize the iodine to make thyroid hormones. The thyroid gland produces two types of thyroid hormones, thyroxine (*tetra*iodothyronine, because it contains four atoms of iodine) and liothyronine (*tri*iodothyronine, because it contains three iodine atoms). Thyroid hormones are made in three steps: first, iodine is removed from the blood that passes through the thyroid; second, the iodine atoms are attached to the amino acid tyrosine; and third, the molecules are coupled to form the three- and four-atom iodine hormones. These hormones are then stored in the thyroid gland in a mucoprotein molecule, called *thyroglobulin*, until they are split off and secreted into the blood when needed.

Thyroid gland disorders are broadly classified either as hypothyroidism, resulting from a decrease in thyroid hormone, or as hyperthyroidism, resulting from an increase in thyroid hormone. Simple nontoxic goiter is another disorder, characterized by an enlarged thyroid gland but normal secretion of hormone. This "euthyroid" or essentially normal thyroid state occurs because the gland has enlarged to compensate for conditions which would otherwise result in deficient secretion. The most common cause of simple goiter is lack of dietary iodine; this condition is now rare in the United States because of the availability of iodized table salt.

HYPOTHYROIDISM

Hypothyroidism is a condition characterized by signs and symptoms of a depressant or decreased nature: sleepiness; lethargy; emotional dullness; hypoactive reflexes; bradycardia; hypotension; anemia; pale, coarse, dry, thickened skin; low body temperature; intolerance to cold; decreased appetite; and a tendency toward menorrhagia, sterility, or habitual abortion. Cretinism and myxedema are the two deficiency syndromes associated with hypothyroidism.

Cretinism

Cretinism is the result of glandular deficiency in infancy. It is a congenital hypothyroidism that may result from an inborn enzymatic defect that interferes with iodine uptake and utilization. More commonly, it occurs when a child is born without a thyroid gland (athyreosis) or with one that has failed to develop properly. Lack of iodine in the mother's diet may still account for some cases of cretinism in some isolated areas of the world.

Growth and development of the nervous and skeletal systems are retarded in congenital hypothyroidism. If the child is hypothyroid during fetal development or if the condition is not diagnosed and treated early, permanent mental retardation usually occurs. Initial treatment consists of relatively large doses of thyroid preparations; maintenance doses are determined by periodic blood studies of protein-bound iodine.

Myxedema

Myxedema results from thyroid deficiency in adults or older children (juvenile myxedema). It usually develops slowly, but occasionally follows acute or chronic inflammatory destruction of the gland. Overtreatment of hyperthyroidism with drugs, radiation therapy, or surgery may also lead to myxedema. Myxedema is considered "primary" if the disorder occurs within the thyroid gland, and "secondary" if the disorder results from failure of the pituitary gland to secrete thyrotropin. Thyrotropin (Thytropar) can be prepared from the pituitary glands of animals; it is used to differentiate between primary and secondary myxedema. If the disorder is secondary to pituitary dysfunction, injection of thyrotropin will cause a measurable increase in the uptake of radioactive iodine. If the disorder is primary, the radioactive iodine uptake will continue to be low despite the injection of thyrotropin.

The Therapeutic Use Of Thyroid Preparations

The aim of treatment for myxedema is to provide the greatest possible improvement with the lowest dosage of thyroid; that is, to help the patient be as close to normal as possible without causing *hyperthyroidism*. Administration of thyroid hormones will eliminate the generalized puffiness, and the patient will appear more alert and interested and be able to engage in normal physical activity.

Since the presence of thyroid hormone in the blood suppresses the pituitary's secretion of thyrotropin by means of the negative feedback mechanism, thyroid hormones are sometimes used for just this reason—to suppress thyrotropin. This may be useful in the treatment of thyrotropin-dependent cancer of the thyroid. It is also used to decrease the size of the gland, in some cases of simple goiter or when antithyroid drugs are given, as discussed later in this chapter.

Thyroid drugs have been used in the treatment of nonthyroid deficiency conditions such as obesity, gynecological disorders, and various dermatological and musculoskeletal conditions. Thyroid hormones may help in some of these instances, but the dangers involved when thyroid drugs are used in euthyroid patients make other modes of treatment or drug therapy preferable if possible and available.

Thyroid Preparations

Thyroid and thyroglobulin can be made from thyroid glands of animals. These preparations are relatively inexpensive and serve as satisfactory replacement therapy in most cases of hypothyroidism. The specific natural hormones are also available for thyroid therapy. Sodium liothyronine (Cytomel) is the faster acting of the two hormones; it is therefore most useful for emergency treatment of myxedema coma. Its relatively short duration may not make it the drug of choice for maintenance therapy. Thyroxine, the second of the two natural hormones, is available in two forms, sodium levothyroxine (Synthroid) and sodium dextrothyroxine (Choloxin). Sodium dextrothyroxine is the preferred form for reducing plasma cholesterol levels when hyperlipidemia is present. Sodium levothyroxine has a slower onset of action, but once the effects are fully attained, they are longer lasting. Liotrix (Euthroid) is a combination drug containing four parts of levothyroxine to one part liothyronine. This drug is claimed to imitate more closely the effects of the natural thyroid gland secretions. It is said to be more constant in its strength, enabling better interpretation of laboratory tests used to determine the patient's response to treatment.

Adverse Effects Of Thyroid Preparations

The dangerous side effects and symptoms of overdosage of these drugs result from their cardiac effects. Because of the increase in metabolism caused by the thyroid hormones, the heart muscle is forced to work harder. This can result in tachycardia, cardiac arrhythmias, elevated pulse pressure, anginal chest pains from myocardial ischemia, and possible precipitation of congestive heart failure. Other side effects may include excessive sweating, intolerance to heat, fever, flushing, nervousness, irritability, insomnia, headache, abdominal cramping, diarrhea, nausea, and increased appetite.

Administration of thyroid preparations along with adrenergic drugs is not recommended because of the possible combined cardiac effects. If anticoagulants are administered with thyroid drugs, the dosage of the anticoagulant must be reduced to prevent bleeding. Diabetic patients maintained on insulin or oral hypoglycemics may require an adjustment in their diabetic drug dosages after beginning treatment with thyroid drugs. Thyroid drugs are used with caution in patients with a history of angina pectoris, myocardial infarction, congestive heart failure, or hypertension. These drugs are also contraindicated in the presence of adrenal insufficiency (unless the deficiency is first corrected with corticosteroid drugs) or hypopituitarism. A patient with adrenal insufficiency will not be able to cope with the additional physical stress of the increased metabolism imposed by the thyroid hormones.

HYPERTHYROIDISM

Hyperthyroidism (thyrotoxicosis) is a condition characterized by signs and symptoms of a stimulant nature: nervousness; anxiety; hyperactive reflexes; insomnia; tremor; tachycardia; palpitations; increased pulse pressure and systolic hypertension; thin, warm, moist, flushed skin; elevated body temperature; increased appetite, with a tendency to lose weight; goiter; exophthalmos; and amenorrhea. The cause of hyperthyroidism is not known, but it is believed to be a thyroid-stimulating antibody called long acting thyroid stimulator (LATS); unlike the thyrotropic hormone of the pituitary, LATS is *not* suppressed by high plasma levels of thyroid hormone. This theory is demonstrated by the thyroid suppression test, in which sodium liothyronine is administered daily for a week. Euthyroid individuals then show a reduction in radioactive iodine uptake because of the suppression of pituitary thyrotropin. Hyperthyroid individuals, on the other hand, continue to take up radioactive iodine even though the pituitary thyrotropin has been suppressed by the large doses of thyroid hormone.

Treatment of Hyperthyroidism

Symptoms of hyperthyroidism can be controlled by administration of antithyroid drugs; by radiation therapy with the radioactive iodine isotope I [131]; or by subtotal surgical excision of the gland. Antithyroid drugs may be given for six months; if the thyroid suppression test then indicates a decrease in radioactive iodine uptake, chances of remission are good. If the test still indicates the presence of hyperthyroidism, surgery or radiation therapy will probably be needed.

Antithyroid Drugs (goitrogens).   The most commonly used antithyroid drugs are the thiocarbamides, such as methimazole (Tapazole) and propylthiouracil (Propacil). These drugs inhibit the oxidative enzymes that catalyze the second and third steps in the synthesis of thyroid hormones. When the thyroid stops secreting excessive amounts of hormone, the gland goes through a compensatory enlargement. This enlargement may be halted by administering a thyroid drug to suppress the pituitary production of thyrotropin. If a patient takes one of the antithyroid drugs for a year, he may never have a recurrence of the disease. Failure to take the drug regularly at the proper times of day as directed, however, could cause a recurrence of the disease.

Propylthiouracil or a similar drug may also be useful in the preoperative preparation of a patient for a subtotal thyroidectomy. Daily administration of this drug for several weeks helps to bring the patient's metabolism back to normal and to stabilize the cardiovascular system. However, this procedure is likely to cause the gland to grow larger and more vascular, and thus more likely to bleed during surgery. A few drops of an iodine solution, such as Lugol's solution, daily for a week to ten days prior to surgery helps to decrease the vascularity of the thyroid gland.

In addition to their preoperative use, iodine solutions are sometimes used to control mild cases of hyperthyroidism. More severe cases of hyperthyroidism do not respond permanently to iodine, and may actually be made worse by it. The small amounts of iodine solutions such as Lugol's solution and saturated solution of potassium iodide (SSKI) must be carefully measured in drops. The drops are added to fruit juice to disguise the bitter taste; the mixture is best given through a straw to prevent discoloration of the teeth.

Potassium perchlorate is another drug which may be used in the treatment of hyperthyroidism. When administered in several small daily doses with food to reduce gastric irritation, this drug quickly reduces the signs and symptoms of thyrotoxicosis. Potassium perchlorate cannot be used preoperatively because it acts by competing with the iodine ion and keeping it from being taken up by the thyroid. Therefore, it would also keep the patient from profiting from the ability of iodine to decrease the size and vascularity of the thyroid; the patient would be predisposed to bleeding during surgery.

Side Effects.   Side effects of the antithyroid drugs are not usually severe. The thiocarbamides may cause skin rash, gastrointestinal upset, arthralgia, and headache. On rare occasions, these drugs have caused more serious side effects, such as agranulocytosis or hepatitis. The iodine preparations may cause gastric irritation, such as nausea and vomiting, or respiratory tract irritation with symptoms resembling those of the common cold or sinusitis. Potassium perchlorate may cause skin rash and gastric irritation, and may also lead to more serious reactions such as lymphadenopathy, nephrotic syndrome, agranulocytosis, and, rarely, aplastic anemia.

Radioactive Iodine.   I[131] is trapped by the thyroid as though it were ordinary iodine. This isotope gives off beta and gamma radiation useful for diagnosis and treatment of thyroid disease. For the radioactive iodine uptake test, small tracer doses are administered to determine the thyroid's capacity to store iodine. Results are based on a measurable difference between the retention and excretion of the iodine. In myxedema, for example, a small proportion of the iodine is taken up by the thyroid, and most is excreted in the urine. In hyperthyroidism, a large proportion of the iodine is taken up by the thyroid, and very little is excreted in the urine.

Large amounts of I[131] are administered in order to concentrate and destroy thyroid tissue. Therapeutic doses of this isotope are as much as 1000 times as high as the dose for diagnostic testing. Because of the short range of beta rays, cells other than thyroid are not destroyed. The main danger of radiation therapy of this type is that too much thyroid tissue can be destroyed, and the patient can become hypothyroid. Because of the potential hazards of the radiation in the high therapeutic doses, the nurse must observe the necessary precautions, such as the special handling of bedpans, urinals, and excreta.

Table 28-1. Drugs used in treating thyroid disorders.

Generic Name	Trade Name	How Supplied	Routes	Usual Dose	Comments
sodium liothyronine	Cytomel	tablets 5μg.; 25μg.; 50μg.	P.O.	5–100 μg. daily	μg. = mcg.
sodium levothyroxine	Synthroid	tablets 0.025 mg.; 0.05 mg.; 0.1 mg.; 0.15 mg.; 0.2 mg.; 0.3 mg.	P.O.	0.05–0.3 mg.	Parenteral solution to be reconstituted. Use immediately after reconstitution; discard unused portion.
		multiple vial 10 cc. 500 μg./10 cc.	I.V. I.M.	200–400 μg.	
thyroid USP		tablets 1/4 gr.; 1/2 gr.; 1 gr.; 2 gr.; 3 gr.; 4 gr.; 5 gr.	P.O.	1/4 gr.–10 gr. P.O. q.d.	Dosage varies widely depending on the condition, age, and response of the patient.
methimazole	Tapazole	tablets 5 mg.; 10 mg.	P.O.	Initial 15–60 mg. divided into equal doses. Maintenance 5–15 mg. q.d.	Dose is divided into three doses. Take at 8-hour intervals.
liotrix	Euthroid	tablets: *Euthroid 1/2*: thyroid 1/2 gr. sodium levothyroxine 0.05 mg. sodium liothyronine 12.5 μg. *Euthroid 1*: thyroid 1 gr. sodium levothyroxine 0.1 mg. sodium liothyronine 25.0 μg. *Euthroid 2*: thyroid 2 gr. sodium levothyroxine 0.2 mg. sodium liothyronine 50.0 μg. *Euthroid 3*: thyroid 3 gr. sodium levothyroxine 0.3 mg. sodium liothyronine 75.0 μg.	P.O.	1 tablet q.d. (one of the strengths daily)	

REFERENCES

GARDE, SISTER MARIANA. "Cancer of the Thyroid." *American Journal of Nursing* 65:98, November 1965.

MASON, A. S. "The Treatment of Thyrotoxicosis." *Nursing Times* 65:202, February 1969.

NORDYKE, ROBERT. "The Overactive and Underactive Thyroid." *American Journal of Nursing* 63:66, May 1963.

RODMAN, MORTON J. "The Thyroid and Antithyroid Drugs." *RN* 31:52, February 1968.

APPLICATION QUESTIONS

I. *True-False*

For each statement below, write **a** if the statement is true or **b** if it is false.

_____ 1. Euthroid refers to the congenital absence of a thyroid gland.

_____ 2. A nontoxic goiter results in hyperthyroidism.

_____ 3. Iodized salt in a diet provides enough iodine for a normally functioning thyroid gland.

_____ 4. The use of thyroid preparations is contraindicated for infants.

_____ 5. The thyroid gland of a patient with secondary myxedema is capable of producing thyroid hormones.

_____ 6. Patients taking thyroid should not be treated with adrenergic drugs.

_____ 7. Thyrotoxicosis is caused by a pathogenic organism.

_____ 8. The production of long acting thyroid stimulator (LATS) is inhibited by high blood plasma levels of thyroid hormones.

_____ 9. Saturated solution of potassium iodide (SSKI) may be given in orange juice to disguise its taste.

_____ 10. Thyroid and antithyroid drugs are never given in combination.

II. *Multiple Choice*

For each of the following questions, indicate the letter providing the *best* answer.

_____ 1. Symptoms of hyperthyroidism may include which of the following? (a) decreased pulse pressure (b) hypothermia (c) congestive failure (d) bradycardia

_____ 2. Symptoms often demonstrated by patients with hypothyroidism include which of the following? (1) thinning of hair (2) nervousness (3) lethargy (4) intolerance to cold
(a) 1, 2 (b) 1, 3, 4 (c) 1, 3 (d) 2, 4

_____ 3. What is the most common cause of simple nontoxic goiter? (a) a tumor of the thyroid gland (b) a dietary lack of vitamin E (c) a low blood level of iodine (d) congenital absence of the thyroid gland

_____ 4. Which of the following can stimulate the thyroid gland to increase in size? (a) thyroxine (b) thyroglobulin (c) thyrotropin (d) triiodotyrosine

_____ 5. Adequate doses of thyroid hormone for the initial treatment of early myxedema might bring about which of the following? (a) remission of all physical, mental, and emotional symptoms (b) remission of the physical symptoms only (c) no change in the physical symptoms but an improvement in mental or emotional status (d) no change in the symptoms already present but no further deterioration

_____ 6. Primary and secondary myxedema can be differentiated by a radioactive iodine test after administration of which of the following? (a) thyrotropin (b) thyroglobulin (c) liothyronine (d) thyroxin

_____ 7. Which of the following patients would be in the greatest danger if treated for hypothyroidism with thyroid extract? (a) an 85-year-old man with hypotension (b) a 45-year-old man with a history of myocardial infarction (c) a 3-week-old infant (d) a woman 3 months pregnant

_____ 8. Which of the following would be used in the treatment of hyperthyroidism? (1) administration of goitrogens (2) radioisotope I^{131} (3) subtotal thyroidectomy (4) liothyronine
(a) 1, 4 (b) 1, 2, 3 (c) 2, 3, 4 (d) 1, 2, 3, 4

_____ 9. Which of the following signs and symptoms would indicate toxicity from antithyroid drugs? (1) sore throat (2) clubbed fingers (3) jaundice (4) fever
(a) 3 (b) 1, 4 (c) 1, 3, 4 (d) 1, 2, 4

_____ 10. Which of the following medications, given daily for a week to ten days prior to a thyroidectomy, would help decrease the vascularity of the gland? (a) propylthiouracil (Propacil) (b) Lugol's solution (c) potassium perchlorate (d) methimazole (Tapazole)

_____ 11. Which of the following drugs may be given in combination with the thiocarbamides to stop the compensatory enlargement of the thyroid gland? (a) methimazole (Tapazole) (b) radioactive iodine I^{131} (c) propylthiouracil (Propacil) (d) sodium liothyronine (Cytomel)

III. *Matching*

Match each symptom with **a** if it is seen in hypothyroidism or with **b** if it is seen in hyperthyroidism.

_____ 1. moist, warm, thin skin

_____ 2. insomnia

_____ 3. paleness

_____ 4. increased pulse pressure

_____ 5. dry, cold, thick skin

_____ 6. emotional dullness

_____ 7. bradycardia

(a) hypothyroidism

(b) hyperthyroidism

Diabetes Mellitus

Diabetes mellitus is considered to be an endocrine disease because it involves the lack of activity of the hormone insulin. Insulin is secreted by the beta cells (islets of Langerhans) of the endocrine portion of the pancreas. Diabetes is considered to be a disease of carbohydrate metabolism, but most of its complications or disease manifestations actually result from abnormal fat and protein metabolism. Diabetes may be "secondary," resulting from an endocrine disorder or following disease or removal of the pancreas. More commonly, diabetes is of the "primary" type, which involves an inherited tendency. Symptoms may be caused by a partial or total lack of insulin, or by the presence, in normal or above normal amounts, of ineffective insulin. In the latter case, insulin may be protein-bound in the blood, or it may be rendered ineffective by the presence of insulin antagonists such as adrenal steroids (in "steroid diabetes"), somatotropin, ACTH, or thyroxine. Symptoms of diabetes include polyuria, polydipsia, polyphagia, pruritus, glycosuria, and fatigue. Complications or additional manifestations of the disease may include atherosclerosis, renal disease, retinopathy and loss of vision, neuropathies, increased susceptibility to infection, and increased difficulty during pregnancy. Diabetes is *not* acquired from eating too much sugar, and diabetes *cannot* be cured by the avoidance of eating sugar.

Insulin influences the conversion of glucose into its storage form, glycogen, and the rate at which glucose molecules move through cell membranes. Without insulin, glucose remains in the blood and does not move into the cells to be used for energy production. When the cells do not have glucose, fats and proteins are broken down and converted to glucose in an attempt to provide the needed fuel.

Treatment of diabetes involves a prescribed integration of diet, exercise, weight loss, and administration of insulin or oral hypoglycemics when indicated. For further understanding of the disease process and diet therapy, a medical-surgical textbook and a therapeutic nutrition textbook should be consulted.

INSULIN

The hormone insulin can be given parenterally; it is available in the dosage form of units per cc. It is most commonly available in the strengths of 40 units per cc. (U-40); 80 units per cc. (U-80); and 100 units per cc. (U-100). There are 1 cc. insulin syringes available that are calibrated in 40, 80, and 100 units. U-40 insulin bottle labels and syringes are usually color-coded red; and U-80 insulin bottle labels and syringes are color-coded green. The color coding can be used as an aid in avoiding errors by only drawing up insulin with a green-labeled bottle on the green scale, and only drawing the red-labeled insulin on the red scale. A current trend is to attempt to avoid all the potential errors dealing with U-40 and U-80 insulin and syringes by using only U-100 as a universal strength. U-100 doses, of course, can be drawn up in a U-100 syringe or a TB syringe, which is calibrated in hundredths of a cc. The nurse should be aware that *any* strength of insulin may be given with a TB syringe by calculating the dosage in terms of 40 units per cc. or 80 units per cc.

Duration and Peak Action
Times of Insulin

Insulin is available as rapid acting insulin (regular, crystalline), intermediate acting (globin, NPH), and long acting (ultralente). Rapid acting insulin has a duration of 6 to 8 hours, and its peak action occurs 2 to 4 hours after administration. Intermediate acting insulin has a duration of 18 to 28 hours, with its peak action occurring 9 to 12 hours after administration. Long acting insulin has a duration of more that 36 hours; its peak action occurs between 16 and 20 hours after its administration. The nurse should know the times of peak action and duration in order to teach the patient about the interrelationship of his diet and his medication, as well as to aid in determining diabetic extremes. For example, if a patient is maintained on an intermediate acting insulin given once a day at about eight o'clock in the morning, the peak action of his insulin will occur between five and eight o'clock in the evening. Since the peak action is that time when insulin is at its highest concentration in the blood, that would be one of the most critical times for the patient to become hypoglycemic, if there were not enough glucose present. Consequently, for the patient maintained on intermediate acting insulin, the evening meal is very important. To delay the evening meal for this patient could lead to a hypoglycemic reaction. Likewise, to delay the noon meal of a patient who has received a rapid acting insulin at eight o'clock in the morning could lead to a hypoglycemic reaction.

Patient Teaching

Diabetic patients are taught to administer their own insulin injections. The importance of rotating injection sites must be stressed to the patient, because overuse of one site can lead to tissue inflammation, hypertrophy, or atrophy. The patient is told to keep insulin in a cool place, usually the refrigerator, but *not* in the freezer. Absorption may be inhibited and tissue reactions may occur if insulin is taken out of the refrigerator and injected cold. Therefore, it is now believed that the bottle in current use can be stored at room temperature, as long as the temperature does not exceed 90 degrees. Storing the drug in the bathroom should be discouraged to avoid exposure to the heat produced by a shower.

Another factor thought to contribute to tissue reactions is an injection which is not deep enough. The traditional 45-degree angle for injecting a subcutaneous injection may be too shallow for absorption; it may even result in some patients giving intradermal injections. It is now believed that, except for very thin people, patients can give injections at a 90-degree angle with a 1/2-inch or 5/8-inch needle to insure a deep subcutaneous injection.

The patient must also be instructed to check the expiration dates on the insulin bottles and not to use the medication if this date has passed. Insulins which are in suspensions (intermediate and long acting insulins) must not be used if clumps, granules, or solid deposits appear in the solutions. The patient should be told to rotate each bottle of insulin suspension before drawing up an injection to insure that the medication is thoroughly mixed. Insulin should not be shaken vigorously, because the diffuse tiny air bubbles which would result could cause an inaccurate dosage measurement. This is especially noteworthy because of the small doses usually prescribed.

ORAL HYPOGLYCEMICS

Oral hypoglycemics are *not* oral insulin and can never be substituted for insulin. They are never used for cases of juvenile diabetes and are not indicated if the disease can be controlled by diet and weight reduction alone. They may be used in some cases of maturity onset diabetes. Because of recent findings that patients taking these drugs for long periods of time tend to develop cardiovascular complications more often than those treated in other ways, use of these drugs is now discouraged and limited to several special classes of patients: (1) those who are allergic to insulin; (2) those who are unwilling to take insulin because they find injections painful or a cause of disfiguring skin lesions; (3) those who fail to follow directions for correct use of insulin; and (4) those with physical disabilities, such as visual difficulties, arthritis, or other neuromuscular disorders, which would make self-administration of insulin difficult. There are two classes of oral hypoglycemics—the sulfonylureas and the biguanides.

Sulfonylureas

The sulfonylurea drugs include tolbutamide (Orinase), chlorpropamide (Diabinese), acetohexamide (Dymelor), and tolazamide (Tolinase). These drugs act by stimulating production of insulin from the patient's own pancreas. Tolbutamide is shorter acting than chlorpropamide, and hypoglycemia occurs less often with tolbutamide. If a patient taking chlorpropamide has a kidney disorder, hypoglycemia may occur, because this drug depends on renal excretion for elimination. Tolbutamide depends on the liver for metabolism, and therefore must be used with caution for patients with liver disease. Simultaneous administration of the sulfonylureas with drugs such as phenylbutazone, probenecid, salicylates, sulfonamide type antibacterials, and anticoagulants causes an increase in hypoglycemic action. A decrease in the dosage of the sulfonylurea is therefore required. Patients taking drugs such as the thiazide diuretics may require an increase in the sulfonylurea dosage, as the thiazides decrease the hypoglycemic action.

Biguanides

The major drug of this class is phenformin hydrochloride (DBI). This drug also comes in a sustained release form (DBI-TD). Phenformin hydrochloride does *not* stimulate the production of endogenous insulin; rather, it seems to affect tissue cells to force them to absorb and utilize glucose. This drug may be used alone or in combination with one of the sulfonylureas, or it may be used as an adjunct to insulin therapy. Phenformin hydrochloride tends to leave a metallic taste in the mouth and may cause nausea, vomiting, and diarrhea.

DIABETIC EXTREMES

Diabetic extremes result from either *hypo*glycemia or *hyper*glycemia. The hypoglycemic extreme may be referred to as *insulin shock* or *insulin reaction*. The hyperglycemic extreme is, of course, an exaggeration of the disease symptoms; it may be referred to as *diabetic acidosis, ketoacidosis,* or *diabetic coma.* At times it may be difficult to differentiate between diabetic coma and an insidious onset hypoglycemic reaction.

Hypoglycemia

Hypoglycemia may result from too much insulin, too little food, or too much exercise. Symptoms may differ, depending in part on what type of insulin the patient is receiving. If a patient is receiving rapid acting insulin, the drop in blood sugar will most likely be rapid. The body will interpret this as a stressful emergency situation and respond with autonomic nervous system stimulation. Symptoms, then, are predominantly those of sympathetic stimulation: palpitation, tachycardia, blurred vision, and pallor. These may be accompanied by such parasympathetic symptoms as sweating, hunger, nausea, and dizziness.

A patient receiving an intermediate acting or long acting insulin is more likely to experience a more gradual drop in blood sugar and a more insidious onset of vague symptoms. The body may not interpret this gradual drop in blood sugar as an emergency situation and thus may not respond by liberating epinephrine. Instead, symptoms of this type of reaction result from the direct deprivation of glucose to the brain and central nervous system. Symptoms include headache, drowsiness, mental confusion, irritability, and difficulty in concentration and thinking.

Symptoms of insulin shock may vary from one person to another, and may include a combination of both autonomic nervous system *and* central nervous system symptoms. An individual diabetic patient, however, often responds in a similar pattern any time he experiences hypoglycemia. For this reason, it would be helpful for the nurse to inquire about the patient's *usual* symptoms of insulin shock.

Hypoglycemia may be treated by having the patient take some form of glucose by mouth. If he is unable to do this, an intravenous injection of 50 percent glucose may be given. Subcutaneous injections of epinephrine, hydrocortisone, or glucagon may be used to cause an increase in blood sugar by liberating the glycogen storage forms of glucose. This action is dependent, of course, on glycogen stores not yet having been depleted.

Hyperglycemia

Hyperglycemia can result when there is too little insulin, too much food, or too little exercise. Any increase in stress, either emotional or physical, increases the need for insulin; if no adjustment is made, this can lead to hyperglycemia also. A patient may not think he needs to take his insulin during physical illness if he has been vomiting or not eating; however, in this situation he may actually require more than his regular insulin dose, because of the requirements of the physical stress. Symptoms of insulin deficiency hyperglycemia may be insidious in onset or may occur with dramatic suddenness.

Hyperglycemia causes the amount of glucose filtered by the kidneys to be greater than the amount the tubules can absorb. Since water is pulled by the glucose because of osmotic action, polyuria and eventually dehydration can result. Hyperglycemia resulting from lack of insulin is associated with a lack of glucose in tissue cells, even though glucose is abundant in the blood. This lack of cellular glucose stimulates the breakdown of fats and proteins to provide glucose for fuel. This only increases the blood glucose and the polyuria. The intermediary products of fat metabolism—acetone, aceto-acetic acid, and beta-hydroxybutyric acid—are increased, causing the patient to become acidotic. The ketones, metabolic fragments of fat metabolism, are combined with sodium, potassium, and bicarbonate and excreted through the urine. (Some of the ketones are excreted from the lungs by the compensatory Kussmaul-type hyperpnea). The decrease in alkaline reserve through the renal excretion causes the patient to become more acidotic.

Treatment of diabetic ketoacidosis consists primarily of administering rapid acting insulin intravenously. Support of vital signs, replacement of potassium, and correction of acidosis by administering sodium bicarbonate may also be necessary. Insulin may be given in isotonic Ringer's lactate solution or isotonic saline at first. However, to prevent hypoglycemia and to provide a readily available source of glucose for reestablishing glycogen stores, insulin may later be given in 5 percent glucose. The nurse must be aware that when insulin is administered intravenously, there is a tendency for the insulin to adhere to the bottles and tubing, as well as to float on top of the I.V. solution. The infusion bottle should therefore be rotated frequently to insure a consistent infusion of the insulin. Allowing the insulin to float on top and then be administered all at once at the end of the infusion could quite easily cause a dramatic hypoglycemic reaction.

Table 29-1. Insulin for treatment of diabetes mellitus.

Action	Types	Duration	Peak	Comments
rapid	regular crystalline	6–8 hours	2–4 hours after administration	Only rapid acting insulins are clear, and only clear insulins may be given intravenously.
intermediate	NPH globin Lente	18–28 hours	9–12 hours after administration	
long	Ultralente protamine zinc	36 hours or more	16–20 hours after administration	

Table 29-2. Drugs used in hyperglycemia and hypoglycemia.

Generic Name	Trade Name	How Supplied	Routes	Usual Dose	Comments
insulin		rapid, intermediate, and long acting 10 cc. vials: U–40 (40 U./cc.) U–80 (80 U./cc.) U–100 (100 U./cc.)	S.C. I.V. (regular unmodified only)	varies widely individualized	Rotate injection site systematically.
phenformin hydrochloride	DBI DBI-TD	tablets 25 mg. sustained release capsules 50 mg., 100 mg.	P.O.	50–150 mg. q.d.	
tolbutamide	Orinase	tablets 0.5 Gm.	P.O.	0.5–3 Gm. q.d.	Not recommended for management of diabetes during pregnancy.

REFERENCES

A Guide for the Diabetic. Indianapolis: Eli Lilly Company.

GUTHRIE, DIANA, and GUTHRIE, RICHARD. "Coping with Diabetic Ketoacidosis." *Nursing 73* 3:16, November 1973.

LAWRENCE, PATRICIA A. "U-100 Insulin: Let's Make the Transition Trouble Free." *American Journal of Nursing* 73:1539, September 1973.

LAWRENCE, PATRICIA A. "Diabetes Mellitus." *In* Kintzel, Kay, ed. *Advanced Concepts in Clinical Nursing.* Philadelphia: Lippincott, 1971.

LINE, LINDA, et al. "Insulin Reactions in a Brittle Diabetic." *Nursing 72* 2:6, May 1972.

MARTIN, MARGUERITE. "Diabetes Mellitus: Current Concepts." *American Journal of Nursing* 66:510, March 1966.

PORTER, ANNE LYNN, et al. "Giving Diabetics Control of Their Own Lives." *Nursing 73* 3:44, September 1973.

APPLICATION QUESTIONS

I. *True-False*

For each statement below, write **a** if the statement is true or **b** if it is false.

_____ 1. The most dangerous complications of diabetes result from abnormalities in fat and protein metabolism.

_____ 2. The production of insulin is an exocrine function of the pancreas.

_____ 3. Insulin is responsible for the breaking down of muscle protein to amino acids.

_____ 4. Kussmaul-type hyperpnea is a symptom of insulin shock.

_____ 5. The sulfonylureas are oral insulin preparations.

_____ 6. Phenformin (DBI) is often administered along with other hypoglycemic drugs.

_____ 7. Evidence shows that treatment of maturity onset diabetes with oral hypoglycemic drugs raises the risk of cardiovascular complications.

_____ 8. When a diabetic is vomiting, his insulin needs are decreased.

II. *Multiple Choice*

For each of the following questions, indicate the letter providing the *best* answer.

_____ 1. Which of the following types of insulin can be given intravenously? (a) globin (b) NPH (c) crystalline (d) protamine zinc

_____ 2. Which of the following is an intermediate acting insulin? (a) Iletin (b) Ultralente (c) regular (d) NPH

_____ 3. What does "intermediate acting insulin" mean? (a) its peak action occurs in about 4 hours and its action lasts about 12 hours. (b) its peak action occurs in about 10 hours and its action lasts about 24 hours (c) its peak action occurs in about 12 hours and its action lasts about 36 hours (d) its peak action occurs in about 6 hours and its action lasts about 18 hours

_____ 4. A hypoglycemic reaction may occur in which of the following situations? (a) too much food, too little insulin, or too much exercise (b) too much exercise, too much insulin, or too little food (c) too little exercise, too much insulin, or too little food (d) too little food, too little exercise, or too little insulin

_____ 5. You need to give 25 units of U-40 insulin immediately. All you have on hand is U-80 insulin. The doctor tells you to use it. How many *units* of U-80 would you give to obtain the same dosage? (a) 12.5 units (b) 25 units (c) 40 units (d) 50 units

_____ 6. You need to give 45 units of U-80 insulin. What part of a cc. would this be if you must use a TB syringe? (a) 0.56 cc. (b) 1.78 cc. (c) 0.36 cc. (d) 0.60 cc.

_____ 7. What is the correct way to mix a bottle of insulin? (a) shake vigorously (b) rotate between hands (c) invert once (d) turn upside down 5 minutes before use

_____ 8. Which of the following medications would be used if a patient tended toward elevated blood sugar during the night? (a) regular (b) semilente (c) protamine zinc (d) chlorpropamide (Diabinese)

_____ 9. What is the cause of glycosuria associated with diabetes? (a) failure of the renal tubules to reabsorb glucose (b) failure of the glucose to enter the blood stream (c) failure of the bladder to concentrate urine (d) failure of the glucose to combine with urea to form uric acid

_____ 10. What is the appearance of regular insulin? (a) slightly cloudy (b) clear, with a few white granules at the bottom of the bottle before agitation (c) half bluish, half clear until agitation (d) water clear

_____ 11. The osmotic action of glucose has which of the following effects on glomerular filtration? (a) it decreases the amount of urine formed (b) it increases the concentration of urine (c) it increases the amount of urine formed (d) it increases the specific gravity of urine

_____ 12. Which of the following oral hypoglycemic drugs does *not* function by stimulating endogenous production of insulin? (a) acetohexamide (Dymelor) (b) chlorpropamide (Diabinese) (c) tolbutamide (Orinase) (d) phenformin hydrochloride (DBI)

_____ 13. What change should be made in the insulin dose of a diabetic patient when he engages in abnormally strenuous exercise? (a) increase insulin dose (b) decrease insulin dose (c) no change in insulin, but decrease carbohydrate dietary intake (d) test for glycosuria after exercise and take additional insulin accordingly

_____ 14. Which of the following patients would be most likely to be maintained with an oral hypoglycemic? (a) a 21-year-old "swinging" bachelor who has irregular eating, sleeping, and exercise habits (b) a newly diagnosed visually handicapped widow who lives alone (c) a 12-year-old boy who is afraid to give his own injections (d) a 30-year-old "brittle diabetic" businessman who has recurring bouts of ketoacidosis and insulin shock

III. *Symptom–Cause A*

Each of the following statements consists of a symptom of *diabetic acidosis* and an underlying cause for that symptom. Write **a** if both the symptom and the cause are correct; **b** if both the symptom and cause are incorrect; **c** if the symptom is correct and the cause is incorrect; or **d** if the symptom is incorrect and the cause is correct.

_____ 1. Decreased acid reserves, because ketones combine with potassium, sodium, and bicarbonate for excretion

_____ 2. Increased deep respirations, because ketones are carried to the lungs for excretion

_____ 3. Polyuria, because of excessive reabsorption of water by kidney tubules

IV. *Symptom–Cause B*

Each of the following statements consists of a symptom of *insulin reaction* and an underlying cause for that symptom. Write **a** if both the symptom and the cause are correct; **b** if both the symptom and cause are incorrect; **c** if the symptom is correct and the cause is incorrect; **d** if the symptom is incorrect and the cause is correct.

_____ 1. Dry skin, because of polyuria.

_____ 2. Tremors, because of an excess of glucose in the blood

_____ 3. Drowsiness and confusion, because of lack of glucose to the brain

V. *Discussion*

For each patient statement given in next column, write **a** if teaching is needed, or **b** if no teaching is needed. If teaching is needed, outline the content you would include.

_____ 1. "I know it sounds dumb, but I've learned to recognize this strange little pain in my neck as being a warning that I'm hypoglycemic."

_____ 2. "The other day I was at the bank and it was robbed. Golly, was I scared. Funny how my diabetes went out of control afterward, but I'm sure there was no connection."

Drugs Used for Inflammation, Allergy, and Related Disorders

SECTION EIGHT

Adrenocorticosteroid Drugs and Corticotropin (ACTH)

Adrenocorticosteroid drugs are among the most important substances in modern medicine. They are useful in the treatment of many clinical disorders. These drugs are *not* a cure for any disorder, however; they provide only symptomatic relief. The major drawback of these substances is that they can cause very damaging metabolic side effects if large doses are administered over a long period of time.

The secretion of hormones from the adrenal cortex is regulated by the pituitary hormone corticotropin or adrenocorticotropic hormone (ACTH). (See Chapter 26 for an explanation of the negative feedback mechanism between the pituitary and the adrenal glands.) ACTH is believed to be manufactured by the pituitary during the night. The greatest amount is released in the morning, and secretion diminishes throughout the day. Release of the adrenocorticosteroid hormones is also precipitated by physical or emotional stress. Without these hormones, in fact, the body is unable to deal with the demands of stress, and death can result.

Three kinds of natural steroids are secreted by the adrenal cortex: (1) the glucocorticoids (cortisone and cortisol or hydrocortisone), which mainly affect carbohydrate metabolism, but also influence fat and protein metabolism; (2) the mineralocorticoids (aldosterone and desoxycorticosterone), which influence salt and water metabolism by helping the kidneys retain sodium in exchange for potassium ions; and (3) certain male and female sex hormones.

The corticosteroids influence the functioning of most organs and systems in the body. Administration of these hormones has two major clinical uses: as replacement therapy when these hormones are absent or deficient; and as anti-inflammatory agents in almost any condition with inflammation as a symptom. These hormones are sometimes used to increase the body's capacity to withstand stress. Part of this action may have to do with the ability of the corticosteroids to aid circulating vasopressor substances in keeping the blood pressure up.

ADRENAL INSUFFICIENCY

Hypocorticism may occur as a result of adrenal gland damage, atrophy (Addison's disease), or surgical removal. Pituitary failure can also lead to secondary hypocorticism from lack of the pituitary hormone to stimulate production of the cortical steroids.

Large doses of corticosteroid drugs suppress the production of ACTH by the pituitary; the adrenal glands are thus not stimulated to produce the corticosteroids. Long-term therapy with adrenocorticosteroid drugs, then, can actually lead to adrenal atrophy and adrenal insufficiency when the drugs are withdrawn.

Replacement Therapy

Hydrocortisone, a natural glucocorticoid which also has some mineralocorticoid activity, may keep the patient with hypocorticism in metabolic balance. Some patients may require the addition of a pure mineralocorticoid such as desoxycorticosterone acetate to prevent dehydration and hypotension.

The patient on corticosteroid replacement is similar to the diabetic patient in that the replacement hormones are introduced into the body on a regulated schedule, rather than by demand or according to body need. Like the diabetic patient, then, this patient must attempt to adjust his lifestyle to his replacement therapy and take into account any unusual occurrences or stresses. An infection, surgery, or emotional stress can all put demands on the adrenal hormones that the patient on replacement therapy will not be able to meet with his regular daily dosage of hormones. When this patient is hospitalized or experiences any other stress, his drug dosage must be increased accordingly. The nurse must be observant for signs of adrenal crisis, as this can rapidly result in death.

Adrenal Crisis. Adrenal crisis requires intravenous infusion of hydrocortisone sodium succinate (Solu-Cortef) along with large quantities of isotonic fluids. Central venous pressure monitoring is important to prevent overloading. The patient must be kept warm and his vital signs must be observed carefully and supported if necessary. The underlying stressful cause of the crisis—such as an infection—must be treated simultaneously.

INFLAMMATION

Adrenocorticosteroids are most widely used for their effectiveness in suppressing inflammatory and allergic tissue responses. They are used to provide symptomatic relief in the collagen diseases and in some inflammatory musculoskeletal disorders. In such cases, administration of the drug directly into the joint, if practical, decreases the likelihood of systemic effects. Corticosteroids may be used in the treatment of allergic, infectious, and other inflammatory disorders of the skin and of ocular and respiratory mucous membranes. Topical application of corticosteroids may be effective in these situations (see Chapter 33); topical application has the advantage of being less likely to cause systemic toxic reactions. Corticosteroids applied topically to the outer eye tissue have been reported to cause a rise in intraocular pressure and the development of cataracts. Corticosteroids are used in various hematological and neoplastic conditions; they may also be used to decrease inflammation in many types of neuritis. Treatment following organ transplantation usually includes some form of corticosteroid drug to decrease the inflammatory rejection process of the body against the transplanted organ.

TYPES OF ADRENOCORTICOSTEROID DRUGS

Corticosteroid drugs may be administered topically, orally, intra-articularly, intramuscularly, or intravenously. Preparations such as hydrocortisone sodium succinate (Solu-Cortef) and methylprednisolone sodium succinate (Solu-Medrol) are used only for parenteral administration. Preparations such as hydrocortisone acetate (Cortef acetate) and prednisolone acetate (Sterane) are preferred for intra-articular injections.

Corticosteroid drugs vary in their degree of anti-inflammatory potency, their mineralocorticoid activi-

ty, and their duration of action. For example, although all of these drugs exert some anti-inflammatory action, the newer synthetic steroids such as dexamethasone (Decadron) may be as much as 25 to 30 times as potent as the natural hormone hydrocortisone in anti-inflammatory action. The synthetic drugs are also long acting—they may suppress natural adrenal function for as long as two and one-half days. The natural hormones have a short duration of action (about one and one-half days), and drugs such as triamcinolone (Aristocort) and paramethasone acetate (Haldrone) are considered intermediate in activity (about two days). When corticosteroid drugs are used for replacement therapy, the mineralocorticoid activity is desirable. When they are used for other purposes, however, the sodium and fluid retention may be undesirable. This is especially true for patients with hypertension, heart disease, some neurosurgical conditions, and in any other situation in which drug-induced edema could be dangerous. The synthetic steroids such as dexamethasone have very little mineralocorticoid activity; prednisone and prednisolone have moderate mineralocorticoid activity; and the natural hormones, hydrocortisone and cortisone, have the strongest mineralocorticoid activity.

DOSAGE SCHEDULES

The dosage of adrenocorticosteroids needed to produce clinically desirable effects while keeping adverse effects at a minimum varies widely. Dosage must always be individualized and adjusted according to the individual patient's response to the drug. As a rule, these drugs are begun with small doses, which are gradually increased until the desired effect is attained. In *acute* inflammatory situations, however, the opposite dosage schedule would be instituted—a large dose would be given immediately, and the dosage would then be gradually decreased. High steroid dosage does not cause much metabolic toxicity when administered for only a few days before being decreased and then discontinued.

Step-Down Dosage

In conditions that are acutely disabling for a brief period but are not of a chronic nature, one way to bring about rapid symptomatic relief is to use a step-down or cut-down dosage schedule. This involves giving large doses for the first two or three days; then, as symptoms begin to subside, dosage is reduced every few days, and the drug is discontinued after a week to ten days, without having caused any significant side effects.

Intermittent Dosage Schedule

Intermittent dosage schedules are being tried as a means of providing symptomatic relief without causing metabolic toxicity or atrophy of the adrenal glands. Such a schedule may involve taking the dose that would normally be spread over 48 hours, all at once every other morning. Morning is the time recommended to take the drug, because it is thought to interfere less with pituitary production of corticotropin when taken at this time. The importance of taking the drug at the same time every other morning must be stressed to the patient. He must also be helped to understand that this dosage schedule may not bring complete relief of all symptoms; in fact, late on the second day, when the level of steroid falls below the point of effectiveness, he may experience quite noticeable discomfort, but this schedule will help reduce the toxic and metabolic side effects of the drug.

Discontinuing Corticosteroid Drugs

Adrenocorticosteroid drugs should never be discontinued abruptly, because the pituitary-adrenal feedback mechanism may not recover immediately from being suppressed. Dosages are always decreased gradually. When the drugs are being discontinued, the nurse must observe for signs of adrenal insufficiency. Some physicians believe that giving a dose of the pituitary hormone adrenocorticotropin just before the steroids are completely discontinued stimulates the adrenal glands and aids in the recovery of the pituitary-adrenal mechanism.

ADVERSE EFFECTS OF ADRENOCORTICOSTEROID DRUGS

Metabolic Effects

The mineralocorticoid activity of adrenocorticosteroid drugs can lead to excessive retention of sodium and water, as well as to depletion of potassium. These actions can result in edema and some serious electrolyte imbalances.

The glucocorticoid activity of the drugs can lead to Cushingoid symptoms such as the moon-face appearance, buffalo hump, thinning of hair and skin, hirsutism, acne, and abdominal distention. The steroid hormones may also cause an increase in blood sugar (steroid diabetes), because they stimulate gluconeogenesis (the formation of glucose from noncarbohydrate sources, such as proteins and possibly fats), and because they block the effectiveness of insulin.

Peptic ulcer may occur when corticosteroid drugs are given. These ulcers may be referred to as Curling's ulcer, Cushing's ulcer, or stress ulcer. They may occur without administration of these drugs when severe trauma or stress has occurred. For this reason, administration of corticosteroid drugs following massive burns or other trauma that could precipitate development of ulcer anyway must be done with extreme caution. If a patient has a history of ulcer or is highly susceptible to peptic ulcer, adrenocorticosteroid drugs should be given with frequent antacids and perhaps even anticholinergic drugs. The patient's stools should be observed for blood, and gastric X-ray or fluoroscopy should be done. Because of the anti-inflammatory action of the corticosteroids, the patient may experience no pain with the ulcer, even if it is approaching the perforation stage.

Osteoporosis may result from the catabolic activity of the corticosteroids. For this reason, the patient's regimen may include a high protein diet, calcium salt supplements, and anabolic agents. Protein catabolism can also lead to negative nitrogen balance, impaired wound healing, and myopathy with loss of muscle mass.

Adrenocorticosteroid drugs interfere with the body's normal defenses against infection. Healed tuberculosis lesions may be reactivated; therefore, patients with a history of tuberculosis may be given antituberculosis medication along with steroid preparations. The patient must be protected from infection and begun on antibiotics or anti-infective agents at the first sign of infection. Adrenocorticosteroid drugs may be used in the presence of infection if the *inflammatory* process accompanying the infectious process poses a severe threat. The danger of steroid-spread infection is most serious when viruses or fungi are involved, because of the lack of antiviral and antifungal medications.

Central Nervous System Effects

The mental state of a patient taking adrenocorticosteroids is often affected, so that the patient becomes happy and talkative soon after treatment is begun. This euphoric state and feeling of well-being can lead to psychological dependence on the drug. Such dependence, along with the remarkable relief of inflammatory symptoms, may cause the patient to resist reducing the dosage or discontinuing the drug, even when toxicity may become a problem. For this reason, corticosteroids are not recommended for use in chronic inflammatory conditions.

Continued use of the steroid drugs may lead to excessive excitement, restlessness, sleeplessness, and even convulsions. The patient may also begin demonstrating mood swings from manic behavior to agitated depression. The cause of these reactions is uncertain; unlike other types of steroid toxicity, such central effects are not closely related to the length of time patients have been taking large doses. One factor in determining whether a patient is likely to react abnormally is his personality before treatment is begun. Individuals with a history of emotional and psychological difficulties are more likely to develop these kinds of symptoms than other patients. Therefore, it is best to avoid using corticosteroid drugs in such cases.

Endocrine Toxicity

The suppression of the anterior pituitary which occurs when adrenocorticosteroid drugs are taken may account for the fact that children who receive these drugs over a long period of time fail to grow. As discussed, above, the pituitary suppression can lead to atrophy of the adrenal glands. Patients who have been

withdrawn from long-term steroid therapy may show no signs of adrenal insufficiency except in times of stress. Therefore, if such a patient becomes seriously ill within a year after the corticosteroids have been discontinued, he should be placed back on the drugs for the course of his illness. When assessing a patient, it is always important to inquire whether he has ever taken "cortisone" or other adrenocorticosteroid drugs. If he has, the nurse should determine how long ago they were taken and how long the course of treatment was.

ADRENOCORTICOTROPIC HORMONE (ACTH)

The pituitary hormone which stimulates the adrenal glands to produce the steroid hormones has been used for treating most of the same disorders that corticosteroid drug therapy is used for. The corticosteroids are preferred, however, because the foreign protein in ACTH may cause allergic reactions in some

Table 30-1. Adrenocorticosteroid drugs

Generic Name	Trade Name	How Supplied	Routes	Usual Dose	Comments
hydrocortisone	Cortef	oral suspension 10 mg./5 cc. tablets 5 mg.; 10 mg.; 20 mg.	P.O.	individualized	
hydrocortisone acetate	Cortef Acetate	ointment 1%, 2.5% vials 5 cc. 50 mg./cc.	topical intrasynovial		
methylprednisolone sodium succinate	Solu-Medrol	vials 40 mg./cc. when mixed vials 125 mg./2 cc. when mixed vials 500 mg./8 cc. 1000 mg./16 cc. when mixed	I.V. I.M.	individualized	In most indications, initial dosage will be 10–40 mg. q.d. Dosage must be decreased or discontinued after drug has been given for more than a few days.
dexamethasone	Decadron	elixir 0.5 mg./5 cc. tablets 1.5 mg.; 0.75 mg.; 0.5 mg.; 0.25 mg., 4 mg.	P.O.	individualized	
dexamethasone sodium phosphate		vials 1 cc. 4 mg./cc. vials 5 cc. 4 mg./cc. 25 cc. 4 mg./cc. ophthalmic solution (1 mg./cc.) and ointment (0.5 mg./Gm.) aerosol	I.V. I.M. ophthalmic intranasal		

patients. The oral doses of the corticosteroids are more convenient and less expensive than ACTH. In addition, the synthetic steroids produce a much more predictable and potent anti-inflammatory effect and are free of the undesirable mineralocorticoid and sex hormone effects that occur when corticotropin is used.

Adrenocorticotropin may be very useful in determining the level of function of the adrenal glands. If the adrenal glands are functioning properly, plasma steroid levels will increase following an injection of ACTH. This procedure may be used for differentiating between primary hypocorticism (disorder of the adrenal gland) and secondary hypocorticism (pituitary dysfunction). It is also useful for determining whether the adrenals have regained their function after adrenocorticosteroid therapy has been discontinued.

REFERENCES

Blount, Mary, and Kinney, Anna Belle. "Chronic Steroid Therapy." *American Journal of Nursing* 74:1626, September 1974.

Elliott, Diane. "Adrenocortical Insufficiency: A Self-Instructional Unit." *American Journal of Nursing* 74:1115, June 1974.

Hamdi, Mary E. "Nursing Intervention For Patients Receiving Corticosteroid Therapy." In Kintzel, Kay C., ed. *Advanced Concepts in Clinical Nursing.* Philadelphia: Lippincott, 1971.

Mechling, Eileen, et al. "The Patient With Primary Hyperaldosteronism." *Nursing Clinics of North America* 4:165, March 1969.

Shea, Kathleen, et al. "Teaching a Patient to Live With Adrenal Insufficiency." *American Journal of Nursing* 65:80, December 1965.

Strobele, Barbara. "How to Counsel Patients on Cortisone." *RN* 38:57, July 1975.

APPLICATION QUESTIONS

I. *True-False*

For each statement below, write **a** if the statement is true or **b** if it is false.

_____ 1. Large steroid doses do not cause much metabolic toxicity when administered for only a few days.

_____ 2. Corticosteroids should not be given in combination with anti-infective agents.

_____ 3. The use of corticosteroid drugs is never justified for patients who have had tuberculosis, since these drugs may reactivate healed lesions of tuberculosis.

_____ 4. People with a history of emotional and psychological difficulties are not considered likely candidates for steroid therapy.

_____ 5. Patients who become seriously ill during the year after they have been withdrawn from prolonged steroid therapy should be put back on these drugs during the acute illness.

_____ 6. The adrenocorticosteroid drugs have proved useful in curing many diseases.

_____ 7. The adrenal cortex secretes some male and female sex hormones.

_____ 8. The long-term administration of large doses of corticosteroid drugs may cause adrenal insufficiency.

_____ 9. Local administration of steroids lessens the likelihood of systemic toxic reactions.

_____ 10. Continued use of steroids will inevitably cause adverse effects.

II. *Multiple Choice*

For each of the following questions, indicate the letter providing the *best* answer.

_____ 1. Metabolic side effects of corticosteroid drugs include which of the following? (1) moon face (2) thinning hair (3) rounded shoulders (4) acne (a) 1, 2, 3 (b) 1, 3, 4 (c) 2, 3, 4 (d) 1, 2, 3, 4

_____ 2. Which of the following nursing actions would be essential in caring for a patient being treated for acute adrenal insufficiency? (1) frequent vital signs (2) central venous pressure monitoring (3) intake and output (4) hypothermia (a) 1, 3 (b) 1, 3, 4 (c) 1, 2, 3 (d) 1, 2, 3, 4

_____ 3. Which of the following is a primary antistress action of the corticosteroids? (a) its ability to aid in circulating vasodilator substances (b) its ability to aid in destroying microorganisms (c) its ability to aid in circulating vasopressor substances (d) its ability to aid the body reaction by stimulating the pituitary gland

_____ 4. Steroid-induced complications include which of the following? (1) hypotension (2) peptic ulcer (3) osteoporosis (4) diabetes mellitus symptoms (a) 1, 2, 3 (b) 2, 3, 4 (c) 1, 3, 4 (d) 1, 2, 4

_____ 5. What are the disadvantages of utilizing ACTH rather than corticosteroid drugs? (1) ACTH contains foreign protein which may cause an allergic reaction (2) the anti-inflammatory effect of ACTH is less predictable (3) ACTH is more expensive (4) ACTH produces adrenal atrophy more rapidly (a) 1, 2, 4 (b) 1, 2, 3 (c) 2, 3, 4 (d) 1, 2, 3, 4

_____ 6. What is the body's first reaction to a fall in the level of circulating steroids? (a) production of corticotropin (b) production of cortisone (c) retention of fluid (d) increase in carbohydrate metabolism

_____ 7. Mineralocorticoids are used in replacement therapy for patients with chronic adrenal insufficiency to prevent which of the following? (1) hypotension (2) hypertension (3) dehydration (4) edema (a) 1, 4 (b) 2, 4 (c) 1, 3 (d) 2, 3

_____ 8. During periods of stress, the patient being treated for adrenal insufficiency by replacement therapy will require which of the following dosage changes? (a) increase (b) decrease (c) no change (d) omit the drug

III. *Matching A*

Match each function listed below with the hormone responsible for it.

_____ 1. Influences carbohydrate metabolism

_____ 2. Aids in sodium retention

(a) ACTH

(b) glucocorticoids

(c) mineralocorticoids

_____ 3. Controls the production of adrenal cortex hormones

_____ 4. Influences fat and protein metabolism

IV. *Matching B*

Match each clinical condition listed below with the primary purpose of steroid therapy in its treatment.

_____ 1. Addison's disease

_____ 2. Collagen diseases

_____ 3. Poison ivy

_____ 4. Hemorrhage

(a) anti-inflammatory

(b) replacement

(c) antistress

31

Rheumatoid Disorders

In the treatment of rheumatoid arthritis, spondylitis, osteoarthritis, and other rheumatic disorders, drugs are used to provide symptomatic relief. The cause of these diseases is uncertain, and no cure is known. Since rheumatoid arthritis is the most dramatic of the rheumatic disorders, this chapter refers primarily to this disease. The drugs discussed may be used for other rheumatic diseases, but would be used for shorter periods of time or in smaller doses. Gout is a form of arthritis, but it differs from the diseases just mentioned in that drugs are available which can counteract the actual metabolic abnormality involved. Gout is discussed at the end of the chapter.

TREATMENT OF RHEUMATIC DISORDERS

The patient with a chronic, potentially crippling rheumatic disorder must faithfully follow a regimen of rest, special exercises, and drug therapy. Drug therapy is aimed at reducing pain and inflammation. Many types of analgesics and anti-inflammatory drugs may be used, but the salicylates are the mainstay of the conservative management of diseases such as rheumatoid arthritis.

Salicylates

Aspirin is the safest and most effective antirheumatic drug. The salicylates relieve pain and reduce inflammation; they may possibly slow the degenerative processes in the affected joints. Large doses of the salicylates are needed for most effective anti-inflammatory action. Aspirin, for example, may be given in doses as large as four to six grams. These large doses usually bring about symptomatic relief from the hot, red, painfully swollen joints within 24 to 48 hours. Even when symptoms have disappeared, however, it is most important that the patient continue taking the drug. Side effects of the salicylates are much more likely to occur with these large doses than with the small doses (300–600mg.) usually taken for relieving minor pains. The major side effect is gastrointestinal distress; because of the large doses, however, the patient must also be observed for symptoms of salicylism and salicylate poisoning. The salicylate drugs are fully discussed in Chapter 12.

Nonsalicylate-Nonsteroid Drugs

If a patient is hypersensitive to the salicylates, or if the salicylates alone do not adequately control the symptoms of rheumatic disease, other anti-inflammatory agents may be used. The pyrazolon derivative drugs, such as aminopyrine, are potent analgesic, antipyretic, and anti-inflammatory agents. They are rarely used in the United States, however, because of their high toxicity. More commonly used is phenylbutazone (Butazolidin), which is chemically related to the pyrazolon derivatives and shares their toxic properties. However, the potent anti-inflammatory effects of phenylbutazone have been found clinically useful. Phenylbutazone is not only an anti-inflammatory agent, but also has analgesic, antipyretic, and uricosuric actions. It is useful not only in the treatment of arthritis, but also in the treatment of acute gout attacks in patients who cannot tolerate the preferred antigout drug, colchicine. Although use of phenylbutazone for a few days to combat an acute inflammatory process does not usually lead to serious adverse effects, long-term use of the drug can be quite hazardous. Phenylbutazone (Butazolidin) and the related drug oxyphenbutazone (Tandearil) are capable of causing gastrointestinal irritation, bone marrow depression, and fluid retention. The drugs should not be used by patients with a history of peptic ulcer, blood dyscrasias, cardiac conditions, hypertension, or renal disorders. When these drugs are used, the patient must be observed for symptoms such as sore throat, fever, weight gain, and tarry stools. Frequent blood tests must also be done.

Mefenamic acid is an analgesic, antipyretic, anti-inflammatory agent that is neither a salicylate nor a steroid. Like phenylbutazone, it can cause severe adverse reactions, especially gastrointestinal symptoms. Since it is recommended that the drug never be used for a course of treatment lasting more than one week, mefenamic acid is not very useful in the treatment of chronic rheumatoid disorders such as rheumatoid arthritis.

Indomethacin (Indocin) exerts effects similar to the salicylates and phenylbutazone. It has more side effects than the salicylates, but is considered safer and less toxic than phenylbutazone. This drug can cause gastrointestinal, ocular, and central nervous system side effects. Headache, lightheadedness, mental confusion, and vertigo may occur. The patient being treated with indomethacin should be cautioned against activities requiring mental alertness. Because the drug can cause corneal deposits and retinal disturbances, the patient should be questioned about the occurrence of blurred vision and should have frequent ophthalmological examinations.

Treatment with gold salts (chrysotherapy) may be effective for suppressing inflammation in cases of rheumatoid arthritis that do not respond to salicylates. Small doses that cause little toxicity are used in early cases of the disease, before cartilage has been destroyed and joints have degenerated. The treatment regimen with gold salts may last many weeks or months. The dosage is increased only very gradually, and the patient is observed closely for signs of toxicity. Dermatitis, bone marrow damage, and kidney damage may occur. Urinalysis and blood studies are done before each injection.

The antimalarial drugs, chloroquine and hydroxychloroquine, have been of some benefit to some patients with rheumatoid arthritis. The improvement brought about by small doses is slow, but large doses may cause damage to the retina and even permanent blindness. Patients maintained on long-term therapy with these drugs must have frequent ophthalmological examinations and must be observed for gastrointestinal upsets, headache, and skin rashes.

Immunosuppressive drugs such as azathioprine (Imuran) and certain anticancer agents have been used to treat some cases of rheumatoid arthritis that have not responded to other antiarthritic drugs. These drugs are so toxic, however, that their use is reserved mostly for those patients whose disease is very severe or even life-threatening.

Corticosteroid Therapy

Adrenocorticosteroid drugs are highly effective anti-inflammatory agents. They may be administered in massive doses for a few days to combat an acute inflammatory reaction in a rheumatic disorder, giving significant benefits without much toxicity. When these drugs are taken over a long period of time, however, even small doses can cause serious metabolic side effects (see Chapter 30). It is best to avoid long-term use of steroid drugs for patients with chronic rheumatic disorders until the disease does not respond at all to other drug therapy and the patient will be severely disabled if the drugs are not used. Once a patient is begun on treatment with corticosteroids, the relief of symptoms may be so dramatic, and the feeling of well-being that the drugs produce may be so welcome, that the patient may become quite dependent on the drugs and not want to give them up even when threatened with toxicity. For this reason, physicians usually try to regulate the dosage of these drugs so not all of the symptoms are relieved and the patient will not become dependent and reluctant to stop treatment if that becomes necessary.

TREATMENT OF GOUT

Gout is a metabolic disorder characterized by high levels of uric acid in the blood (7 mg. or more per 100 cc. of plasma). The extreme pain associated with the disease results from the settling out of uric acid crystals in the joints, which leads to an inflammatory reaction. Gout may be treated with diet and drug therapy. Drugs used in the treatment of gout act by controlling the acute inflammation of an attack, by increasing the excretion of uric acid by the kidneys (uricosuric agents), or by reducing the production of uric acid by the body. Drugs that affect the metabolism of uric acid are used to prevent attacks, and the anti-inflammatory agents are used to treat and terminate acute attacks that develop despite prophylactic measures.

Prevention of Gout Attacks

Acute attacks of gout can be prevented by keeping the uric acid level below 7 mg. %. The uricosuric drugs probenecid (Benemid) and sulfinpyrazone (Anturane) are most commonly used for this purpose. They prevent the reabsorption of uric acid back into the blood by the kidneys, and thereby cause a reduction in plasma urate levels. Patients receiving these drugs should force fluids to prevent the formation of urate stones in the urinary tract. Sometimes, to aid in preventing these stones, the urine may be alkalinized by having the patient take a teaspoonful of sodium bicarbonate or a dose of potassium citrate several times a day. It is important to observe the patient for signs and symptoms of systemic acid-base imbalance when alkalinizing agents are used.

Side effects such as headache, gastrointestinal distress, and hypersensitivity reactions may occur with the administration of probenecid. Serious adverse reactions such as nephrotic syndrome, hepatic necrosis, and aplastic anemia rarely occur. Salicylate drugs should not be used with probenecid, because the salicylates antagonize the action of the uricosuric.

Probenecid therapy should not be started until an acute attack has subsided. The importance of taking medication daily once this therapy is instituted must be stressed to the patient. If an acute attack occurs *during* treatment with probenecid, daily dosage of the drug should be continued through the attack.

Allopurinol (Zyloprim) is a drug that reduces the production of uric acid, rather than increasing its excretion. This drug is especially useful for treating patients with kidney damage, because it does not involve the demands made on the kidneys by high uric acid

levels. Patients with kidney damage are also more likely to form urate stones when the uricosuric drugs are used. Concomitant administration of allopurinol and one of the uricosuric drugs may be used for prophylactic treatment of gout. The most common side effect occurring with allopurinol is dermatitis. Alopecia and gastrointestinal distress may also occur. Allopurinol should be used with caution when anticoagulants are administered simultaneously, since allopurinol may potentiate the action of the anticoagulants.

Treatment of Acute Gout Attacks

Acute gout attacks are characterized by sudden severe pain. If the drug colchicine is taken immediately, an impending attack may be terminated before it becomes incapacitating. The patient should be instruct-

Table 31–1. Drugs used in treatment of rheumatoid disorders

Generic Name	Trade Name	How Supplied	Routes	Usual Dose	Comments
phenylbutazone	Butazolidin	tablets 100 mg.	P.O.	100–400 mg. q.d. maintenance dose. Initial doses vary.	Also available in combination with aluminum hydroxide gel and magnesium trisilicate.
indomethacin	Indocin	capsules 25 mg., 50 mg.	P.O.	25–200 mg. b.i.d. or t.i.d.	Always give the drug with food, after meals, or with antacids. Not recommended for children. Doses above 200 mg. do not generally increase the effectiveness of this drug. Contraindicated in pregnant women and nursing mothers.
probenecid	Benemid	tablets 0.5 Gm.	P.O.	0.25–0.5 Gm. b.i.d.	Usually not to exceed 2 Gm. daily. Contraindicated in children under two.
allopurinol	Zyloprim	tablets 100 mg. 300 mg.	P.O.	200–600 mg. daily	Not to exceed 800 mg. daily.
colchicine (phenanthrene derivative)		tablets 0.6 mg. 0.5 mg.	P.O.	1–2 tablets initially followed by 1 tablet every hour until pain has subsided or until nausea, vomiting, or diarrhea occurs.	This drug's anti-inflammatory action is not understood. Maintenance dose varies with the severity of the disease. I.V. dose given to decrease GI effects or when attack cannot be treated promptly. I.V. dose not to exceed 4 mg. q. 24h.
		ampuls 2 cc. 0.5 mg./cc.	I.V.	Initial dose of 2 mg. followed by 0.5 mg. q. 6h. until satisfactory response is achieved.	

ed to carry colchicine with him at all times. One or two tablets are taken at the first indication of the attack, followed by one tablet every hour until the pain is relieved or until gastrointestinal symptoms develop. The patient may take paregoric or an antiemetic to control the diarrhea, nausea, and vomiting that the colchicine may cause. Colchicine may also be injected intravenously to decrease its gastrointestinal effects and to treat attacks that do not respond to oral doses. Large doses of the drug administered in this manner may cause kidney and bone marrow damage. Other anti-inflammatory drugs may also be used to treat the acute attack, such as phenylbutazone (Butazolidin), corticotropin (ACTH), or indomethacin (Indocin). The corticotropin may be administered by intramuscular injection or by an injection directly into the involved joint. The patient should rest in bed during the acute attack, but when the pain subsides, he should be encouraged to walk about and exercise the joints.

REFERENCES

JOHNSON, S. B. "Understanding Hyperuricemia." *Nursing Clinics of North America* 7:399, June 1972.

MacGINNISS, OSCIA. "Rheumatoid Arthritis–My Tutor." *American Journal of Nursing* 68:1699, August 1968.

WALIKE, BARBARA, et al. "Rheumatoid Arthritis." *American Journal of Nursing* 67:1420, July 1967.

APPLICATION QUESTIONS

I. *True-False*

For each statement below, write **a** if the statement is true or **b** if it is false.

_____ 1. The antimalarial drugs sometimes used for patients with rheumatoid arthritis may cause deafness.

_____ 2. Immunosuppressive drugs are used early in the treatment of degenerative rheumatoid arthritis.

_____ 3. Indomethacin (Indocin) is less toxic than aspirin.

_____ 4. Chrysotherapy (gold salts) is best used in early cases of arthritis, before joint damage has taken place.

_____ 5. The most common adverse reaction of gold salts is dermatitis.

II. *Multiple Choice*

For each of the following questions, indicate the letter providing the *best* answer.

_____ 1. How often should blood tests and urine tests be done for a patient receiving chrysotherapy (gold salts)? (a) before each dose (b) monthly (c) prior to dose change (d) only if toxic symptoms occur

_____ 2. Which of the following is the drug of choice for treatment of rheumatoid arthritis? (a) gold salts (b) steroids (c) salicylates (d) immunosuppressives

_____ 3. Which of the following statements are true regarding phenylbutazone (Butazolidin)? (1) it has uricosuric actions (2) it is potentially highly toxic (3) it may be used by patients with peptic ulcer (4) it is useful in short-term anti-inflammatory therapy (a) 1, 2, 3, 4 (b) 1, 2, 4 (c) 2, 3, 4 (d) 1, 4

_____ 4. Which of the following diagnostic test results could be noted to detect adverse reactions to phenylbutazone (Butazolidin)? (1) urinalysis (2) gastrointestinal series (3) CBC (4) blood pressure (a) 1 (b) 2, 3 (c) 1, 2, 4 (d) 1, 2, 3, 4

_____ 5. Which of the following examinations is the most essential for patients being maintained on long-term indomethacin (Indocin) therapy? (a) chest X-ray (b) IVP (c) ophthalmological examination (d) EEG

III. *Matching A*

Match the following drugs with their clinical purpose in the treatment of gout.

_____ 1. Colchicine

_____ 2. Probenecid (Benemid)

_____ 3. Allopurinol (Zyloprim)

(a) controls inflammation

(b) increases excretion of uric acid

(c) reduces production of uric acid

IV. *Matching B*

Match each drug classification with its pharmacological effect.

_____ 1. Anti-inflammatory

_____ 2. Anti-pyretic

_____ 3. Analgesic

_____ 4. Uricosuric

(a) reduces fever

(b) increases uric acid excretion

(c) relieves pain

(d) suppresses connective tissue reaction

V. *Discussion*

Suppose that each of the statements below is made by a patient with *rheumatoid arthritis* who has been taking *adrenocorticosteroid* drugs. For each patient statement, write **a** if teaching is needed or **b** if no teaching is needed. If teaching is needed, outline the content you would include.

_____ 1. "I intend to take these pills *forever*, because they help me so much."

_____ 3. "That shot he put in my knee should prevent it from breaking down like the other joints have, right?"

_____ 2. "It really upsets me that I must cut down on these pills when it makes me feel worse, but I understand why the doctor says I must, so I'll do as he says."

32

Antihistamine Drugs

Most people who suffer from allergic disorders are *atopic*—that is, they have inherited a tendency toward allergic reactions. These disorders mainly involve reactions in the skin, the mucous membranes of the nose, and the bronchial smooth muscle.

Exposure to an antigen stimulates the production of specific antibodies. If the antigen is an organism, the antibody will destroy the bacteria. If the antigen is a foreign protein such as those in food, plants, or other substances, the antibody (or reagin) belongs to the immunoglobulin E (IgE) family of body proteins and acts similarly to other antibodies. When a previously exposed or sensitized individual with large amounts of IgE in his body is again exposed to the same specific antigen, an antigen-antibody reaction occurs that is damaging to the involved tissues. As a result of this reaction in the target tissues, certain chemicals or *autacoids* are released, including histamine, bradykinin, and SRS-A (slow-reacting substance A). This chapter deals with drugs used to combat signs and symptoms which are believed to result from the liberation of histamine.

All three of the autacoids can cause bronchoconstriction. Histamine and bradykinin can also cause vasodilation and increase the permeability of capillaries. The increased permeability of the arterioles and venules, with the resultant leaking of fluid out into the surrounding tissues, accounts for the reddened wheals on the skin, and the nasal and lung congestion seen in allergic disorders. Histamine also increases lacrimal and gastric secretions, which leads to the increased tearing, reddened eyes, and epigastric distress seen in allergic disorders.

TREATMENT OF ALLERGY

There are no drugs available that "cure" allergy. Agents available merely relieve the signs and symptoms of the disorder. Sympathomimetic drugs (Chapter 16) produce effects that are directly opposite to the effects of histamine, and corticosteroid drugs (Chapter 30) reduce the responsiveness of the sensitized person's tissues to the actions of histamine. Both of these drugs may be utilized in the management of allergic disorders.

Antihistamines are the most commonly used drugs for the treatment of allergy; they act by competing with histamine at the reactive tissue receptor sites. When the antihistamine drug molecules have occupied these receptor sites, histamine cannot become attached to cause the signs and symptoms of allergy.

Hyposensitization

Hyposensitization is a procedure used to make allergic patients less reactive when they are exposed to the antigens to which they have become sensitized. This procedure consists of regular, frequent injections of dilute extracts of the antigen. The injections are believed to stimulate the production of "blocking" antibodies, IgG, which then compete with the IgE antibodies and prevent allergic symptoms.

The patient must understand the importance of receiving *every* injection in the series. The strength of the injected antigen is gradually increased, and if the patient misses an injection or two he could experience a severe allergic reaction when the next injection is given. Missing an injection, then, may require that the entire process of hyposensitization be restarted from the beginning.

The nurse must understand that the patient could experience an allergic reaction after any of the injections. For this reason the patient is asked to remain in the clinic or office for about twenty minutes after the injection is given; during this time he is observed for any untoward reaction. The nurse should be sure emergency drugs such as epinephrine and corticosteroids, as well as antihistamines, are available if needed. Oxygen and tracheotomy equipment should be available in case of a severe reaction. A tourniquet

180

should also be available, because it can be applied to the extremity above the injection site to prevent further systemic absorption of the antigen.

USE OF ANTIHISTAMINE DRUGS

Antihistamine drugs are most useful, of course, in those allergic reactions caused mainly by the liberation of histamine. They are *not* effective, for example, in the treatment of bronchial asthma, because this persistent bronchospasm is believed to be caused mainly by the release of SRS-A and bradykinin. The more severe and immediate symptoms of anaphylactic shock are also believed to be caused by the other autacoids; antihistamines would therefore be administered only after adrenergic drugs have been given and the vital signs have stabilized. The most significant indications for antihistamines are allergic rhinitis and allergic skin disorders.

Allergic Rhinitis

Allergic rhinitis results when the histamine target tissue is the mucous membranes of the nose. Some people suffer from "seasonal rhinitis," which is the occurrence of allergy at certain seasons of the year, as occurs with hay fever. Other people suffer from "perennial rhinitis," which can be precipitated at any time from exposure to certain foods, from chilling, or from emotional factors. Patients with perennial rhinitis tend to develop pathological changes of the nasal mucosa as a result of chronic inflammation and frequent secondary infections.

Allergic Skin Disorders

Antihistamine drugs are more effective for treating acute urticaria than for chronic urticaria. The histamine blocking effects of the drugs prevent the edema and itching (pruritus) characteristic of acute urticaria. Antihistamines with sedating or tranquilizing effects may be helpful in chronic urticaria and contact dermatitis by decreasing the patient's awareness of pruritus. Some antihistaminic agents such as tripelennamine (Pyribenzamine) exert a local anesthetic effect when applied topically. Patients with atopic dermatitis, however, may develop an allergy to any substance applied to the skin, including these drugs.

Common Cold

Antihistamines may provide relief for the symptoms of the common cold. It must be remembered that the drugs do not *cure* the cold, but only provide symptomatic relief. Those antihistamines that exert the atropine-like drying effect tend to be most beneficial in treating this condition.

TYPES OF ANTIHISTAMINES

There are many types of antihistamines; some of them have other actions in addition to the blocking of histamine. Diphenhydramine hydrochloride (Benadryl), for example, is one of the more sedating drugs of this class. It is useful when sedation is also desirable, such as at night when pruritus might keep the patient awake, or for relief or pruritus in contact dermatitis or chronic urticaria. Moderately sedating antihistamines useful for daytime therapy include tripelennamine (Pyribenzamine) and chlorpheniramine maleate (Chlor-Trimeton). The antihistamines with tranquilizing effects, such as hydroxyzine pamoate (Vistaril), promethazine hydrochloride (Phenergan), and cyproheptadine hydrochloride (Periactin), may be helpful for relieving the anxiety and apprehension that may accompany an allergy. There are antihistamine-tranquilizers that are actually phenothiazine drugs, such as trimeprazine (Temaril) and methdilazine (Tacaryl). Of course, all the cautions, contraindications, and side effects of phenothiazines apply to these drugs (see Chapter 7).

Combination Products

There are numerous proprietary and prescription products available that combine an antihistamine with a decongestant. This combination is used in treatment of the common cold and for some cases of allergic rhinitis. One such product is Ornade, which combines chlorpheniramine maleate with phenylpropanolamine hydrochloride and also contains isopropamide, an iodide used as a drying agent. Another example is Neotep, which combines chlorpheniramine maleate with phenylephrine hydrochloride. Most of the decongestants utilized are adrenergic drugs; therefore, the side effects, cautions, and contraindications of any adrenergic must be considered when these products are used (see Chapter 16). A possible advantage of combining these two drugs is that the adrenergic stimulation might help to overcome the sedation caused by the antihistamine, and the patient would experience less drowsiness than if the antihistamine were given alone. If the preparation (such as Ornade) contains an iodide as a drying agent, it should not be used by patients allergic to iodine. It must be remembered that the iodide in these preparations could interfere with results of diagnostic tests based on iodine determination, such as thyroid tests.

In the past, some allergy-provoking substances such as penicillin were available in combination with antihistamines. The presence of the antihistamine did, however, *mask* the early warning symptoms of anaphylaxis and offer no assistance in overcoming the serious symptoms of cardiovascular and respiratory collapse.

SIDE EFFECTS AND CAUTIONS WHEN USING ANTIHISTAMINES

The main drawback of many of the antihistamines is the drowsiness they tend to produce. Patients should not drive an automobile or operate machinery while taking these drugs until it is certain that drowsiness is not a problem. Patients should also be warned against drinking alcohol or taking other depressants such as barbiturates or opiates, because these would have additive depressant effects when taken with an antihistamine.

Since patients differ in their response to antihistamines, trial and error may be the only way to find the least sedating drug for any one individual. The patient should be encouraged to tell the physician if his medication is making him drowsy and interfering with his daily living patterns. The physician may then change the antihistamine order and attempt to find one that is less sedating. Sometimes a small dose of a psychomotor stimulant such as caffeine or an amphetamine may be added to overcome daytime drowsiness.

Some antihistamines have a strong anticholinergic effect. The atropine-like actions of drugs such as diphenhydramine and tripelennamine may be useful for relieving symptoms of rhinitis, but the dryness of mouth, nose, and throat, and the thickening of mucus

Table 32–1. Antihistamine drugs.

Generic Name	Trade Name	How Supplied	Routes	Usual Dose	Comments
chlorpheniramine	Chlor-Trimeton	tablets 4 mg.	P.O.	4 mg. t.i.d. or or q.i.d.	Also available in combination forms for expectorant.
		sustained release tablets 8 mg., 12 mg.		8–12 mg. h.s. or q. 8–10h. during day.	
		syrup 2 mg./5 cc.		1 tsp. q.i.d.	
		ampuls 1 cc. 10 mg./cc.	I.M. I.V.	10–20 mg. I.V.	100 mg./cc. injection for I.M. or S.C. use only.
		vials 2 cc. 100 mg./cc.	S.C.		
diphenhydramine hydrochloride	Benadryl	capsules 25 mg., 50 mg.	P.O.	50 mg. P.O. t.i.d. or q.i.d.	Contraindicated for premature or newborn infants.
		elixir 12.5 mg./5 cc.		2–4 tsp. t.i.d. or q.i.d.	
		vials 10 cc., 30 cc. 10 mg./cc.	I.M. I.V.	10–50 mg. I.M. I.V.	Maximum daily dose 400 mg.
		ampuls 1 cc. 50 mg./cc.			
trimeprazine	Temaril	tablets 2.5 mg.	P.O.	2.5 mg. q.i.d.	
		syrup 2.5 mg./5 cc.			
		sustained release capsules 5 mg.			
chlorpheniramine maleate	Neotep	sustained release capsules: chlorpheniramine 9 mg.	P.O.	1 capsule q. 12h.	
phenylephrine hydrochloride		phenylephrine 21 mg.			

could cause the patient discomfort. These effects could be dangerous for the patient with bronchial asthma, because the thick, dry mucus may obstruct the air passages. Other anticholinergic side effects would include blurred vision, difficulty in urinating, and gastrointestinal distress. Like other anticholinergic drugs, these would be contraindicated for patients with prostatic hypertrophy, acute glaucoma, and those taking drugs of the monoamine oxidase inhibiting class.

Although antihistamines are relatively safe drugs, they may be dangerous if taken in overdosage. Children may ingest excessive amounts of these drugs and suffer convulsions, coma, cardiovascular collapse, and respiratory failure. Both the higher dosage prescription products and the lower dosage proprietary products must be kept out of the reach of children. To prevent toxicity to the fetus and the newborn baby, antihistamines should not be used during pregnancy or lactation except under a physician's direction.

REFERENCES

Craven, Ruth, and Lester, Joan. "Anaphylactic Shock." *American Journal of Nursing* 72:718, April 1972.

DiPalma, Joseph R. "Histamine and Antihistamine Drugs." *RN* 37:49, June 1974.

Johnson, Kenneth J. "Allergen Injections." *American Journal of Nursing* 65:121, July 1965.

Rodman, Morton J. "Drugs for Allergic Disorders: Part 1, Anaphylaxis and Asthma." *RN* 34:63, June 1971.

Rodman, Morton J. "Drugs for Allergic Disorders: Part 2, Pollinosis, Perennial Rhinitis, Dermatitis." *RN* 34:53, July 1971.

APPLICATION QUESTIONS

I. *True-False*

For each statement below, write **a** if the statement is true or **b** if it is false.

_____ 1. Atopic individuals have a tendency to develop allergic reactions.

_____ 2. Histamine stimulates the flow of gastric juices.

_____ 3. Corticosteroid drugs increase the responsiveness of the sensitized patient's tissues to the actions of the autacoids.

_____ 4. For some patients with allergic skin disorders, antihistamines may be safely combined with tranquilizers.

_____ 5. Antihistamines cure colds.

_____ 6. The drying effects of antihistamines are especially therapeutic in asthma.

_____ 7. Determining the best antihistamine for daytime therapy may be done on a trial and error basis.

_____ 8. Antihistamines may not be combined with a psychomotor stimulant.

_____ 9. Antihistamines can be taken over long periods of time with no ill effects.

_____ 10. Antihistamines can be used to treat symptoms caused by any of the autacoids.

_____ 11. Combining antihistamines with an allergy-provoking substance such as penicillin will prevent serious allergy reactions from occurring.

_____ 12. Antihistamines are the drug of choice for the immediate treatment of anaphylactic shock.

II. *Multiple Choice*

For each of the following questions, indicate the letter providing the *best* answer.

_____ 1. Which of the following autacoids bring about capillary permeability? (1) SRS-A (2) bradykinin (3) histamine
(a) 1, 3 (b) 2, 3 (c) 1, 2, 3 (d) none of the above

_____ 2. Which of the following statements best explains the allergic response of wheals and congestion? (a) an increase in capillary permeability leads to fluid leakage to interstitial spaces (b) an increase in cellular permeability leads to intracellular fluid leakage to extracellular spaces (c) a generalized vasodilation leads to fluid stasis within the vessels (d) an increase in capillary and cellular permeability results in a shift from plasma to intracellular fluid

_____ 3. Sympathomimetic drugs produce which of the following body responses? (a) bronchodilation (b) increased gastric secretion (c) increased bronchial secretions (d) capillary dilation

_____ 4. Antihistamines with atropine-like peripheral effects are contraindicated in which of the following conditions? (1) acute glaucoma (2) enlarged prostate (3) hay fever (4) asthma
(a) 1, 2, 4 (b) 1 (c) 3 (d) 2, 3

_____ 5. What is the *primary* reason antihistamine drugs are often undesirable for patients with bronchial asthma? (a) the drying action of the drug leads to mucus plug formation (b) the antitussive action leads to accumulation of secretions (c) the drugs cause a reduction in respiratory rate (d) the drugs cause drowsiness and the patient becomes inactive

_____ 6. Which of the following best describes the action of antihistamines? (a) they destroy the molecules of histamine (b) they prohibit the release of histamine (c) they compete with histamine for receptor sites (d) they produce a chemical effect neutralizing histamines

_____ 7. What is hyposensitization? (a) administering increasing doses of an antigen to decrease the allergic response (b) administering decreasing doses of an antigen to minimize the allergic response (c) giving repeated doses of an autacoid to block the allergic response to an antigen (d) decreasing the number of antigens within the environment

_____ 8. Arrange the following steps of an allergic process in their proper sequence: (1) release of autacoids (2) production of reagins (3) exposure to antigen (4) reaction in target tissues
(a) 3—2—4—1 (b) 4—1—2—3 (c) 1—2—3—4 (d) 3—1—4—2

_____ 9. What is histamine? (a) a reagin (b) an antibody (c) an autacoid (d) an antigen

III. *Discussion*

For each patient statement given below, write **a** if teaching is needed, or **b** if no teaching is needed. If teaching is needed, outline the content you would include.

_____ 1. "I know this mask looks funny, but it sure keeps me from sneezing when I clean house."

_____ 2. "It seems my asthma gets lots worse when my mother-in-law visits. I must be allergic to her."

_____ 3. "I sure do get sleepy with those new allergy pills, but that's just something I'll have to live with, I guess."

_____ 4. "I'm going to ask the druggist if he has an antihistamine in a bigger pill. You know, with my glaucoma, these little things are hard to see."

_____ 5. "I'm just starting to feel better now after that prostate surgery and this cold has to come along. I don't think I'll bother the doctor about it, I'm just going to get some antihistamines from the store and take some aspirin."

_____ 6. "Do you have any of those 'cold pills'? Something to make me feel better and clear up my head? I've been looking forward to this cocktail party for a month, and it's really important to me; I sure don't want this cold to mess up the evening."

_____ 7. "My poor little son—this is his very first week in school and he's so excited about what's happening in first grade. His cold is really getting to him, though. Do you think if I gave him half of one of these antihistamines, it would be okay?"

_____ 8. "I can't get to the doctor's tomorrow for that allergy shot. Since I'm getting them three times a week, though, I guess missing one won't hurt any."

_____ 9. "The doctor told me to take two of these allergy pills a day. I've been taking one in the morning after I get to work, then I don't take the other one until I get home in the evening. That way I'm not taking them before I drive the car."

IV. *Discussion*

You are a camp nurse. Make a list of the drugs and equipment you will need for a kit labeled "Allergic Reactions."

V. *Calculation*

_____ 1. A child is ordered to have 20 mg. of Benadryl I.M. for an allergy reaction. The drug on hand is labeled Benadryl 50 mg./cc. How many cc. would you give?

Topical Drugs Used in Dermatology

Many types of drugs and chemicals can be applied topically to treat dermatological conditions. Topical agents come in many different preparations, such as ointments, pastes, creams, lotions, liniments, emulsions, paints, powders, wet dressings, and baths. This chapter discusses four broad categories of dermatological preparations: (1) those used to decrease inflammation, irritation, and itching; (2) those used for their irritating effects; (3) those used to treat thermal burns, alter pigmentation, or act as sunscreens; and (4) those used in the prevention and treatment of infection.

DRUGS USED TO DECREASE INFLAMMATION, IRRITATION, AND ITCHING

Topical corticosteroids probably account for about half of all of the ordered preparations for treating skin disorders. These drugs relieve acute and chronic inflammation and are safe from systemic steroid toxicity. Patients may fear that they will develop Cushingoid symptoms from using topical steroids, but the nurse can offer reassurance that this rarely occurs.

Triamcinolone acetonide (Aristocort, Kenalog) and other topical steroids are available in creams, ointments, lotions, and sprays. Sprays and cream-based steroids are used for leaving a thin film over reddened and oozing denuded areas. Lotions are used on hairy areas of the body and on the face. Greasy ointments are not used on hairy areas but are used mainly for dry, scaly lesions.

These preparations, used in the conditions discussed below, do not directly "heal" the lesions. The purpose of using these drugs is to help the skin's natural healing mechanisms bring about recovery. If the patient does not rub the lesions, scratch the itching areas, or pick at the protective crusts, the skin disorder will heal completely. Drug therapy is used to relieve itching, dry up oozing areas, and protect the damaged skin from further injury or infection.

Dermatitis

Dermatitis is a term applied to any inflammation of the skin. Signs and symptoms may vary from slight redness (erythema) to massive blisters (bullae), with destruction to underlying tissues. The nurse must remember that the most common complication of dermatitis is secondary infection, usually brought about by scratching the area and contaminating it with organisms from under the fingernails. The nurse can easily explain to the patient that he should not scratch the affected areas, and it is usually easy for the patient to understand the reason for this. However, the sensation of itching has the ability to override both intelligence and will power. When applying topical preparations, it is important to use a firm touch, as touching the skin only lightly or dabbing on a drug can increase the sensation of itching. The nurse should also remember that applying a topical preparation in too copious quantities is untidy, uncomfortable for the patient, and unnecessarily expensive.

Acute Contact Dermatitis. This condition results from exposure of skin to a substance that elicits an inflammatory response. The substance may be an irritant that would cause a response in most people, or it may be a substance to which an individual has become allergic. One of the most familiar causes of contact dermatitis is poison ivy. Scratching the lesions of poison ivy does not spread the poison. Treatment for the itching in this condition is for the same reason as in other forms of dermatitis—to prevent secondary infection.

In the acute stages of contact dermatitis, itching is best controlled by wet dressings followed by application of a protective lotion. Evaporation of water from the compresses has a cooling effect. Solutions such as aluminum acetate or potassium permanganate add a desirable astringent effect that aids in drying the oozing areas and allows crusts to form. Compresses are usually applied for about twenty minutes. Following the compresses, the area is daubed with a drying lotion, and then a thin layer of a skin protectant such as zinc oxide or calamine lotion is applied to soothe the skin and relieve itching. The addition of phenol, menthol, or camphor to calamine lotion adds to its antipruritic action. Topical steroids are not very useful until the acute stage has subsided, because they are washed away by the serous fluid from broken vesicles.

In later stages of contact dermatitis, when skin becomes dry and cracked, calamine *ointment* or another greasy emollient substance may be preferred. Topical steroids may be used in the later stages, but they are not as necessary in these conditions as in other pruritic dermatoses, and they may be very expensive if large areas of the body are involved. Systemic steroids may be preferred for severe, extensive contact dermatitis. Some topical antihistaminic agents such as tripelennamine are effective for relieving itching. Oral antihistamines such as cyproheptadine hydrochloride (Periactin) may also help relieve itching.

Atopic Dermatitis. This is a chronic skin condition that often appears in infancy and lasts into adult life. Atopic dermatitis, like other skin conditions, is often referred to as eczema.

The treatment of this condition is aimed at relieving itching and inflammation. The most effective agents are topical corticosteroids in creams, lotions, or ointments. Hydrocortisone preparations are the least expensive of the corticosteroids, but the new synthetic compounds, such as triamcinolone acetonide (Aristocort, Kenalog), are much more potent.

Anesthetic creams can relieve itching, but a patient with atopic dermatitis may easily become sensitized to these drugs. Actually, these patients have very sensitive skin, and *any* drug or chemical can be a source of irritation. For this reason, oral antihistamines may be preferred to topical ones for reducing the awareness of itching.

DRUGS USED FOR THEIR IRRITATING EFFECTS

Irritating chemicals are used to speed the peeling of epithelial cells and thereby permit healing. One way to cause this desquamation is by softening skin keratin; therefore, some of these agents are referred to as keratolytics. Some of these substances may be irritating enough to cause skin ulcers in patients with poor local circulation. Patients with peripheral vascular disease or diabetes should thus be warned against the use of proprietary products containing salicylic acid or other keratolytic agents to treat corns and calluses.

Three common conditions requiring the use of irritants will be discussed here: acne, psoriasis, and seborrheic dermatitis. In addition to these, however, caustic chemicals are sometimes applied to warts to remove them. Silver nitrate sticks may be moistened and simply touched to granulation tissue, wounds, or warts that require cauterization. Whenever corrosive agents such as formaldehyde or trichloroacetic acid are employed, care must be taken to avoid contact with normal skin. This is usually done by applying petrolatum to surrounding areas.

Acne

Acne is one of the most common of all skin disorders; it affects 80 to 90 percent of all adolescents to some extent. The lesions develop during adolescence, when androgens stimulate growth and secretion of the sebaceous glands. At the same time, the pores that open onto the skin surface become plugged with cellular debris; the resulting comedones (blackheads) cause local inflammation.

The basis of any acne treatment program is thorough cleansing of the skin with soap and water. Even nonpathogenic skin bacteria can cause irritation and inflammation. Alcohol sponges and detergent liquids such as hexachlorophene may be useful for reducing bacterial flora. Reducing bacteria is also the rationale for administering broad-spectrum antibiotics such as tetracycline in some instances.

Topical preparations containing mild keratolytic agents such as resorcinol, salicylic acid, and sulfur are used in less severe cases of acne. For deeper pustules and cysts, hot compresses made with sulfurated lime solution (Vleminckx's solution) or a lotion of zinc sulfate and sulfurated potash (White lotion) may be used.

Tretinoin (Retin-A), an acid derivative of vitamin A, has recently been introduced for use in place of traditional peeling agents. The patient swabs his face with this solution at bedtime for four to six weeks. At first, the skin may look worse, but redness and peeling are prerequisite to improvement.

Girls who have not responded to topical treatment or systemic antibiotics may be given small doses of an estrogen drug such as mestranol to antagonize androgens and decrease sebum secretion. A progestin may be added and then withdrawn to avoid menstrual irregularities.

Psoriasis

This is a chronic skin condition characterized by reddish papules covered by dry, silvery scales, or squama. This condition responds to treatment, but the lesions almost inevitably recur.

Mildly irritating materials such as ammoniated mercury ointment are applied to remove psoriatic scales and stimulate healing of underlying tissues. A somewhat more irritating substance such as coal tar or anthralin may be added later. Anthralin is less likely to stain the skin and clothing. Most of these substances lose their effectiveness after a period of time, but withholding treatment during remissions may delay tolerance.

Topical corticosteroids are relatively ineffective when simply rubbed into the skin; when covered with an occlusive dressing, however, drugs such as triamcinolone acetonide and flurandrenolide (Cordran) are often quite effective. The dressings keep moisture from evaporating from the skin and allow the steroid to diffuse down into deeper skin layers. Systemic corticosteroid therapy is sometimes used; however, the large doses required often cause hypercorticism, and the skin condition may become worse when the steroids are finally withdrawn. Continued use of corticosteroids is undesirable in a chronic condition such as psoriasis, which is not potentially fatal (see Chapter 30).

Methotrexate, an anticancer drug, has recently been used for treating selected cases of severe psoriasis that can no longer be controlled by topical therapy or systemic steroids. Although the drug may help produce remissions, it is very toxic (see Chapter 39).

Seborrheic Dermatitis

The most common form of this condition is dandruff of the scalp. Dandruff can be kept under control with frequent shampooing, particularly with a medicated detergent suspension such as selenium sulfide (Selsun) or cadmium sulfide (Capsebon). Selenium salt may cause arsenic-like systemic toxicity if ingested; therefore, it is important to keep this medication (as well as all other household products and drugs) away from children.

More severe forms of chronic seborrheic dermatitis are treated by rubbing the same irritant-keratolytic agents used for psoriasis into the scalp at bedtime and then shampooing in the morning. Care must be taken to avoid allowing the solution to run into the eyes or ears.

DRUGS USED FOR THERMAL, SOLAR, AND PIGMENTATION CONDITIONS

Burns

The pain of sunburn may be relieved by tepid baths containing cornstarch or other colloids. Severe sunburn with blistering may be treated with mildly astringent and cooling liquids such as aluminum acetate solution, or with corticosteroid sprays to control pain and itching. Phenolated calamine lotion, zinc oxide, or creams containing topical anesthetics or antihistamines can be used to cover and protect the healing areas.

Topical medication is only one aspect of the care necessary in treating acute thermal burns. Mafenide (Sulfamylon), silver nitrate, and gentamicin sulfate (Garamycin) may be used topically for treating these burns. All of these drugs are discussed in Chapters 35 and 36. Topical corticosteroids are sometimes used after the healing of a burn or grafted area to reduce hypertrophic scars.

Sun Sensitivity

Sun-induced skin damage of a chronic nature often occurs in light-skinned people whose occupations demand prolonged exposure to sunlight. Chronic skin damage of this type can lead to skin cancer or to the development of precancerous growths called keratoses. Fluorouracil (Efudex), when applied topically as a cream or solution, is often effective in clearing up solar keratoses and preventing their progress to the malignant stage. During the two- to four-week course of treatment, the patient's skin first seems to get worse, but redness, blistering, ulcer formation, and necrosis are necessary preliminaries to healing. The patient must avoid exposure to sun during treatment with this drug; care must be taken not to allow the drug to contact uninvolved areas.

Sunscreen chemicals are available for protecting the skin of sun-sensitive patients. Zinc oxide, titanium oxide, and red veterinary petrolatum may all be used for completely excluding light rays from the skin. Other products available now are cosmetically more attractive, such as benzophenone, oxybenzone, and sulisobenzone.

Para-aminobenzoic acid (PABA) is preferred for use by people who want to tan without burning. A 5 percent solution of PABA in 75 to 90 percent ethyl alcohol is said to be more effective for this purpose than any of the commercially available products.

Pigmentation Conditions

Vitiligo is a hypopigmentation disorder caused by loss of melanin in scattered patches of skin. This condition has been treated with oral drugs of the psoralen type, such as trioxsalen (Trisoralen) and methoxsalen (Meloxine). Full pigmentation may require several years of carefully regulated treatment.

Hyperpigmentation may be managed by local application of chemicals such as hydroquinone and monobenzone. When applied as a lotion or ointment to heavily freckled skin, these substances often lighten the spots. These preparations may also be used for treating melasma (chloasma), which is a hyperpigmentation condition that sometimes develops during pregnancy or when oral contraceptives are used. These agents must be used with care to avoid removing melanin from normal skin.

DRUGS USED IN THE PREVENTION AND TREATMENT OF INFECTION

Skin is an effective natural barrier against the entrance of microbes into the body. When the natural resistance of the skin is reduced, organisms can cause skin infections as well as breaking through the skin and causing infections within the body. Topical antiseptics are not very effective for treating skin infections, but agents that kill or control the growth of skin microbes are useful for preventing infection or for limiting its spread.

Skin Cleansing and Disinfecting

Soap has little effect as an antibacterial agent, but as a detergent, it removes skin debris and most of the contaminating bacteria contained in the debris. Soaps and certain synthetic "wetting agents" permit water to penetrate better and thus float out some of the flora that hides in the crypts and crevices of the skin. Friction also plays an important role in cleansing the skin. Alcohols are often used to rinse residual soap from the skin. Alcohols can kill bacteria but not their spores. The longer the alcohols are in contact with the skin, the greater their germicidal effect.

Iodine dissolved in diluted alcohol is used in preoperative skin preparation. The iodine-scrubbed area is usually swabbed with alcohol before the operative area is draped, because residual iodine may cause damage to the skin. Some people are sensitive to even small amounts of iodine, and severe skin reactions may result. It is important to ask the patient specifically before he goes to surgery if he knows whether he is sensitive to iodine. If he is, this information should be posted on the front of the patient's chart.

Compounds such as benzalkonium chloride (Zephiran) have both antiseptic and detergent properties; they may be used preoperatively for handwashing or for disinfecting the patient's skin. The antibacterial action of these substances is almost completely neutralized by the presence of even small traces of soap on the skin. The surgical field, then, must be rinsed thoroughly with water and then swabbed with alcohol before benzalkonium or other cationic detergent antiseptics are applied.

Hexachlorophene, a phenol derivative, is an effective antibacterial agent that does not usually damage skin as phenol does. If hexachlorophene is to be used preoperatively, the patient should be instructed to wash the area daily for four days to one week before surgery, in order to build up a bacteriostatic residue on the skin. The patient should also be told not to rinse the area with alcohol, as this would remove the hexachlorophene film that is being built up. Hexachlorophene was used in many commercial products until it was found to cause nerve tissue damage when absorbed through the skin. The agent is still available and is used in some instances in the hospital (for patients and personnel allergic to iodine, for example); it may be prescribed by a physician for the treatment of acne.

Most of the antiseptics available to the public for treating cuts and abrasions have little value. Most scratches and abrasions are best treated by washing with soap and water. Some of the available antiseptics are actually toxic or irritating to the skin; others merely interfere with the skin's natural defenses. Boric acid, for example, is a topical antiseptic with weak antibacterial and antifungal effects. At one time it was widely used for treating diaper rash in babies, but applying boric acid as a full strength powder has actually caused toxicity and death.

Fungal Infections of the Skin

Fungal infections of the skin are caused by two types of organisms: dermatophytes that burrow into the skin to cause athlete's foot (tinea pedis), ringworm of the scalp (tinea capitis), or ringworm of the groin (tinea cruris); and *Candida albicans*, which is a yeast-like organism.

Griseofulvin, administered orally, is the most effective treatment for advanced cases of dermatophytosis affecting the skin and nails. Topical antifungal chemicals may be used for treating less severe ringworm infections. Some of these topical agents are single chemicals such as tolnaftate, acrisorcin, haloprogin, and zincundecate (Desenex). Others are combinations of chemicals, such as carbon-fuchsin solution, which combines agents to relieve pruritus, to dry the area, and to stop further fungal growth directly; and Whitfield's ointment, which combines the keratolytic agent salicylic acid with an antifungal agent, benzoic acid.

Candida albicans infections (moniliasis) are not limited to the skin. During treatment with systemic antibiotics, overgrowths of this organism may develop in the mouth, anogenital region, and vaginal tract. These infections are best treated by topical application of one of the antifungal antibiotics such as nystatin or amphotericin B (see Chapter 35). Candicidin is a newer antibiotic reserved for treating vaginal candidiasis.

Parasitic Infestations of the Skin

Infestations by mites and lice lead to itching and scratching that can result in secondary skin infections. These conditions, scabies and pediculosis, are best treated with insecticides such as chlorophenothane (DDT), benzyl benzoate, and gamma benzene hexachloride. Prolonged bathing in warm soapy water and vigorous shampooing are also important. Clothing and bedding should always be laundered, sterilized, or fumigated to avoid reexposure.

Table 33–1. Topical drugs used in dermatology

Generic Name	Trade Name	How Supplied	Routes	Usual Dose	Comments
triamcinolone acetonide	Aristocort	topical cream 0.1%, 0.5%, 0.025% topical ointment 0.1%, 0.5%	topical	apply to affected area t.i.d. or q.i.d.	
salicylic acid; colloidal sulfur	Acne-dome	lotion or cream	topical	use t.i.d.	Massage for five minutes, then rinse.
selenium sulfide	Selsun	4 oz. bottles lotion shampoo	topical	1–2 tsp. massaged into scalp twice a week as shampoo	Allow to remain on scalp 2–3 minutes, then rinse.
trioxsalen	Trisoralen	tablets 5 mg.	P.O.	10 mg. q.d.	
hydroquinone	Eldoquin / Eldoquin Forte	2% cream tubes 2% lotion bottles 4% lotion bottles	topical	apply q. 12h.	If rash develops, discontinue use. Avoid contact with eyes or open cuts. Do not use on children under 12.
benzalkonium chloride	Zephiran	solutions 1:750 tinted tincture 1:750 spray 1:750	topical	as directed	Dilute with distilled water; rinse all soap from skin.
hexachlorophene	pHisoHex	bottles 5 oz., 1 pt., 1 gal.	topical	as directed	Should not be used routinely for bathing infants or for routine total body bathing of adults. Rinse thoroughly after use.

REFERENCES

Barrett, Daniel, and Klibanski, Aron. "Collagenase Debridement." *American Journal of Nursing* 73:849, May 1973.

DiPalma, Joseph. "Enzymes Used As Drugs." *RN* 35:53, January 1972.

Leider, Morris. "Some Principles of Dermatologic Nursing." *RN* 35:48, May 1972.

Rodman, Morton J. "Systemic and Topical Drugs for Psoriasis and Acne." *RN* 38:63, April 1975.

Rodman, Morton J. "Preventing and Treating Skin-Sun Reactions." *RN* 32:63, April 1969.

APPLICATION QUESTIONS

I. *True-False*

For each statement below, write **a** if the statement is true or **b** if it is false.

1. Vitiligo is best treated with topical hyperpigmentation agents.
2. Only pathogenic bacteria can cause the local irritation and inflammation of acne.
3. Birth control pills may be used for young adolescent females to treat acne.
4. Benzalkonium chloride (Zephiran) has both antiseptic and detergent properties.
5. Phenol is commonly used as a preoperative skin preparation agent.
6. Merthiolate and mercurochrome are very effective in preventing infections in cuts.
7. Diaper rash may be treated with pure boric acid powder.
8. Apply keratolytic agents in copious quantities when treating the scalp for seborrheic dermatitis.
9. Systemic toxicity rarely occurs with the use of topical steroid preparations.
10. Greasy ointment bases are used in hairy areas.
11. Massive blisters involving deep destruction of the dermis are termed *bullae*.
12. Scratching poison ivy spreads the poison.
13. Local anesthetic creams are rarely used for atopic dermatitis because of the possibility of the patient becoming sensitized to the drug.
14. Oral antihistamines are rarely used for atopic dermatitis because of their central depressant effects.
15. Sunscreen lotions are used for completely excluding light rays from the skin.
16. The only effective treatment for psoriasis is the long-term use of systemic steroids.
17. A keratolytic agent is used as a protectant.
18. Keratolytic agents must be discontinued if the patient's skin begins to look worse.
19. The most important aspect of acne treatment is cleansing the skin with soap and water.
20. Psoralen-type agents are used to treat the hyperpigmentation of chloasma.

II. *Multiple Choice*

For each of the following questions, indicate the letter providing the *best* answer.

1. Topical steroid application is *not* very useful in which of the following conditions? (a) atopic dermatitis (b) sunburn (c) acute stage of contact dermatitis (d) psoriasis
2. In what order are the following treatments usually used for contact dermatitis? (1) wet dressings (2) application of drying lotion (3) application of protective lotion
(a) 1—3—2 (b) 3—1—2 (c) 1—2—3 (d) 2—3—1
3. Which of the following drug therapies may be used in the treatment of pruritus? (1) oral antihistamine (2) aspirin (3) anesthetic ointment (4) thiamine
(a) 1, 3 (b) 1, 2 (c) 3, 4 (d) 2, 4
4. Which of the following drugs are keratolytic agents? (1) hydrocortisone (2) salicylic acid (3) calamine lotion (4) silver nitrate
(a) 2 (b) 1, 3 (c) 2, 4 (d) 1, 3, 4
5. Which of the following substances would be most effective in protecting the surrounding tissue when using caustic chemicals to remove warts? (a) talcum powder (b) petrolatum (c) mineral oil (d) water
6. Tolerance to irritants in the treatment of psoriasis may be delayed by which of the following actions? (a) withholding drug during remission (b) administering drug in combination with antihistamine (c) administering two or more irritants simultaneously (d) applying drug continuously and consistently throughout periods of remission and exacerbation
7. Which of the following must be done before using benzalkonium chloride (Zephiran) as a preoperative skin preparation? (a) swab area with alcohol to remove all traces of soap (b) shave the area (c) dry the area thoroughly (d) determine whether the patient is allergic to iodine

_____ 8. When teaching a patient about using hexachlorophene for treating acne, which of the following should be included? (1) wash the area daily (2) scrub for several minutes (3) rinse with alcohol (4) maintain separate linen
(a) 1, 2 (b) 3, 4 (c) 1, 2, 4 (d) 1, 2, 3, 4

_____ 9. Which of the following substances is never used in the treatment of acne? (a) sulfurated potash (b) alcohol (c) baby oil (d) tetracycline

_____ 10. When topical corticosteroids are being used in the treatment of psoriasis, the nurse would need to apply the drug in which of the following ways? (a) with a gauze cover to avoid staining of clothes (b) with an airtight dressing to avoid skin evaporation (c) with a nonmetallic spatula to avoid chemical interaction (d) mixed with baby oil, then rubbed vigorously and left open to dry

_____ 11. The pain of sunburn can be relieved by which of the following substances? (1) cornstarch bath (2) aluminum acetate solution (3) alcohol (4) coal tar
(a) 1 (b) 1, 2 (c) 2, 4 (d) 1, 2, 3, 4

_____ 12. If a patient receiving fluorouracil (Efudex) asks why blisters and ulcers have appeared, what would be the best response for the nurse to give? (a) "It would seem that you're having a reaction to the drug." (b) "You should stop using the drug." (c) "It is a necessary preliminary to healing." (d) "You should ask your doctor."

_____ 13. Which of the following dermatological preparations does not completely exclude sunlight? (a) para-aminobenzoic acid (PABA) (b) oxybenzone (c) red veterinary petrolatum (d) zinc oxide

III. *Discussion*

For each patient statement given below, write **a** if teaching is needed, or **b** if no teaching is needed. If teaching is needed, outline the content you would include.

_____ 1. "I've gotten what the doctor calls solar keratosis from being out in the sun so much with my job. I'm using this Efudex now to treat it, and the doctor said not to go out to the construction site, but I feel fine so I'm still putting in my eight hours."

_____ 2. "One thing I remember they told me when I first had my leg trouble was not to use corn plasters, so I just soak my feet and rub them with a towel."

Bronchodilators, Expectorants, and Mucolytic Agents

Although there are many chronic disabling pulmonary diseases, they are characterized by similar symptoms and treated with similar drugs. This chapter deals specifically with bronchial asthma; however, the usefulness of the same drugs in other pulmonary conditions should be apparent.

BRONCHIAL ASTHMA

This disease is referred to as either extrinsic or intrinsic. Extrinsic asthma occurs in allergic or atopic individuals; their asthmatic attacks are in response to a specific antigen in the environment. Intrinsic asthma is caused by microorganisms and occurs in patients with chronic respiratory infections. A person with extrinsic asthma may try to avoid exposure to the causative allergen as much as possible or may undergo hyposensitization treatments (see Chapter 33). The person suffering from intrinsic asthma may experience fewer attacks if maintained on prophylactic doses of broad-spectrum antibiotics.

Bronchodilator Drugs

During an acute asthmatic attack, the smooth muscle of the bronchioles constricts in spasm and occludes the air passages. Either adrenergic drugs or theophylline-type bronchodilators may be used to relieve spasm. Because adrenergic drugs are discussed in Chapter 16, only the theophylline-type drugs are discussed here.

Theophylline and its derivatives, such as aminophylline, diphylline, and oxtriphylline, may be used to treat acute asthmatic attacks or to prevent attacks.

When taken orally in doses high enough to be effective, these drugs are quite irritating to the gastrointestinal tract. To prevent this distressing side effect, certain theophylline derivatives may be given by intramuscular or intravenous injection, by rectal suppository, or by retention enema. The drug may be irritating to the anorectal mucosa, and a patient receiving suppositories or retention enemas should be observed for irritation in this area. Injected theophylline derivatives may cause pain and irritation at the injection site.

Aminophylline is the most versatile of the theophylline derivatives; it can be given by various routes. Aminophylline may be given by slow intravenous injection for treatment of status asthmaticus. Too rapid intravenous administration of this drug can cause hypotension and cardiac irregularities. The heart-stimulating side effect of the drug may be an advantage in patients with pulmonary edema or left-sided heart failure.

Drug Combinations

Bronchodilating drugs are often given in combination. For example, combining an adrenergic drug such as ephedrine with a theophylline derivative causes a greater bronchodilation than either drug alone. The combination also delays the development of tolerance to the adrenergic drug. Since both drugs provide central stimulation and could cause restlessness, hyperactivity, and insomnia, a barbiturate may be added to the combination to decrease these symptoms.

Control of Mucus

When mucus secretions become thick and hardened, they are difficult to remove and predispose to complications. The easiest way to keep mucus from becoming viscid and hardened is to promote good hydration. Asthmatic patients need large quantities of water, so the nurse should be sure to force fluids. Two types of drugs used to help liquefy secretions are expectorants and mucolytic agents. The main difference between these drugs is that expectorant drugs act systemically, whereas mucolytic agents act locally.

The Expectorant Drugs.   These drugs include potassium iodide, ammonium chloride, and syrup of ipecac; they are taken orally. They irritate the gastric lining in such a way as to stimulate secretion in the respiratory tract of a natural lubricating fluid called RTF (respiratory tract fluid).

Mucolytic Agents.   These are wetting agents applied to the respiratory tract that break down mucus plugs by chemical or enzymatic action and draw water into the mucus. These agents, such as acetylcysteine (Mucomyst) and tyloxapol (Alevaire), are very irritating and are therefore reserved for short-term use. Because these drugs must come directly in contact with the mucus deep in the pulmonary tree, they are often nebulized into very fine particles and given with the force of an intermittent positive pressure machine.

Drugs such as adrenocorticosteroids, antibiotics, antihistamines, and antitussives are also used in the treatment of chronic lung disease. These drugs are discussed in other chapters.

Special Consideration

It is important to remember that any time a narcotic is given to a patient with a lung condition, the side effects of decreasing respiration and depressing the cough center must be carefully considered. Narcotic antitussives are contraindicated for the patient with asthma because breathing will become more difficult and the patient will not be coughing up the mucus as it collects.

REFERENCES

LANSER, J., et al. "Caring for the Asthmatic at Home, in School, and on the Job." *Nursing 73* 3:62, November 1973.

Table 34–1. Bronchodilators, expectorants, and mucolytic agents.

Generic Name	Trade Name	How Supplied	Routes	Usual Dose	Comments
aminophylline	Somophyllin	rectal instillation: 60 mg./cc.	rectal	adult: 120 mg.–300 mg. q. 6h.	Aminophylline is included in many compounds not mentioned here. It should be used with extreme caution for children weighing less than 25 pounds.
	Lixaminol	elixir: 250 mg./Tbsp.	P.O.	adult: 250 mg. q. 8h. child: 0.1 cc./lb. of body weight q. 8h.	
	Aminodur other manufacturers	tablets: 300 mg. 100 mg. 200 mg.		adult: 1–2 tablets q. 8h.	
potassium iodide	Pima Syrup	5 gr./tsp.	P.O.	adult: 1–2 tsp. q. 4–6 h. child: 1/2–1 tsp. q. 4–6h.	Included in many compounds.
saturated solution of potassium iodide	SSKI	dropper bottle 1 oz., 300 mg./0.3 cc. bottle 8 oz., 300 mg./0.3 cc.	P.O.	0.3 cc./day in orange juice	
acetylcysteine	Mucomyst	vials 4 cc., 10 cc., 30 cc. 10% and 20% solution	nebulization	3–5 ml. of 20% sol. or 6–10 ml. of 10% sol. t.i.d. or q.i.d.	Mucomyst should not be placed in the chamber of a heated nebulizer.
tyloxapol	Alevaire	vials 60 cc.	nebulization	Continuous inhalation of mist for a few days or intermittently for longer periods.	

Moody, L. "Asthma—Physiology and Patient Care." *American Journal of Nursing* 73:1212, July 1973.

Rodman, Morton J. "Drugs For Allergic Disorders: Part 1, Anaphylaxis and Asthma." *RN* 34:63, June 1971.

Rodman, Morton J. "Drugs Used Against Chronic Airway Obstruction." *RN* 37:45, February 1974.

APPLICATION QUESTIONS

I. *True-False*

For each statement below, write **a** if the statement is true or **b** if it is false.

_____ 1. Most patients with extrinsic asthma have a history of allergy from early childhood.

_____ 2. Theophylline derivatives are central nervous system stimulants.

_____ 3. Theophylline may be combined with ephedrine and a barbiturate for the treatment of asthma.

_____ 4. Rectal irritation is a common untoward effect of aminophylline suppositories.

_____ 5. An advantage of the adrenergic bronchodilator aerosols is that the patient rarely becomes resistant to their action.

_____ 6. Expectorants can be taken orally but are more effective when inhaled.

_____ 7. Mucolytic agents help liquefy bronchial secretions, and expectorants stimulate the cough center, causing the patient to cough.

_____ 8. Codeine is used as an antitussive agent in the treatment of asthma.

II. *Multiple Choice*

For each of the following questions, indicate the letter providing the *best* answer.

_____ 1. How much water should the asthmatic patient drink? (a) large quantities of water to keep sputum less viscid (b) small amounts of water to avoid stomach pressure on the diaphragm (c) moderate amounts of water to prevent overload on the cardiovascular system (d) water intake does not influence the condition

_____ 2. Which of the following drugs is not an expectorant? (a) potassium iodide (b) ammonium chloride (c) theophylline (d) syrup of ipecac

_____ 3. Theophylline-type agents may be administered through which of the following routes? (1) intravenous (2) oral (3) rectal (4) intramuscular (a) 1, 2, 3 (b) 2, 3, 4 (c) 1, 3, 4 (d) 1, 2, 3, 4

_____ 4. What would be the most effective means of removing a solid mucus plug causing respiratory obstruction? (a) instill an expectorant into the respiratory tract (b) instill a mucolytic agent into the respiratory tract (c) administer an expectorant drug orally (d) administer I.V. aminophylline (e) suction the air passages with high suction

_____ 5. Which of the following side effects might be exhibited by a patient receiving epinephrine? (a) nervousness, trembling, and heart palpitation (b) drowsiness and mental confusion (c) visual disturbances and gastrointestinal hyperactivity (d) breathlessness, hypotension, and rapid, weak pulse

III. *Matching A*

Match each antigen with the type of asthma it produces.

_____ 1. Goldenrod   (a) intrinsic

_____ 2. Pseudomonas   (b) extrinsic

_____ 3. Eggs

_____ 4. Horse hair

_____ 5. Streptococcus

IV. *Matching B*

Match each drug listed below with its classification.

_____ 1. Epinephrine   (a) bronchodilator

_____ 2. Hydrocortisone   (b) expectorant

_____ 3. Aminophylline   (c) mucolytic

_____ 4. Tyloxapol   (d) adrenocorticosteroid
         (Alevaire)

_____ 5. Syrup of ipecac

V. *Matching C*

Match each mode of action to the appropriate drug classification.

_____ 1. Stimulates natural   (a) bronchodilator
         respiratory
         tract fluid   (b) expectorant

_____ 2. Draws water into   (c) mucolytic
         the mucus, making
         it less viscid   (d) adrenocorticosteroid

_____ 3. Breaks down
         mucus with
         enzyme action

_____ 4. Reduces
         inflammation

_____ 5. Acts on smooth
         muscles to relax
         spasms

Drugs Used for Treating Infections

SECTION NINE

35

Antibiotics

Drugs of many types are available for treating infections. There are agents specific for bacterial, fungal, and some viral and parasitic infections. By literal definition, however, only compounds of natural origin that eliminate or destroy organisms are termed *antibiotics.* Synthetic anti-infective agents are not considered antibiotics. This chapter discusses the antibiotics, except for those used in tuberculosis. In the following chapter, all other anti-infective agents will be discussed, along with management of tuberculosis.

Antibiotics are available for many bacterial and fungal infections. An antibiotic is considered to be *bactericidal* if it is capable of killing organisms. The penicillins and their related drugs are bactericidal. Some antibiotics do not kill organisms, but rather inhibit the growth and multiplication of organisms and thereby allow the body's own defenses to eliminate them. Antibiotics acting in this manner are called *bacteriostatic.*

ACTION AND SPECTRUM OF ANTIBIOTICS

Specificity of Antibiotics

Before administering an antibiotic, it is important to identify the organism it is to eliminate. This is done by taking a culture of the infected area. Since many drugs are specific ("narrow-spectrum") for *either* gram-negative *or* gram-positive organisms, making this determination is important. In addition to identification of the organism, sensitivity studies may be done to aid in selecting an antibiotic. Organisms may be or become resistant to antibiotics; therefore, it is important to determine an antibiotic to which the organism is susceptible. If time does not permit a culture and sensitivity study to be done, a patient may begin therapy with one of the "broad-spectrum" antibiotics. These are drugs such as tetracycline (a bacteriostatic agent) and some of the newer synthetic anti-infective agents which are effective against many gram-posi-

tive, gram-negative, rickettsial, and even some viral infections.

Administration of Antibiotics

As a general rule, oral antibiotics are better absorbed if taken between meals. A constant blood level can best be maintained if the drug is given at equal intervals throughout the twenty-four-hour day. Therapy with antibiotics is continued until systemic signs of infection (fever, white blood count) have remained within normal limits for several days. The usual course of treatment is from seven to ten days. If treatment of an infection is not continued for an adequate amount of time, relapse or sensitivity may occur, or resistant strains of the organism may develop. Resistance may also occur when an antibiotic is used over an extended period of time. Combining two antibiotics may slow the development of resistant strains; however, this process may work in reverse and actually encourage the emergence of resistant strains, especially if one of the combined antibiotics is given in very small doses. The individual situation, then, is the determinant for whether combination therapy should be used.

Adverse Reactions

Antibiotics are capable of causing adverse reactions, which tend to fall into three general catagories: direct toxicity, allergic reactions, and superinfections. *Direct toxic effects* may cause damage to gastrointestinal tissue, the kidney, or the liver; specific nerves may also be damaged, such as the auditory, optic, or various peripheral nerves. *Allergic reactions* may cause varying skin conditions, depress bone marrow, lead to blood dyscrasias, or cause severe and life-threatening reactions such as anaphylactic shock. *Superinfection* is caused by the overgrowth of resistant bacteria or fungi that are normally present. Many of the side effects of antibiotics, such as nausea, vomiting, anorexia, diarrhea, and vaginal or anal pruritus, are caused by superinfection of the gastrointestinal or vaginal tract. The most serious superinfections occur with an overgrowth of pseudomonas or other gram-negative organisms.

THE PENICILLINS

All of the penicillins are bactericidal; they are therefore the preferred treatment for many infections. It is important to encourage patients to complete the prescribed course of treatment with any of the penicillins. Patients should also be warned not to medicate themselves with leftover pills to avoid developing resistance or hypersensitivity to the drugs.

Penicillin G

When penicillin is indicated, the first drug of choice is penicillin G. This is a narrow-spectrum drug which is useful against many of the common gram-positive organisms: streptococci, staphylococci, gonococci, and *Treponema pallidum.*

Penicillin G is effective in treating venereal diseases such as gonorrhea and syphilis. Early treatment of syphilis consists of injections of 2.4 million units at weekly intervals. Gonorrhea may be treated with a single high dose injection, such as 4.8 million units. A patient may be given an oral dose of probenecid (an antigout drug) thirty minutes before the penicillin injection. Probenecid has been found to delay the elimination of penicillin from the body; it thus aids in keeping a high tissue level of the drug over a longer period of time.

Although penicillin G is usually administered parenterally, it may be given in daily oral doses for long-term prophylactic therapy, as for patients with a history of rheumatic fever. Long-term prophylaxis may also be maintained by monthly injections of the long-acting benzathine penicillin G (Bicillin).

Penicillin V

Penicillin V has a range of activity similar to penicillin G, but since it is more stable in gastric juices, it can be given by mouth in smaller doses. Penicillin V is an exception to the rule of giving antibiotics on an empty stomach. This drug actually is better absorbed if given after a meal.

Penicillinase Resistant Drugs

Some organisms, specifically strains of staphylococci, produce an enzyme called penicillinase which is capable of breaking penicillin down into inactive fragments. In this way the organism is resistant to penicillin. Some specific penicillin drugs are penicillinase resistant; these are used against penicillinase-producing organisms. Examples of these drugs are: sodium methicillin (Staphcillin); sodium nafcillin (Unipen); sodium oxacillin (Prostaphlin); sodium cloxacillin (Tegopen); and sodium dicloxacillin (Dynapen). These drugs are used only against penicillinase resistant organisms, because they are not as effective as other penicillins against other gram-positive organisms.

Semisynthetic Penicillins

Ampicillin is a semisynthetic penicillin with a broader spectrum of activity than penicillin G or V. It is not as effective against most gram-positive organisms, and it is ineffective against penicillinase-producing organisms, but it has been shown to be effective against some gram-negative organisms. Ampicillin can be used for urinary tract infections caused by *E. coli* and *Proteus mirabilis,* and for meningitis and respiratory tract infections caused by *Hemophilus influenzae.* In comparison wiith other broad-spectrum antibiotics, ampicillin does not carry the potential of causing severe toxicity, as chloramphenicol does; in addition, it is bactericidal, whereas tetracycline is bacteriostatic. Ampicillin is not effective against rickettsial organisms, as tetracycline is, and except for those mentioned, it has no effect against other gram-negative organisms such as Klebsiella, Enterobacter, and *Pseudomonas aeruginosa.*

Carbenicillin (Geocillin, Geopen) is another new broad-spectrum semisynthetic penicillin. It is effective against many gram-positive and gram-negative organisms, including *Pseudomonas aeruginosa.* It is especially useful against gram-negative urinary tract infections because of the high concentration reached in the urine as the drug is being excreted. Unlike other antipseudomonal antibiotics, carbenicillin is not toxic to kidney tissue and may therefore be used when chronic kidney disorders are present, but the dose should be lowered. Because of the sodium in the injectable disodium carbenicillin (Geopen), patients who need to restrict sodium should be watched for retention.

Adverse Reactions of the Penicillins

The penicillins are capable of bringing about all three types of general adverse reactions. Direct tissue toxicity and superinfection occur less frequently with the penicillins than with other antibiotics. Hypersensitivity and allergic reactions are the most common adverse reactions.

Direct tissue toxicity may occur when large doses are used, causing high concentrations in the nervous system. Disodium carbenicillin has been reported to cause occasional convulsive seizures. Intrathecal injections (into the spinal fluid) of any of the penicillins may also precipitate convulsive seizures.

Allergic reactions may range from mild skin reactions to severe reactions which can cause death in minutes. Allergic reactions occur in 1 to 10 percent of patients receiving penicillin. Always ask a patient if he has ever had a reaction to penicillin or if he has a history of allergy in general, such as asthma, hay fever, or food allergies. A patient who is allergic to *any* of the penicillins will probably have a cross sensitivity to the others. If uncertain about whether a patient will have a reaction, skin testing may be done with the drug before it is administered for therapy. If a severe anaphylactic reaction occurs, epinephrine, corticosteroids, parenteral antihistamines, and oxygen are employed quickly.

ALTERNATIVES TO PENICILLIN

If a person is allergic to penicillin, he can often be given an alternative drug. Erythromycin is similar to penicillin in its effectiveness against gram-positive and gram-negative organisms. It may be used to treat gonorrhea or primary syphilis in patients allergic to penicillin.

Lincomycin is an alternative to penicillin in that it is effective against the same gram-positive organisms. It is not, however, effective against gonorrhea, and it is not considered a first choice antibiotic for any infection.

The cephalosporin family of antibiotics, cephalothin (Keflin) and cephaloridine (Loridine), are very similar to the penicillins in action. For that reason, they may be called alternatives. They are sometimes used for patients who are allergic to penicillin. There may be a cross-tolerance, however, and patients who are allergic to penicillin may have some hypersensitive reaction to the cephalosporins. These drugs are usually reserved for use against the most serious infections caused by gram-positive, gram-negative, and penicillinase-producing organisms. Cephalothin may cause local reactions when given in repeated intramuscular or intravenous injections. Cephaloridine is less likely to cause these reactions, but is more likely to cause kidney toxicity. Several oral cephalosporin

drugs are now available; two examples are cephalexin monohydrate (Keflex), and cephaloglycin dihydrate (Kafocin).

THE TETRACYCLINES

The tetracyclines are broad-spectrum antibiotics which are bacteriostatic, not bactericidal. Many strains of organisms have acquired resistance to these drugs. The tetracyclines are second choice drugs for gram-negative and gram-positive infections (including venereal disease) that do not respond to first choice bactericidal antibiotics. The tetracyclines are uniquely effective against rickettsial infections, including Rocky Mountain spotted fever. The only other antibiotic effective against this disease is chloramphenicol; tetracycline is the drug of choice. The tetracyclines are also very effective against psittacosis, trachoma, lymphogranuloma venereum, and primary atypical pneumonia caused by *Mycoplasma pneumoniae.*

Adverse Reactions of the Tetracyclines

The tetracyclines are relatively safe drugs, although all three types of adverse reactions can occur. The most common side effect of these drugs is abdominal discomfort with nausea and vomiting. It is not advisable to give milk or food with the tetracyclines, because absorption is inhibited. Antacids, if given for the gastric discomfort, also impair absorption. Diarrhea may occur due to superinfection. Superinfection may also lead to inflammation of the mouth, tongue, throat, and anogenital area.

A side effect that may occur with the tetracyclines is a phototoxic reaction if the patient is exposed to sunlight. Patients taking the drugs should be warned against exposure to the sun and told of the severe sunburn that may occur.

Discoloration of the teeth may occur when these drugs are taken during periods of tooth development, such as the last months of pregnancy, during infancy, and up to eight years of age. Because of the effect on the teeth as well as the possibility of skeletal growth retardation, these drugs are not used for infants or children if at all possible.

If the drug is improperly stored or given after its expiration date, kidney damage may occur. If kidney damage is present which interferes with the excretion of tetracycline, a buildup of the drug could lead to liver damage.

OTHER ANTIBIOTICS

Chloramphenicol

Chloramphenicol (Chloromycetin) has broad-spectrum activity but is reserved for treating serious infections that do not respond to any other anti-infective agent. This drug is not first choice for any infection because of its potential for causing bone marrow depression and leading to blood dyscrasias, including fatal aplastic anemia. Chloramphenicol may be used for treating patients with typhoid fever, rickettsial infections, *Hemophilus influenzae*, and other conditions due to gram-negative organisms.

Gentamicin-Kanamycin-Neomycin-Polymycin Group

These drugs may be applied topically against many gram-negative and gram-positive organisms, taken orally for concentrated local effect in the gastrointestinal tract, or administered parenterally for serious systemic infections. They are particularly effective against gram-negative sepsis and gram-negative urinary tract infections. Gentamicin is the most widely used drug of this group, because it has the broadest spectrum of activity and the least toxicity. Neomycin and kanamycin are used cautiously because of toxicity to the kidney and the acoustic nerve.

None of these drugs cause nephrotoxicity or ototoxicity when applied topically, however; they are therefore often used in ointments, creams, and ophthalmic solutions. When these drugs are taken orally, very little is absorbed; therefore, they may be used to treat diarrhea caused by *E. coli* and Shigella, or to prepare the bowel before abdominal surgery. Kanamycin and neomycin are given orally in hepatic coma to suppress intestinal bacteria that produce ammonia. If fecal spillage occurs during abdominal surgery, kanamycin may be used for instillation directly into the abdominal cavity. This cannot be done however, until after recovery from anesthesia, as the neuromuscular blocking properties of kanamycin could lead to respiratory depression.

Bacitracin and tyrothricin are two more drugs of this group that are used for topical use only. Spectinomycin, another drug of this group, is useful when given in a single large-dose intramuscular injection, for treating acute gonorrheal urethritis, cervicitis, or proctitis which is resistant to penicillin, tetracycline, or other anti-infective agents. Spectinomycin is not effective against syphilis, so serology results must be watched carefully if both diseases are suspected.

Antifungal Antibiotics

Amphotericin B (Fungizone) can be used to treat systemic or local fungus infections. Nystatin (Mycostatin) is used topically only for fungal infections. Neither is effective against dermatophytic fungi (ringworm), which can be treated by oral griseofulvin.

Table 35-1. Antibiotics

Generic Name	Trade Name	How Supplied	Routes	Usual Dose	Comments
potassium penicillin G		vials 5,000,000 U. for reconstitution	I.M. I.V.	varies greatly with severity of infection	With refrigeration, drug retains its potency for 1 week after reconstitution.
		tablets 125 mg., 250 mg., 500 mg. syrup 125 mg. or 250 mg./5 cc.	P.O.		
potassium phenoxymethyl penicillin	V-Cillin K	tablets 125 mg., 250 mg., 500 mg. oral solution 125 mg./5 cc. 250 mg./5 cc.	P.O.	varies greatly with severity of infection	After mixing, store oral solution in refrigerator.
benzathine penicillin	Bicillin	vials 300,000 U./cc. 600,000 U./cc.	I.M.	dosage varies with age and condition	Shake vials vigorously. For deep I.M. injection only. Vary injection site.

procaine pen. G. - gonorrhea I.M.

Generic Name	Trade Name	How Supplied	Routes	Usual Dose	Comments
ampicillin	Polycillin *Penbritin*	suspension 125 mg., 250 mg., or 500 mg./5 cc. capsules 250 mg., 500 mg. chewable tablets 125 mg. pediatric drops 100 mg./cc. vials 125 mg., 250 mg., 500 mg., 1.0 Gm., 2.0 Gm. for reconstitution	P.O. I.M. I.V.	250–500 mg. 3–4 times/day. Large doses may be needed for severe infections. Children's doses should be calculated according to weight.	Patients should continue the medication at least 48–72 hrs. after all symptoms have subsided. I.V. solution should be given slowly to avoid the untoward reaction of seizures.
sodium cephalothin	Keflin	ampuls 1 Gm., 2 Gm., 4 Gm., for reconstitution	intra-peritoneal I.V. I.M.	adult: 500 mg.–1 Gm. q. 4–6h. children: 100 mg./kg. body weight daily, in divided doses	With refrigeration, drug maintains its potency for 48 hrs. after reconstitution. All cephalosporins will cause a false positive reaction for glucose with Clinitest tablets but *not* with Tes-Tape.
cephalexin monohydrate	Keflex	capsules 250 mg., 500 mg., 1 Gm.	P.O.	250 mg. q. 6h.	If daily dose greater than 4 Gm. is required, parenteral cephalosporins should be considered.
tetracycline hydrochloride	Achromycin	capsules 500 mg., 250 mg., 100 mg. syrup 125 mg./5 cc. pediatric drops 100 mg./20 gtts. or 1 cc. ophthalmic ointment 1% in 1/8 oz. tubes topical ointment 3% in 1/2 and 1 oz. tubes vials 100 mg., 250 mg. for reconstitution vials 100 mg., 250 mg., 500 mg. with vitamin C for reconstitution	P.O. ophthalmic topical I.M. I.V.	P.O.: adult: 1–2 Gm. daily divided in two or four equal doses. child: 25–50 mg./kg. of body weight I.M.: adult: 250 mg. given in divided doses at 8–12h. intervals. children: 15–25 mg./kg. up to 250 mg. daily I.V.: adult: 250–500 mg. q. 12h. children: 12 mg./kg. daily	Therapy should continue at least 24–48 hours after symptoms subside. After reconstitution of parenteral solutions, store at room temperature. I.M. solutions retain potency for 24 hours. I.V. solutions retain potency for 12 hours. Dosage I.V. should never exceed 2 Gm. per 24 hours.

Generic Name	Trade Name	How Supplied	Routes	Usual Dose	Comments
gentamicin sulfate	Garamycin	vials 2 cc. 10 mg./cc. 40 mg./cc. disposable syringes 1.5 cc. syringe 60 mg. 2 cc. syringe 80 mg.	I.M. I.V.	I.M., I.V.: adults over 60 kg. body weight: 80 mg. t.i.d.; adults under 60 kg. body weight; 60 mg. t.i.d.; children: 3–5 mg./kg./24h.	Patients treated with gentamicin injectable should be observed closely for vestibular and auditory toxicity, particularly those with preexisting renal damage.
		topical 0.1% cream 0.1% ointment	topical	topical: small amount applied gently t.i.d. or q.i.d.	
		ophthalmic solution 0.3% in 5 cc. bottles ophthalmic ointment 0.3% in 1/8 oz. tubes	ophthalmic	solution: 1 or 2 gtts. q. 4h. ointment: applied b.i.d. or t.i.d.	
nystatin	Mycostatin	tablets 500,000 U. oral suspension 100,000 U./cc.	P.O.	1–2 tablets t.i.d. 4–6 cc. q.i.d.	Suspension should be retained in the mouth for as long as possible before swallowing.
		vaginal tablets 100,000 U.	vaginal	1–2 tablets q.d.	Appliance for placing the tablets high in the vagina should be used.
		cream 100,000 U./Gm. in 15 Gm. or 30 Gm. tubes. ointment 100,000 U./Gm. in 15 Gm. or 30 Gm. tubes powder 100,000 U./Gm. in 15 Gm. bottles.	topical	Apply liberally b.i.d.	

REFERENCES

Brown, William J. "Acquired Syphilis—Drugs and Blood Tests." *American Journal of Nursing* 71:713, April 1971.

Lee, Richard V. "Antimicrobial Therapy." *American Journal of Nursing* 73:2044, December 1973.

Rodman, Morton J. "Drugs for Respiratory Tract Infection." *RN* 34:55, September 1971.

Rodman, Morton J. "Drugs for Bacterial Pneumonia." *RN* 34:55, November 1971.

APPLICATION QUESTIONS

I. *True-False*

For each statement below, write **a** if the statement is true or **b** if it is false.

_____ 1. Bacteriostatic drugs are used to kill bacteria which cause infection.

_____ 2. A broad-spectrum antibiotic can be used to treat any gram-positive or gram-negative organism.

_____ 3. If an organism fails to grow on agar that has been treated with a specific antibiotic, the organism is considered resistant to that drug.

_____ 4. Patients should be instructed to stop taking antibiotics as soon as symptoms of the infection subside.

_____ 5. Combining a large amount of one antibiotic with a small quantity of another antibiotic tends to result in the emergence of resistant strains of organisms.

_____ 6. Long-term administration of penicillin G has proved effective in preventing repeated streptococcal infections in patients subject to recurrent attacks.

_____ 7. The only antibiotic effective against the common cold virus is penicillin G.

_____ 8. Instilling kanamycin into the abdominal cavity during surgery can cause further respiratory depression.

_____ 9. Kanamycin and neomycin are poorly absorbed when taken orally and can therefore be used to control organisms in the bowel.

_____ 10. Penicillin G is most effective against gram-positive organisms but has no effect on gram-negative organisms.

_____ 11. A penicillinase-resistant penicillin should be used if a patient is allergic to penicillin G.

_____ 12. Kidney toxicity rarely occurs with tetracycline therapy unless there is a preexisting kidney impairment.

II. *Multiple Choice*

For each of the following questions, indicate the letter providing the *best* answer.

_____ 1. Which of the following drugs is bacteriostatic and not bactericidal? (a) penicillin G (b) penicillin V (c) ampicillin (d) tetracycline

_____ 2. What are the most common adverse reactions to occur with the penicillins? (a) direct tissue toxicity (b) allergic reactions (c) superinfections

_____ 3. What is the advantage of penicillin V over penicillin G? (a) it has a more prolonged action (b) it is more stable in gastric juice (c) it has fewer side effects (d) it can be given intravenously

_____ 4. Which of the following drugs cannot be used safely for a patient who is allergic to penicillin? (a) lincomycin (b) cephalosporin (c) carbenicillin (d) erythromycin

_____ 5. Ampicillin could be used in treating which of the following situations? (a) a urinary tract infection by *E. coli* (b) Rocky Mountain spotted fever (c) a pseudomonas infection in a third degree burn (d) a systemic fungus infection

_____ 6. What percentage of patients experience allergic reactions to penicillin? (a) less than 1 percent (b) 1 to 10 percent (c) 20 to 30 percent (d) 30 to 50 percent

_____ 7. Why is probenecid sometimes given with massive doses of penicillin? (a) to reduce toxic effects of penicillin (b) to slow the absorption of penicillin (c) to delay the elimination of penicillin by the kidney (d) to prevent organisms from becoming resistant to penicillin

_____ 8. Which of the penicillins listed below is claimed to be better absorbed after a meal than on an empty stomach? (a) dicloxacillin (b) penicillin V (c) cloxacillin (d) carbenicillin

_____ 9. The nurse is about to give an injection of penicillin when the patient comments, "I was allergic to penicillin once, but it doesn't seem to be bothering me this time." Which of the following would be an appropriate nursing action? (a) withhold the injection (b) give the injection with an antihistamine (c) give the injection and record the comment

_____ 10. Which of the following best describes an anaphylactic reaction? (a) there is a generalized fluid shift from intracellular to extracellular spaces, resulting in congestive heart failure (b) there is a relative loss of blood due to peripheral vascular collapse, leading to inadequate tissue perfusion (c) there is diffuse vasoconstriction, resulting in hypertension and poor tissue perfusion (d) vascular collapse in the brain leads to cerebral edema, seizures, and coma

_____ 11. Which of the following drugs is *not* considered useful in treating gonorrhea? (a) penicillin G (b) tetracycline (c) erythromycin (d) Chloromycetin

_____ 12. Why is tetracycline rarely given to children under 8 years of age? (a) it may cause discoloration of the teeth (b) it may increase the rate of bone growth (c) it may cause chronic kidney damage (d) it may cause vision impairment

_____ 13. When advising a patient about the phototoxic reactions that may occur with the tetracyclines, which of the following cautions would be relevant? (a) wear dark glasses (b) avoid prolonged skin exposure to sunlight (c) don't drive a car at night (d) wear dark clothing in preference to colors which reflect light

_____ 14. What action would you take if an order was written for tetracycline 250 mg. P.O. q.i.d., and you observed the medicine ticket written as: "Tetracycline P.O. 250 mg. 9AM—1PM—5PM—9PM"? (a) change the times of the medicine ticket to 12MN—6AM—12N—6PM (b) call the doctor and question the dose (c) add on the ticket, "after meals and with h.s. snack" (d) no change needed

_____ 15. Rickettsial infections are most quickly controlled with which of the following antibiotics? (1) tetracycline (2) chloramphenicol (3) cephaloridine (4) gentamicin (5) penicillin (a) 4 (b) 1, 3 (c) 1, 2 (d) 2, 5 (e) 3, 4, 5

_____ 16. What is the most dangerous side effect of chloramphenicol? (a) kidney toxicity (b) liver toxicity (c) aplastic anemia (d) anaphylactic reaction (e) electrolyte imbalance

_____ 17. Which of the following drugs is *not* considered nephrotoxic when used systemically? (a) neomycin (b) penicillin G (c) cephalothin (Keflin) (d) kanamycin

_____ 18. Of the following, which would be the drug best suited for treating sepsis caused by a gram-negative bacillus? (a) penicillin G (b) amphotericin B (c) gentamicin

_____ 19. Which of the following organisms is a gram-negative organism? (a) Streptococcus (b) Staphylococcus (c) Pseudomonas (d) Gonococcus

_____ 20. Oral kanamycin and neomycin would be used in which of the following clinical situations? (a) gram-positive sepsis (b) gram-positive meningitis (c) hepatic coma (d) Pseudomonas urinary tract infection

_____ 21. Which of the following drugs is useful in controlling ringworm infections? (a) amphotericin B (b) nystatin (c) griseofulvin (d) bacitracin

III. *Discussion*

For each patient statement given below, write **a** if teaching is needed, or **b** if no teaching is needed. If teaching is needed, outline the content you would include.

_____ 1. "This antibiotic upsets my stomach some, so I just take it with a glass of milk."

_____ 2. "The doctor said I should stop by for a renewal of my tetracycline prescription. I've got to hurry, though, the kids are waiting for me—we're going to the beach."

_____ 3. "You know, the antibiotic sure has seemed to clear up this chest infection, but now I have an awful vaginal infection. You'd think the antibiotic would clear that up too, wouldn't you?"

_____ 4. "My four-year-old seems to have gotten my respiratory infection. I think I'll just give her some of that tetracycline the doctor gave me."

IV. *Calculation*

_____ 1. An order reads, "Weigh child and administer tetracycline 15 mg./lb. daily, divided into 4 doses." You weigh the child and record the weight at 80 pounds. (a) What is the total daily dose of tetracycline? (b) If the daily dose is given in four equal doses, how much would be given at one time? (c) If tetracycline syrup is on hand labeled 125 mg./5 cc., how much syrup would you give for one dose?

_____ 2. The doctor orders penicillin G 600,000 units I.V. On hand you have a vial of powdered penicillin G labeled 1,000,000 units. You want to give an injection of 1.5 cc. How much diluent would you add to the powder to achieve the dosage of 600,000 U./1.5 cc.?

36

Synthetic Anti-infectives

This chapter deals with eight categories of synthetic anti-infective drugs: (1) the sulfonamides; (2) other drugs for treating urinary tract infections; (3) drugs for treating tuberculosis (including the antibiotics and nonantibiotics used for this disease); (4) drugs used in the treatment of leprosy; (5) antiviral chemotherapy; (6) antimalarial drugs; (7) antiamebic drugs; and (8) anthelmintics.

THE SULFONAMIDES

The sulfonamides were the first significant chemicals developed for treating systemic infections. The sulfonamides are now rarely the first choice for treating systemic infections, because of the introduction of antibiotics; because many bacteria are now resistant to sulfonamides; and because these drugs are bacteriostatic, not bactericidal. They are useful for patients who are allergic to penicillin and in some other specific situations.

Uses for Sulfonamides

The most common use for sulfonamides today is in the treatment of urinary tract infections, especially those caused by the gram-negative organism E. coli. In these infections, drugs such as sulfisoxazole (Gantrisin) are given by mouth and rapidly excreted. Because of their rapid excretion, they quickly reach high levels in the urine. In fact, the drug may reach such high concentrations as to be bactericidal in the urine.

Some chronic urinary tract infections may be treated with more slowly excreted sulfonamides such as sulfamethoxypyridazine (Kynex). The main disadvantage to long-lasting sulfonamides is that if allergy or toxicity develops, the untoward effects may last for several days until all of the drug is excreted.

The sulfonamides may also be used in the treatment of some cases of meningitis caused by meningococci or *Hemophilus influenzae*. In addition, drugs such as succinylsulfathiazole (Sulfasuxidine) may be given orally to prepare the bowel before surgery. The latter drug is very poorly absorbed and therefore reaches high concentrations in the intestines.

Although topical sulfonamides were widely used at one time, they are not used frequently any more. They have been found to be a common cause of allergy and sensitization to the chemical. Their only topical use now is for the mucous membranes of the vagina, rectum, eye, and ear. Mafenide acetate (Sulfamylon) has been found particularly useful in treating second and third degree burns. This drug retains its antibacterial properties even in the presence of pus and necrotic tissue. It is effective against *Psuedomonas aeruginosa,* which is a common cause of infection in burn areas. Close monitoring of the patient's acid-base balance is necessary when using mafenide acetate, as it can lead to metabolic acidosis. Impaired pulmonary or renal function tends to exaggerate the carbonic anhydrase inhibition, and metabolic acidosis may develop more rapidly in such cases.

Sulfonamides are sometimes effective against fungal and protozoal infections. They may be used to treat chloroquine-resistant cases of malaria.

Adverse Reactions to Sulfonamides

The sulfonamides can cause severe and even fatal reactions in some patients. Various gastrointestinal disturbances may occur with these drugs. Periodic kidney function tests may be ordered to detect renal damage. Because these drugs can cause crystalluria, the nurse should *always* force fluids for any patient receiving a sulfonamide drug. Other adverse reactions include blood dyscrasias, which may be serious; laboratory studies should be done to detect the possibility of agranulocytosis, thrombocytopenia, aplastic anemia, or acute hemolytic anemia.

Dermatological reactions of many kinds may occur with sulfonamides. The patient should be cautioned against excessive exposure to sunlight while taking these drugs, because they may cause photosensitivity. A more serious dermatologic reaction, the Stevens-Johnson syndrome, is manifested as blisters on the skin or mucous membranes. Bleeding may occur into the center of these lesions, giving them a bulls-eye appearance. These blisters, if present in the respiratory tract, may be severe enough to cause death. Another complication is exfoliative dermatitis, which may occur with or without periods of fever.

Special cautions are raised for infants and for patients with impaired liver function. Since such patients lack the enzyme necessary for detoxification of the drugs, toxic levels could occur quickly. Sulfonamides are also used with caution for pregnant women, because the drugs may cross the placental barrier.

OTHER DRUGS FOR TREATING URINARY TRACT INFECTIONS

Because of the frequent emergence of resistant strains of organisms and the possibility of sensitization and subsequent allergic reactions, there is a need for alternative drugs to the sulfonamides, especially in the treatment of chronic urinary tract infections. Methenamine mandelate and nitrofurantoin are two such alternative drugs. Organisms do not usually become resistant to these drugs. Methenamine breaks down in acid urine to form the bactericidal substance formaldehyde. Methenamine is given in combination with an acidifier such as mandelate, hippurate, or sulfosalicylate. If the patient's urine is difficult to acidify, these drugs may need to be supplemented with additional urine acidifiers such as ammonium chloride or ascorbic acid. Patients should test urine pH regularly, as formaldehyde will not form in a pH higher than 5.5.

Phenazopyridine hydrochloride (Pyridium) has a very weak urinary antiseptic action; however, its usefulness in treating urinary tract infections lies in its anesthetic effect on urinary tract mucosa. This drug is usually given in combination with another drug indicated for urinary tract infections, in order to relieve pain, burning, and urgency accompanying the disorder. Patients should be told that this azo dye drug will cause their urine to be colored orange or red, so that they do not become alarmed at the color and believe there is blood in the urine. Patients with urinary tract infections maintained on medications containing azo dye should have their urine checked for the presence of blood, as hematuria may not be noticeable on gross observation of the urine.

TREATMENT OF TUBERCULOSIS

Although tuberculosis is not as prevalent in the United States as it is in many other countries, several hundred thousand Americans have the disease, many of whom remain undiagnosed. Pharmacology has played an important role in changing the treatment for this disease and removing the stigma it once carried. People are no longer sent to sanitariums for long periods of time, nor do they undergo surgery for collapsing and resting the lungs.

Tuberculosis can usually be controlled with longterm drug therapy at home after only a brief stay at the hospital. Clinical improvement may occur rapidly when the patient begins medical therapy. He may be symptom free and believe he is cured. The challenge to the health team is to encourage the patient continually to take his medication for many months as prescribed, even though he is feeling fine. The patient needs to be informed that cessation of his drug will not only cause a personal danger by allowing the disease to become active again, but will also threaten those he lives with and comes in contact with daily.

Tuberculosis Management With Primary Drugs

There are five first-line drugs for tuberculosis: isoniazid (INH); aminosalicylic acid (PAS); streptomycin; ethambutal hydrochloride; and rifampin. These drugs are the most effective against the disease and have a wide margin of safety. Antituberculosis drugs are never given singly; they are given in combinations of two or more to slow the development of strains resistant to any one drug.

Isoniazid.   Isoniazid (INH) is the single most effective antituberculosis drug. It is usually given orally in small daily doses, in combination with PAS or ethambutal hydrochloride. It is not expensive for the patient and may be used prophylactically to prevent subclinical cases or healed cases from flaring up.

Chemoprophylaxis is recommended for children under six who have been exposed to the disease, because they are more likely to develop tuberculosis meningitis or miliary tuberculosis (generalized or "extrapulmonary" tuberculosis). Chemoprophylaxis should also be given to people with positive tuberculosis skin tests whose normal body defenses may be disturbed by such conditions as poorly controlled diabetes, any severe or chronic disease state, or therapy with corticosteroid drugs.

A few patients are hypersensitive to INH and may develop hepatitis. Initial and periodic liver function tests are advisable. In addition, INH should be kept out of the reach of children, as an overdose can cause convulsions and coma.

Aminosalicylic Acid.   A patient who is taking aminosalicylic acid (PAS) as one of his antituberculosis drugs may need much encouragement to continue taking the medication. This drug may cause heartburn, nausea, and other gastrointestinal discomforts. Encourage the patient to take the drug after meals to minimize some of its unpleasant effects.

Ethambutol Hydrochloride. This drug is now substituted for PAS in many instances, because its side effects do not seem as bothersome. This drug has the potential to cause optic neuritis when taken in large doses. This effect seldom occurs with ordinary doses, but the patient taking this drug should be encouraged to seek periodic ophthalmoscopic exams.

Streptomycin. This antibiotic is reserved for use when cavities are in the lung, for miliary tuberculosis, or for triple drug therapy if needed. Resistance to streptomycin develops very quickly, and the drug may cause acoustic nerve damage. Patients should have their hearing checked frequently if they are maintained on this drug. Another disadvantage of streptomycin is that it cannot be given orally, and intramuscular injection may be painful.

Rifampin. This is the newest of the antituberculosis drugs; it has been found very effective in combination with INH. The disadvantages of this drug include its high cost to the patient as well as the fact that not enough time has passed to determine whether resistant strains will develop.

Alternative Drug Therapy for Tuberculosis

Second-line drugs have a smaller safety margin and are used to treat tuberculosis only when those in the first choice group fail. Viomycin can cause kidney damage and hearing loss, and has the potential for developing allergies. Cycloserine causes a central toxicity that may lead to such symptoms as headache, drowsiness, confusion, tremors, and convulsions. Capreomycin can cause sterile abscesses if not administered very deep into the muscle. It is also toxic to the kidney and the acoustic nerve.

DRUGS USED IN THE TREATMENT OF LEPROSY

Leprosy (Hansen's disease) can be cured today. Some signs and symptoms improve immediately after drug therapy is initiated, and healing of all lesions can be completed in two to three years if the disease is diagnosed early.

The Sulfones

Drugs in this class are chemically related to the sulfonamides and are the most effective drugs for treating leprosy. Dapsone, considered the most useful leprostatic drug, is taken orally in small doses. Gastrointestinal disturbances and allergic skin rashes may occur as side effects when small doses are taken. Large doses may cause hemolysis of red blood cells.

In some patients, the sulfones may trigger a severe form of the disease. If the disease appears to be worsening as a result of drug therapy, the drug is discontinued and corticosteroids are given for a few days. After the inflammation subsides, the sulfones are again administered, but in very small doses which are increased very cautiously.

Nonsulfone Drugs

Some nonsulfone leprostatic drugs are available, such as clofazimine and thalidomide. Clofazimine has been found to cause red and black pigmentation in light-skinned people. Thalidomide is the drug found to cause severe birth defects when taken by pregnant women during the first trimester. These drugs are reserved for treating the rare cases that become resistant to the sulfones.

ANTIVIRAL CHEMOTHERAPY

Viral diseases are difficult to treat with drugs. Some viruses mutate so frequently that drugs quickly become ineffective.

Amantadine hydrochloride (Symmetrel) is a drug proved effective for preventing influenza by certain strains of A_2 type virus. It is not useful after influenza symptoms develop, but it may be used prophylactically after a person has been exposed to the virus. It should be taken for ten days or more during an epidemic year. Side effects of the drug include difficulty in concentrating, ataxia, lightheadedness, giddiness, blurred vision, slurred speech, and feelings of being "drunk." With large doses or in individuals with a history of arteriosclerosis or epilepsy, more serious side effects may develop, including insomnia, nervousness, depression, feelings of depersonalization, hallucinations, and convulsions. Patients with Parkinson's disease may require lower doses of antiparkinsonism drugs when taking amantadine hydrochloride to prevent central nervous system toxicity.

Idoxuridine is a topical antiviral drug used for treating eye infections caused by the herpes virus. It is most effective when viral invasion is still only superficial on the cornea.

All antiviral drugs are potentially quite toxic. A drug that interferes with a virus may also interfere with the metabolism of the cell the virus has invaded.

Because the body can produce a substance called interferon, which is a natural defense against viral invasions, scientists are searching for a means of stimulating production of this substance. However, no such agents are available for therapeutic use at this time.

ANTIMALARIAL DRUGS

Four species of protozoa can cause the parasitic disease, malaria. We shall discuss two of them here: *Plasmodium vivax*, the cause of benign tertian malaria; and *Plasmodium falciparum*, the cause of malignant tertian malaria. *P. vivax* is less severe, less likely to have an explosive course, and less likely to be fatal than *P. falciparum*.

The female anopheles mosquito ingests protozoan gametocytes from an infected person. They mate in the mosquito's stomach and form zygotes, which in turn become sporozoites and find their way to the mosquito's salivary glands. The next person bitten by the mosquito is thus injected with sporozoites. These go directly to the individual's liver, where they reproduce by cell division. They burst forth from the liver, invade red blood cells, and continue their cell division, bursting from cells and invading more red cells. When red cells rupture, the infected person feels chills. The body's response to the liberated spores then brings about fever. *P. vivax* malaria can have relapses as some schizonts make their way back to the liver and tissue cells and periodically send forth more invaders. These are called exo-erythrocytic forms. *P. falciparum* does not cause relapses, because no exo-erythrocytic schizonts persist.

Antimalarial drugs are capable of controlling plasmodial parasites at one or more stages in their life cycle. Theoretically, this disease could be prevented if everyone took an antimalarial pill every week. This, of course, is not practical in view of difficulties in achieving individual cooperation, in addition to problems of expense and toxicity. Instead of using drugs, public health practitioners are trying to control the disease by controlling mosquitoes and encouraging individuals to protect themselves from mosquito bites.

Small doses of chloroquine, hydroxychloroquine, or amodiaquin given to a person infected by the mosquito will suppress symptoms and prevent destruction of erythrocytes. These same drugs can be used for a clinical cure by quickly terminating an acute attack, but they do not cure the disease, and people infected with *P. vivax* are subject to relapses. Primaquine, pyrimethamine, and chlorguanide can

destroy or sterilize the gametocytes, as well as kill schizonts. A radical cure—killing exo-erythrocytic schizonts—can occur with primaquine.

If malaria becomes resistant to chloroquine, drugs such as quinine and certain sulfonamides may be used.

Travelers to areas in which malaria is prevalent cannot keep from being bitten. Such people should take, on a weekly basis, a tablet that combines one of the drugs used for suppressive or clinical treatment with a small dose of primaquine. Treatment should begin at least one day before arrival in the area and continue for eight weeks after departure from the area.

ANTIAMEBIC DRUGS

Amebiasis is caused by the protozoan *Entamoeba histolytica*. It occurs in the United States in residential institutions and in areas in which sanitary conditions are substandard. A person can be affected with amebiases in one of several ways. He may be an asymptomatic carrier. He may have mild intestinal symptoms. He may have acute amebic dysentery, with bowel movements so frequent and severe that dehydration and death quickly occur. He may have extraintestinal amebiasis, including amebic hepatitis and liver abscess. Extraintestinal amebiasis occurs when amebae break through the intestinal wall and travel through the blood to the liver, lungs, and other organs.

The disease is spread by amebic cysts passed in the feces of infected persons. The cysts are very resistant to the environment and can survive for several weeks. They are picked up by other people or by flies and ingested on contaminated food. In the small intestine, the amebae break out of the cysts and form trophozoites, which in turn set up large colonies in the colon and rectum.

Some drugs used in the treatment of amebiasis are poorly absorbed and concentrate in the intestines. These drugs are not useful, of course, for treating extraintestinal amebiasis. Acute amebic dysentery may be treated with a broad-spectrum antibiotic such as oxytetracycline, in combination with an organic iodide such as di-iodohydroxyquin or an aresenical such as carbarsone.

Emetine and dehydroemetine are reserved for treating severe dysentery that does not respond to other drugs, and for extraintestinal infections. These drugs are very toxic and can cause severe heart damage as well as aching at the injection site. Patients usually require hospitalization during treatment. Emetine does not actually cure the disease.

Metronidazole (Flagyl) was recently the drug of choice only for trichomonas vaginitis. It has now been found useful for all forms of amebiasis; it may be the drug of choice, because it can cure intestinal amebiasis and is much safer than emetine.

Amebic hepatitis and liver abscess are treated with emetine, chloroquine, or metronidazole (Flagyl). Asymptomatic carriers may be treated with di-iodohydroxyquin or metronidazole.

Travelers to areas where amebiasis is prevalent may take drugs such as di-iodohydroxyquin or iodochlorhydroxyquine for prophylaxis. This practice is questionable because its effectiveness has not been proven, and peripheral and central nerve damage can occur, including inflammation and atrophy of the optic nerve.

ANTHELMINTICS

When a person is infected with worms, it is important to determine the kind of worm involved. Specific drugs used for pinworms, roundworms, threadworms, hookworms, tapeworms, and trichinosis are discussed below.

Pinworms (Enterobiasis). This condition may be treated with piperazine citrate, pyrvinium pamoate, or pyrantel pamoate. Although a single dose of pyrvinium pamoate usually eradicates pinworms, many physicians still prefer daily doses of piperazine citrate for a week. Taking the drug over a period of time may serve as a reminder about health habits. The patient and all members of his household need to be instructed about frequent handwashing, the importance of taking a shower in the morning to wash away eggs laid around the anus during the night, and the importance of disinfecting the bathroom, bedclothes, and toilet seats.

Roundworms (Ascariasis). These worms are very susceptible to piperazine citrate taken daily for one week. If other worms are present, it is important to treat the roundworms first or use a drug to treat both types of worms. Hexylresorcinol is one drug used to treat both roundworms and hookworms.

Threadworms (Strongyloides). These worms are seen in the southern parts of the United States, as well as the tropics. At one time, it was difficult to treat this parasite, but a new broad-spectrum antibiotic, thiabendazole (Mintezol), has proved to be effective for threadworm. This drug has also demonstrated effectiveness against pinworm, roundworm, and both types of hookworm.

Whipworm (Trichuriasis). Whipworms localize in the mucosa of the cecum and rarely burrow deeper. Mildly infected patients may require no treatment, but those requiring treatment may use the drug hexylresorcinol.

Hookworm (Uncinariasis). This is a debilitating condition because it causes damage to the intestine as well as anemia. Correction of anemia and fluid and electrolyte imbalance must be done before beginning treatment with anthelmintics. There are two types of hookworm, *Necator americanus,* the most common in the western hemisphere, and *Ancylostoma duodenale. Necator americanus* is readily treated by tetrachloroethylene. This drug increases the chances of complications with roundworms, however, if they are present. Therefore, in the presence of roundworms or for treatment of *Ancylostoma duodenale,* the drug bephenium hydroxynaphthoate is preferred. However, this drug is so bitter to the taste that it may cause gagging and even vomiting.

Tapeworms. This worm may be found in beef, fish, or pork. Infection with beef or fish tapeworm is not usually serious, and treatment is instituted more for psychological reasons. Pork tapeworm, which is not common in the United States, is potentially more serious, because the larvae may be carried by the blood to other organs and tissues of the body. The drug of choice for tapeworm is quinacrine.

Trichinosis (Trichinella). The most damaging effects of trichinosis occur when the larvae reach the skeletal muscles. There are no chemotherapeutic agents effective against this parasite. Corticosteroids may be used to treat the inflammatory process in the muscle, but this is only symptomatic treatment.

REFERENCES

DiPalma, Joseph R. "Drugs for Malaria." *RN 30:*77, January 1967.

Hughes, Sr. Ann Elizabeth, et al. "Nurses at Carville." *American Journal of Nursing 68:*2564, December 1968.

Rodman, Morton J. "Combating Urinary Tract Infections." *RN 31:*59, November 1968.

Burns

Henley, Nellie L. "Sulfamylon for Burns." *American Journal of Nursing 69:*2122, October 1969.

Jacoby, Florence. "Current Nursing Care of the Burned Patient." *Nursing Clinics of North America 5:*563, December 1970.

Table 36–1. Synthetic anti-infectives

Generic Name	Trade Name	How Supplied	Routes	Usual Dose	Comments
sulfisoxazole	Gantrisin	tablets 0.5 Gm. pediatric suspension and syrup 0.5 Gm./5 cc. chocolate and raspberry flavors lipogantrisin 1 Gm./5 cc. vanilla-mint flavor	P.O.	pediatric: 150 mg./kg./24h. to be divided into 4–6 doses; adult: 4–8 Gm. q.d., to be divided in 4–6 doses	Force fluids. Contraindicated in infants under 2 months of age, pregnancy at term, and lactating mothers.
		ampuls 5 cc. 2 Gm./5 cc. 10 cc. 4 Gm./10 cc.	S.C. I.M. I.V.	100 mg./kg./24h. divided into 3 doses for S.C., 4 doses for I.V., and 2 or 3 doses for I.M.	Maximum: 6 Gm./24 hrs.
sulfamethoxypridazine	Kynex	tablets 500 mg. suspension 250 mg./5 cc.	P.O.	adult: 1 Gm. initially, 0.5 Gm. q.d. thereafter; child: 30 mg./kg. of body weight initially, 15 mg./kg. of body weight q.d. thereafter	Force fluids.
Amino-salicylic acid (PAS)	Pamisyl	tablets 500 mg.	P.O.	12 Gm. divided into 4 doses after meals and at bedtime	Given in combination with other tuberculosis drugs.
isoniazid (INH)	Nydrazid	tablets 100 mg. syrup 10 mg./cc. in 1 pt. bottles vials 10 cc. 100 mg./cc.	P.O. I.M.	adult: 5 mg./kg. daily up to 300 mg.; child: 10–30 mg./kg. body weight daily, up to 300–500 mg. total	Given in combination with other tuberculosis drugs.
streptomycin sulfate		multiple dose vials 0.5 Gm./cc.	I.M.	1 Gm. twice weekly or daily	Given in combination with other tuberculosis drugs.
rifampin	Rifadin	capsules 300 mg.	P.O.	adult: 600 mg. in single daily dose; child: 10–20 mg./kg., not to exceed 600 mg.	Should be taken one hour before or two hours after meals.
ethambutol hydrochloride	Myambutol	tablets 100 mg., 400 mg.	P.O.	15 mg./kg. body weight daily; varies with condition of patient.	Not recommended for use in children under 13. Given in combination with other tuberculosis drugs. May produce decrease in visual acuity.

Generic Name	Trade Name	How Supplied	Routes	Usual Dose	Comments
chloroquine phosphate	Aralen	tablets 500 mg.	P.O.	Dependent on the diagnosis, ranging from daily doses to weekly doses.	Also available in combination with primaquin. P.O. must be taken on same day each week.
piperazine	Antepar	syrup 500 mg./5 cc. in 1 pt. bottles wafers 500 mg. tablets 500 mg.	P.O.	70 mg./lb. body wt. single dose, or adult: 3.5 Gm. q.d.x2; children: 75 mg./kg. q.d.x2	Maximum dose: 3 Gm. for single dose, 3.5 Gm. q.d. for multiple dose regimen.
metronidazole	Flagyl	tablets 250 mg. vaginal inserts 500 mg.	P.O. vaginal	oral 250 mg. b.i.d. or t.i.d.x10 days, vaginal 500 mg. q.d.x10	Contraindicated in first trimester of pregnancy.
hexylresorcinol	Crystoids	gelatin-coated pills 100 mg., 200 mg.	P.O.	adult: 1 Gm.; children: 8–12 yr., 800 mg.; 6–8 yr., 600 mg.	To be followed by saline cathartic 2–4 hours after dose is taken. Treatment may be repeated in 3 days if required.

MINCKLEY, BARBARA B. "Expert Nursing Care for Burned Patients." *American Journal of Nursing* 70:1888, September 1970.

Tuberculosis

HLOHINEC, EILEEN. "Hospital Care for the Tuberculosis Child." *American Journal of Nursing* 68:1913, September 1968.

KOONZ, FRANCES P. "Nursing in Tuberculosis." *Nursing Clinics of North America* 3:403, September 1968.

McINNIS, JANET K. "Do Patients Take Anti-Tuberculosis Drugs?" *American Journal of Nursing* 70:2152, October 1970.

APPLICATION QUESTIONS

I. *True-False*

For each statement below, write **a** if the statement is true or **b** if it is false.

____ 1. The sulfonamides are useful adjuncts to antibiotic therapy.

____ 2. Reactions to sulfonamides occur most commonly in patients who are allergic or sensitive to other drugs.

____ 3. Sulfonamide drugs may cross the placenta.

____ 4. Uropathogens that are initially sensitive to the urinary antiseptic methenamine mandelate do not ordinarily become resistant.

____ 5. Urine pH must stay at or below 5.5 in order for methenamine mandelate to break down into formaldehyde.

____ 6. The sulfonamides are most useful against gram-positive urinary tract infections.

____ 7. Sulfasuxidine is rapidly absorbed and excreted, thereby reaching a high concentration in the urine.

____ 8. Isoniazid is the most effective drug for the treatment of tuberculosis.

____ 9. Secondary drugs or minor tuberculostatic drugs are safer than primary or major tuberculosis drugs.

____ 10. Viomycin is similar to streptomycin, except that its toxic effects are less.

____ 11. In order to prevent resistance to streptomycin, the drug should be given every other week.

____ 12. Leprosy is also called Hansen's disease.

____ 13. Leprosy is seen only in the tropical parts of the world.

_____ 14. Leprosy can be arrested with chemotherapeutic agents now available.

_____ 15. Large doses of dapsone may lead to hemolysis of red blood cells.

_____ 16. Many antiviral agents are available for the prevention and treatment of specific viral infections.

_____ 17. Symmetrel is effective for treating A_2 type virus influenza.

_____ 18. Amebiasis is a disease found only in the tropics.

_____ 19. In the cyst phase of development, the E. histolytica can survive for several weeks.

_____ 20. E. histolytica cysts are usually destroyed by acid gastric juices.

_____ 21. Emetine is a cure for amebiasis.

_____ 22. Travelers in areas where amebiasis is prevalent should take a drug such as di-iodohydroxyquine to prevent diarrhea.

_____ 23. Metronidazole (Flagyl) has been found to be useful in treating all forms of amebiasis, including extraintestinal infections.

II. *Multiple Choice*

For each of the following questions, indicate the letter providing the *best* answer.

_____ 1. Sulfonamides may be used today to treat which of the following? (a) acute gonorrhea (b) skin infections (c) meningococcal meningitis (d) pneumococcal pneumonia

_____ 2. Patients receiving sulfonamides should follow which of the following regimens regarding fluid intake? (a) drink enough to produce a minimum of 1200 cc. of urine daily (b) drink at least 500 cc. daily (c) limit all fluid intake to water (d) drink enough water to produce 5000 cc. of urine daily

_____ 3. The Stevens-Johnson syndrome, a serious reaction to the sulfonamides, has which of the following characteristic skin lesions? (a) red blotches with raised edges (b) clear blisters with bloody centers (c) fine nondescript rash on chest (d) pus-filled weeping lesions

_____ 4. Which of the following substances acidify urine? (1) ammonium chloride (2) ascorbic acid (3) methenamine mandelate (4) sodium bicarbonate (a) 1, 3 (b) 2, 3 (c) 1, 2, 3 (d) 1, 2, 4 (e) 2, 3, 4

_____ 5. Which of the following electrolyte imbalances may occur when mafenide (Sulfamylon) is used topically in the treatment of burns? (a) respiratory acidosis (b) metabolic acidosis (c) respiratory alkalosis (d) metabolic alkalosis

_____ 6. Which of the following drugs are classified as primary chemotherapeutic agents for tuberculosis? (1) rifampin (2) cycloserine (3) isoniazid (4) capreomycin (a) 1, 3 (b) 2, 4 (c) 1, 4 (d) 2, 3

_____ 7. Which of the following diagnostic tests would be done to detect the dangerous side effects of maintenance therapy with isoniazid? (a) pulmonary function tests (b) BSP (c) EEG (d) myelogram

_____ 8. The danger of tuberculosis meningitis and miliary infections is greatest in which age group? (a) from infancy to school age (b) school age (c) young adults (d) middle-aged adults

_____ 9. Patients being maintained on ethambutol hydrochloride (Myambutol) should be given which of the following examinations frequently to detect the drug's side effects? (a) sigmoidoscopy (b) bone scan (c) EKG (d) ophthalmic examination

_____ 10. Adverse reactions to dapsone (Avlosulfon) can be avoided by beginning treatment in which of the following ways? (a) start with large doses and decrease slowly until adverse reactions disappear (b) start with small dose and increase the weekly intake gradually (c) give high doses of corticosteroid drugs in combination (d) alternate the dosage from large to small weekly

_____ 11. Ill effects from prophylactic doses of amantadine (Symmetrel) include which of the following? (1) depression (2) feelings of depersonalization (3) insomnia (4) convulsions (a) 4 (b) 3, 4 (c) 1, 2, 3 (d) 1, 2, 3, 4

_____ 12. When a person is injected with sporozoites through a mosquito bite, how do the organisms behave? (a) they stay in the bloodstream (b) they go directly to liver (c) they attack the lungs (d) they travel in the bloodstream to human saliva

_____ 13. Which of the following statements would help most to encourage an asymptomatic amebiasis carrier to continue therapy? (a) "Remember, Mr. Jones, you have a responsibility to those around you—you can give them this disease." (b) "Mr. Jones, this disease could really destroy your liver and kill you if you don't take your pills." (c) "It must be difficult to have to take medicine when you don't feel sick, Mr. Jones, but do you remember what this disease could do to you and your family?" (d) "Now, Mr. Jones, I know you are smart enough to realize the importance of taking these drugs."

_____ 14. Hygienic measures directed toward avoiding reinfection with pinworms include which of the following? (1) keeping fingernails short and clean (2) covering mouth when coughing (3) disinfecting toilet seats (4) showering at bedtime (a) 1, 4 (b) 1, 3 (c) 2, 3 (d) 2, 4

____ 15. Which of the following worm infestations is most likely to cause serious complications if left untreated? (a) whipworms (b) hookworms (c) tapeworm (d) pinworm

____ 16. Which of the following worm infestations would most likely be treated first if a patient was infested with all of them simultaneously? (a) hookworm (b) pinworm (c) roundworm (d) threadworm

____ 17. Which of the following clinical pictures might occur in amebiasis? (1) no symptoms at all (2) mild intestinal symptoms (3) acute dysentery (4) hepatitis
(a) 1 (b) 1, 2 (c) 2, 3, 4 (d) 1, 2, 3, 4

____ 18. Which of the following statements regarding activity would be the most therapeutic in beginning to plan for discharge of Mr. Jones, who has just completed a course of emetine therapy? (a) "You'll have to take it easy for awhile, Mr. Jones." (b) "Have you thought about what activities you are going to be able to do, Mr. Jones?" (c) "Be sure to ask your doctor what you can and can't do when you go home." (d) "Have your wife come in and talk to me, Mr. Jones, so we can plan your activities after you go home."

III. *Discussion*

For each patient statement given below, write **a** if teaching is needed, or **b** if no teaching is needed. If teaching is needed, outline the content you would include.

____ 1. "It's awfully hard to get Dad to take his TB medicines. Now that he feels better, it's hard to convince him he's still sick."

____ 2. "I thought only people in the ghettoes got worms —I hope my friends don't find this out."

____ 3. "I guess the worst part of this worm bit is the itching around my rectum, but I've found that my baby's diaper rash medicine helps relieve it."

____ 4. "The doctor said to shower Tracy in the mornings to help get rid of these pinworms. Mornings are so hectic around the house, so I've been giving her a bath at night—it really doesn't make any difference, does it?"

____ 5. "I just found out I have a tapeworm from eating fish. I sure hope the doctor can get it out before it eats up my intestines!"

____ 6. "Actually, I kind of like the taste of rare pork, and if I get that trichinosis worm, I'll just have the doctor give me a pill."

Miscellaneous Therapeutic and Diagnostic Agents

SECTION TEN

Drugs Affecting Gastrointestinal Function

Gastrointestinal symptoms are among the most common patient complaints. Several types of drugs used in the treatment of gastrointestinal symptoms are discussed in previous chapters: the cholinergic drugs for stimulating motility, discussed in Chapter 15; paregoric and opiates for reducing motility, discussed in Chapter 12; and anticholinergics and antacids for peptic ulcer, discussed in Chapter 16. This chapter discusses other drugs used in the treatment of constipation, diarrhea, nausea and vomiting, and indigestion.

THE USE OF CATHARTICS OR LAXATIVES

Cathartics may be used to clear the bowel of fecal material before bowel surgery, abdominal X-ray, or procedures such as proctosigmoidoscopy. They may also be administered before and after administration of anthelmintic medication to aid the action of the anthelmintic and to remove the worms from the intestines. In cases of ingested poisons which have passed the pylorus and can no longer be removed by gastric lavage, cathartics may be employed to flush the poison from the intestine.

The use of laxatives or stool softeners may be indicated in conditions where straining at stool could be very painful or dangerous. These conditions would include myocardial infarction, aneurysm, embolus, and anorectal lesions or surgery. Patients who are immobile or confined to bed may profit from the administration of laxatives or stool softeners, because the lack of exercise, loss of appetite, and the effects of other medications such as narcotic analgesics, all tend to cause a decrease in bowel motility.

Physicians do not order routine laxatives as frequently as they used to; if nurses encourage the use of other measures to prevent constipation, a great many hospitalized patients will have no need for drug-induced bowel evacuation. Ambulation is very important in preventing constipation. Early ambulation is encouraged after surgery, and the nurse should provide regular times for ambulating to the bathroom. The impossibility of natural positioning and the lack of privacy can lead to constipation, so aiding the patient to get to the bathroom or to sit on a bedside commode and providing for his privacy are useful measures. Encouraging a regular, varied diet including fresh fruits and vegetables and insuring adequate hydration will also greatly aid in preventing constipation.

The routine or habitual use of cathartics should be discouraged; this practice is actually one of the most common *causes* of constipation. People need to be taught that infrequent bowel movements do not necessarily indicate poor health, and that *all* people do not need to have a daily bowel movement. However, it is not always easy (or wise) to change the habits of a habitual laxative user. An elderly person who has taken a daily laxative for many years, and who is using a relatively safe agent, may cause no harm by continuing his habit. To judge, reprimand, or shame a patient will not help in changing his habits. The nurse may explain to the patient that when a laxative is taken, the entire intestinal tract is usually emptied. This prevents the colon from filling again for a day or two, so another bowel movement will not occur during this time. If the patient becomes alarmed because of the absence of a bowel movement and takes another cathartic, he begins a vicious cycle whereby he may become psychologically dependent on the laxative and the bowel can become accustomed to the external stimulation. Instead of achieving "natural regularity," then, this patient will have a difficult time ever achieving a natural bowel movement.

Treatment of Chronic Constipation

Any patient with chronic constipation should be

encouraged to see a physician. Although most constipation is caused by irregular dietary and living patterns, a change in bowel habits could indicate intestinal pathology. If there is no pathology, the patient
should be encouraged to eat a regular diet including
foods that leave a bulky residue. One of the bulk-
producing agents discussed below may also be used to
help form a bulkier stool. If the patient drinks plenty
of fluids and establishes regular dietary habits which
include fresh fruits and vegetables, as well as establishing regular daily patterns of living with a decrease
in emotional tension, he should have no further need
for cathartics.

Types of Cathartics

Some cathartics act chemically to stimulate the intestinal muscle directly to contract more forcefully
and frequently. Other agents increase intestinal bulk,
which in turn causes mechanical stimulation of peristalsis. The stool softeners and lubricants do not cause
an increase in bowel activity, but rather, they act to
soften the fecal matter and make it easier to pass.

Irritants.   Castor oil is the only potent irritant presently in clinical use that is capable of emptying the
entire intestinal tract. In the intestines, castor oil is
broken down by fat-splitting enzymes to release ri-
cinoleic acid, a substance which stimulates gastrointestinal motility. This agent leads to the evacuation
of both the small and large intestines; it may be particularly useful prior to X-ray examinations. Castor oil
should never be given at bedtime, because its strong
actions usually occur within several hours and would
cause the patient to have a very uncomfortable and
restless night.

Another class of irritants with a milder action is the
anthraquinone class. These drugs are not useful for
emptying the entire tract, because they act only on the
large intestines. Drugs of the anthraquinone class include cascara sagrada, phenolphthalein, oxyphenisatin acetate, and bisacodyl (Dulcolax). The administration of cascara sagrada can lead to the formation of
a single soft stool about eight hours after it is given.
Oxyphenisatin acetate is usually given rectally to
avoid systemic absorption, because oral administration of this drug sometimes causes jaundice. Bisacodyl
can be given orally at night to produce a bowel
movement in the morning. This drug is also available
in suppository form; it can cause stimulation of colon
motility within minutes after the chemical is brought
in contact with the mucosa of the colon. Phenolphthalein is a common component in many proprietary laxatives, including the popular chocolate and

gum medications. Severe toxicity is rare even if it is
eaten in large quantities by children. Overdose may,
however, lead to a dehydrating diarrhea. Hypersensitivity reactions to phenolphthalein are characterized
by a colorful dermatitis. The itchy, burning patches
may blister and ulcerate. Occasionally, the pink or purple patches retain their color for many months, even
after the condition has cleared up. "Fixed eruption"
may also occur, which is the appearance of identical
lesions in the same places on subsequent exposure to
the drug.

Bulk-forming Laxatives.   Saline cathartics such as
sodium sulfate, sodium phosphate (Fleet enema), and
magnesium sulfate (Epsom salts), are poorly absorbed
salts which cause an increase in intestinal bulk when
given with large amounts of water. Saline cathartics
are best administered in the morning or afternoon, as
they act within one to two hours after their administration.

Hydrophilic colloids and other indigestible fibers
act by forming a bulky, jellyish mass in the intestine.
They have an effect similar to the food residues that
normally stimulate peristalsis. These bulk formers,
such as plantago seed, methylcellulose, psyllium hydrophilic mucilloid (Metamucil), and sodium carboxymethylcellulose, are the most natural and least irritating laxatives. Patients should be told never to take
these products without water, because if they are
swallowed dry, they may pick up just enough water in
the esophagus to swell and obstruct the esophagus.
These agents should be mixed with water and followed by plenty of fluid.

Stool Softeners and Lubricants.   Retention enemas of
olive oil or cottonseed oil can soften and moisten dry,
hardened fecal masses and enable them to be passed
or washed out with a cleansing enema. Mineral oil
may be taken orally or rectally. If it is taken orally, the
oily aftertaste may be decreased by having the patient
suck on an orange slice. Flavored emulsions of mineral oil are available, but these agents are not only
expensive, but they may also lead to systemic absorption of the oil. Mineral oil is best taken at bedtime
and *not* with meals, as it can interfere with the absorption of fat-soluble vitamins. Rectal administration
would, of course, prevent the possible interference
with the absorption of these vitamins and would also
avoid the possibility of aspiration into the lungs.
Mineral oil is unabsorbable; once it gets into the
tissues, it acts as a foreign body. Pneumonia could
therefore result if mineral oil were aspirated into the
lungs.

Surface-active agents act like detergents; they soften stool by reducing the surface tension of fecal contents, permitting water and fatty materials to penetrate to make a more moist and bulky mass. Dioctyl calcium sulfosuccinate (Surfak) and dioctyl sodium sulfosuccinate (Colace) are the most commonly used stool softeners.

Contraindications for Laxatives

As mentioned previously, habitual use of cathartics is undesirable, because it can lead to chronic constipation. Habitual use may also lead to chronic colitis, dehydration, and electrolyte imbalances.

Patients should be warned never to medicate themselves with cathartics when they have abdominal pain, cramps, or are nauseated and vomiting. Drug-induced stimulation of bowel motility may lead to perforation of the inflamed intestinal wall, which in turn can cause peritonitis if the gastrointestinal symptoms are caused by acute appendicitis, enteritis, ulcerative colitis, diverticulitis, or organic bowel obstruction.

DRUGS USED FOR THE RELIEF OF DIARRHEA

Diarrhea may be a symptom of many diseases. Serious complications may result from diarrhea, such as dehydration, electrolyte imbalance, hemoconcentration, and cardiac irregularities. Even when the cause of diarrhea cannot readily be found, the patient is usually provided with symptomatic relief. In addition to the centrally acting opiates and anticholinergic drugs discussed in other chapters, there are locally acting agents that are useful in the control of diarrhea.

Locally Acting Antidiarrheal Drugs

Kaolin and pectin are two commonly used antidiarrheal drugs; they are often given in combination (Kaopectate). Kaolin is an adsorbent which picks up, binds, and removes bacteria, toxins, and other irritants from the intestines. Kaolin also forms a protective coating over the mucosa of the bowel while its adsorptive properties filter out toxins that may be absorbed into the blood. Pectin is a demulcent which soothes the irritated mucosa. It also aids in adsorption.

Attapulgite (Claysorb) is several times more effective than kaolin in adsorptive action. This agent is sometimes suspended in aluminum gel, which also has adsorbent, demulcent, and astringent properties.

Other substances such as activated charcoal and salts of magnesium, aluminum, and bismuth are also used in antidiarrheal preparations. Activated charcoal, although useful for treating poisoning (see Chapter 3), is not really very effective for controlling diarrhea. Magnesium and aluminum salts are more effective as antacids (see Chapter 16) than for controlling diarrhea; and there is little proof of the effectiveness of bismuth salts when taken internally for diarrhea.

Hydroabsorptive Substances.   Ordinarily, most of the fluids in the intestinal contents are absorbed in the large intestine. Excessive peristalsis permits little time for the absorption of fluid as the contents are rushed through; liquid stools thus result. Hydrophilic substances absorb some of the intestinal moisture. The same indigestible fibers used as bulk formers in the treatment of constipation may be used to absorb intestinal fluids in the treatment of diarrhea. Polycarbophil is claimed to act in the alkaline medium of the intestine and not to swell in the stomach to cause an uncomfortable feeling of fullness.

ANTIEMETIC DRUGS

Nausea is a common and very distressing symptom, often accompanied or followed by vomiting. Although vomiting can be useful when it occurs to remove toxins or poisons from the stomach, it often occurs when emptying the stomach contents is not necessary. Vomiting can lead to severe fluid and electrolyte imbalances.

The stimulus for vomiting may originate in the gastrointestinal tract, but it may also originate in other parts of the body. The stimulus may be chemical or psychological in origin. Locally acting or centrally acting antiemetics may be used to provide symptomatic relief of nausea and vomiting regardless of the cause.

Locally Acting Antiemetics

Benzocaine and procaine may be used to reduce the number of afferent impulses arising from the gastrointestinal tract. These short acting topical anesthetics may not be as effective as the longer acting anesthetic, lidocaine. Lidocaine is available as a viscous solution which may control vomiting for several hours when taken in a dose of one tablespoonful. Oxethazine is an anesthetic suspended in alumina gel; it provides a prolonged effect because the gel coats the irritated mucosa.

Volatile oils such as peppermint, clove, ginger, and cinnamon may be given as alcoholic solutions (spirits) or as waters; they give a feeling of warmth in the stomach. They may also help expel gas by causing a reflex increase in gastric motility. Other commonly used antinauseants include Coca Cola syrup and phosphorylated carbohydrate solution (Emetrol), which is similar to Coca Cola syrup. These agents are taken in tablespoonful doses without any other fluids.

Centrally Acting Antiemetics

The first centrally acting antiemetic drugs were the barbiturates and scopolamine. Because of their side effects, these have largely been replaced by other, more specifically acting antiemetics. Centrally acting antiemetics are usually classified as the phenothiazines and the nonphenothiazines. The phenothiazines include agents used as major tranquilizers, and the nonphenothiazines include drugs used as antihistaminic and anticholinergic agents.

Phenothiazines. The phenothiazines, such as chlorpromazine hydrochloride (Thorazine) and prochlorperazine maleate (Compazine), seem to act by reducing the responsiveness of certain brain cells to the emetic stimulus. These brain cells make up an area called the chemoreceptor trigger zone (C.T.Z.), which is especially sensitive to circulating chemicals that cause nausea and vomiting. The phenothiazines block the stimulation of the C.T.Z. Most of the adverse effects of the phenothiazines that occur when they are used in the treatment of mental illness do not occur when they are used as antiemetics, because of the much smaller doses used in the latter situation. The drugs *may* cause muscle spasms and extrapyramidal system reactions, however; since children and young adults are especially susceptible to these reactions, the drugs are not recommended for children under twelve years of age.

Nonphenothiazines. A commonly employed nonphenothiazine drug is dimenhydrinate (Dramamine) which is related to the antihistamine diphenhydramine (Benadryl). The antiemetic effect does not stem from the histamine antagonistic action, but rather from the ability of the drug to block nerve impulses passing between the vestibular portion of the inner ear and the vomiting center in the brain stem. These drugs are thus more effective than the phenothiazines for controlling nausea and vomiting associated with conditions such as Meniere's disease and labyrinthitis, as well as following surgical procedures on the inner ear.

Drowsiness is the most common side effect of dimenhydrinate and diphenhydramine. The more recent drugs such as trimethobenzamide hydrochloride (Tigan), cyclizine (Marezine), and meclizine hydrochloride (Bonine) are claimed to cause less drowsiness and fewer side effects such as dry mouth and

blurred vision. Cyclizine and meclizine hydrochloride are contraindicated for use by pregnant women, because they are teratogenic in experimental animals.

DRUGS USED FOR CONTROLLING INDIGESTION

The terms *indigestion* and *dyspepsia* are used to describe many vague abdominal symptoms. These symptoms may be caused by gastrointestinal irritation or by emotional tension. They are occasionally caused by an actual lack of the chemical substances secreted into the gastrointestinal tract during digestion.

Hydrochloric Acid

Deficiency of gastric acid may occur in various conditions, including pernicious anemia. The administration of dilute hydrochloric acid is said to relieve the vague symptoms of stomach distress in patients with hypochlorhydria or achlorhydria. This solution, when given during and after meals, must be well diluted; it should be given through a glass straw to protect the patient's teeth. After administration, the patient should be offered an alkaline mouthwash. Preparations of betaine hydrochloride or glutamic acid hydrochloride (Acidulin) may be taken in capsules or tablets; these release hydrochloric acid in the stomach. Although these agents do not release much acid, they are safer and more convenient to use.

Digestive Enzymes

Pepsin. Hydrochloric acid is present in the stomach to furnish an optimal medium for the action of pepsin, the enzyme which begins the breakdown of proteins into simpler compounds. If a patient is lacking both pepsin and hydrochloric acid, they are given together. Pepsin alone is not ordinarily lacking, however, and even if it is, the pancreatic and intestinal enzymes can break down protein when it has not been acted upon by pepsin.

Pancreatic Enzymes. Pancrelipase (Cotazym) is a concentrated mixture of pancreatic enzymes recommended for replacement therapy in patients whose pancreas has been surgically removed, or for patients with cystic fibrosis, chronic pancreatitis, or pancreatic duct blockage secondary to neoplastic disease.

Bile Salts and Other Choleretics

Although it contains no enzymes, bile plays an important part in the digestion of fats and is essential for the absorption of the fat-soluble vitamins A, D, E, and K. Bile salts are sometimes useful as replacement therapy for patients with partial biliary obstruction or biliary fistulas, or after cholecystectomy or other surgical procedures on the biliary system which have led to a deficiency of natural bile.

Bile salts also have choleretic action; that is, they stimulate the liver to secrete increased quantities of whole bile. A substance such as dehydrocholic acid that stimulates a flow of *thin, fluid* bile may help to flush out the biliary tract when it is only partially obstructed by mucus or small stones, and keep the passages free of infection and calculi. The sodium salt of this solution, sodium dehydrocholate, is used in some types of biliary tract roentgenography and for the determination of circulation time.

Chenodeoxycholic acid (CDC) is a natural constituent of human bile which has been prepared synthetically; it is being tested in the treatment of patients with gallstones of the cholesterol type. It is thought that this substance may keep cholesterol from becoming supersaturated and crystallizing out in the gallbladder.

Cholestyramine resin (Cuemid, Questran) is a substance that binds bile acids in the intestine before they can be reabsorbed. This drug may be used to lower plasma bile levels in jaundiced patients.

Simethicone

Simethicone (Mylicon) helps to eliminate gastrointestinal gas. It is a defoaming agent which causes small gas bubbles to coalesce, making it easier to expel the gas.

REFERENCES

BESSKEN, P., and MILLER, W. "A Family Copes with Cystic Fibrosis." *American Journal of Nursing* 67:341, February 1967.

Table 37-1. Drugs affecting gastrointestinal function.

Generic Name	Trade Name	How Supplied	Routes	Usual Dose	Comments
oleum ricini	Castor oil	bottles	P.O.	15 cc.	Usually given during waking hours. Give with fruit juice to disguise the taste. Ice held in the mouth before taking dulls the taste.
bisacodyl	Dulcolax	tablets 5 mg.	P.O.	two tablets	Tablets should not be taken within one hour of antacids or milk. Tablets should be swallowed whole, not chewed or crushed.
		suppositories 10 mg.	rectal	one suppository	
kaolin mixture with pectin	Kaopectate	liquid	P.O.	4–30 cc. p.r.n.	
psyllium hydrophilic mucilloid	Metamucil	powder 7 Gm./tsp.	P.O.	one tsp. t.i.d.	Stir powder into glass of cool water. Best results are obtained if followed by another glass of water.
		instant mix 6.4 Gm./packet		1 packet t.i.d.	
dioctyl sodium sulfosuccinate	Colace	capsules 50 mg., 100 mg.	P.O.	50–200 mg. P.O.	Dose should be adjusted to individual response. Liquid may be given orally in milk or juice to mask the taste, or rectally in retention enema.
		syrup 20 mg./tsp.			
		liquid 1% sol. 10 mg./cc.	rectal	50–100 mg. in retention enema	

Generic Name	Trade Name	How Supplied	Routes	Usual Dose	Comments
dimenhydrinate	Dramamine	tablets 50 mg.	P.O.	50 mg. P.O. q. 4h.	I.V. to be given in 10 cc. saline over a two minute period
		liquid 12.5 mg./4 cc.			
		ampuls 1 cc. 50 mg./cc.	I.M. I.V.	50 mg. I.M. and I.V.	
		vials 5 cc. 50 mg./cc.			
		suppository 100 mg.	rectal	one suppository q.d. or b.i.d.	
trimethobenzamide hydrochloride	Tigan	capsules 100 mg., 250 mg.	P.O.	250 mg. t.i.d. or q.i.d.	Deep injection recommended. Not recommended for I.V. use. Injectable form contraindicated in children. Suppositories contraindicated in premature and newborn infants.
		suppository 200 mg.	rectal	one suppository t.i.d. or q.i.d.	
		pediatric suppository 100 mg.			
		ampuls 2 cc. 100 mg./cc.	I.M.	200 mg. I.M. t.i.d. or q.i.d.	
		vials 20 cc. 100 mg./cc.			
thiethylperazine	Torecan	tablets 10 mg.	P.O.	10–30 mg. q.d.	The route which seems practical may be chosen for administration (for example, if a patient is vomiting, the rectal or I.M. route would be preferable). I.V. route is contraindicated. Phenothiazine derivative precautions should be considered. Safety for use in children under 12 has not been established.
		ampuls 2 cc. 5 mg./cc.	I.M.		
		suppository 10 mg.	rectal		
pancrelipase	Cotazym	capsules: lipase: 8,000 U. protease: 30,000 U. amylase: 30,000 U.	P.O.	1–3 capsules just prior to meals or snacks	Use with caution in patients sensitive to pork protein.
		packets: lipase: 16,000 U. protease: 60,000 U. amylase: 60,000 U.		1–2 packets just prior to meals or snacks	
		packets (cherry flavored): lipase: 40,000 U. protease: 150,000 U. amylase: 150,000 U.			

CORMON, MARVIN, et al. "Cathartics." *American Journal of Nursing* 75:273, February 1975.

DOWNS, H. S. "The Control of Vomiting." *American Journal of Nursing* 66:76, January 1966.

MCKITTRICK, JOHN, and SHOTKIN, JANE. "Ulcerative Colitis." *American Journal of Nursing* 62:60, August 1962.

OLSEN, E., ed. "The Hazards of Immobility: Effects on Gastrointestinal Function." *American Journal of Nursing* 67:785, April 1967.

APPLICATION QUESTIONS

I. *True-False*

For each statement below, write **a** if the statement is true or **b** if it is false.

_____ 1. Irritant laxatives are indicated for treating habitual constipation.

_____ 2. A daily bowel evacuation is necessary to maintain bowel muscle tone.

_____ 3. Habitual use of cathartics may cause chronic constipation.

_____ 4. Failure to empty the colon results in toxins being reabsorbed into the body.

_____ 5. Cascara sagrada exerts a strong action on both the small and large intestines.

_____ 6. Antihistaminic antiemetics are more effective than the phenothiazines in treating nausea and vomiting caused by inner ear conditions.

_____ 7. Phenothiazine antiemetics are contraindicated for children under 12 years of age.

_____ 8. When the phenothiazines are being used as antiemetics, the doses are larger than when these drugs are used in the treatment of mental disorders.

II. *Multiple Choice*

For each of the following questions, indicate the letter providing the *best* answer.

_____ 1. It is *imperative* that fluids be forced when which of the following laxatives is given? (a) cascara sagrada (b) psyllium hydrophilic mucilloid (Metamucil) (c) castor oil (d) mineral oil

_____ 2. Which of the following side effects may occur with phenolphthalein? (a) alopecia (b) hiccups (c) thick nails (d) purple skin patches

_____ 3. Which of the following situations would indicate the most urgent need for medical attention? (a) a 40-year-old man who has recently developed an alternating constipation and diarrhea pattern (b) an 80-year-old woman whose bowels rarely move more than 2 or 3 times a week (c) an 18-year-old girl whose bowel habits change only during her menstrual periods (d) a 20-year-old football player who develops diarrhea just prior to each game

_____ 4. Which of the following could result if psyllium hydrophilic mucilloid (Metamucil) were taken in powder form without any fluid? (a) indigestion (b) obstruction of the esophagus (c) dehydration (d) diarrhea

_____ 5. What possible complications might result from taking mineral oil after meals? (1) bleeding gums (2) aspiration (3) irritation of the intestine (4) prevention of vitamin C absorption (a) 2 (b) 1, 3 (c) 1, 2 (d) 2, 3, 4

_____ 6. Which of the following would be the drug of choice for severe reflex vomiting? (a) pepsin (b) lidocaine (c) Maalox (d) benzocaine

_____ 7. Hydrochloric acid should be taken in which of the following ways? (a) after meals (b) before meals with water (c) mixed with food (d) at bedtime and upon rising

_____ 8. How do bile salts function? (1) they aid in fat digestion (2) they increase fat absorption (3) they decrease peristalsis (4) they assist in absorption of vitamin K (a) 1, 2 (b) 3, 4 (c) 1, 2, 3 (d) 1, 2, 4

_____ 9. Which of the following patients would be likely to receive a cathartic or stool softener? (1) a man recovering from a myocardial infarction (2) a woman with abdominal cramps (3) a man scheduled for a barium enema (4) a girl with ulcerative colitis (a) 1, 3 (b) 3, 4 (c) 2, 3 (d) 1, 4

_____ 10. Which of the following responses would be most appropriate when an elderly patient tells you he takes a laxative every night? (a) "We don't let you do that, because we don't want your bowels to get used to having one." (b) "Okay, tell me what you take and I'll get it for you." (c) "That's a *very* bad habit. When you do that, you keep your intestine from acting naturally." (d) "I'm glad you mentioned that. We'll get you something for tonight, and then tomorrow we can talk about some alternatives."

_____ 11. Which of the following questions would be the most helpful to ask when assessing the bowel activity of an immobilized orthopedic patient? (a) "Have your bowels moved today?" (b) "When did your bowels move last?" (c) "Are you constipated?" (d) "Are your bowels moving with the same frequency and consistency as before your hospitalization?"

III. *Discussion*

For each patient statement given below, write **a** if teaching is needed, or **b** if no teaching is needed. If teaching is needed, outline the content you would include.

_____ 1. "Mother is bedridden now, and despite our efforts with fluid and foods, we have to give her a laxative every now and then."

_____ 2. "I know it's a bad habit to take laxatives, so I don't, even though I have a lot of constipation and bad hemorrhoids."

_____ 3. "Since I gave Susie that strong laxative before her worm medicine, I just don't have the heart to give her another one."

_____ 4. "I'm so excited—John said that before the baby is born next spring, we're going to fly to Paris for a last fling. I'm going to take some Bonine before I get on the plane to keep me from getting sick."

38

Drugs Used in Labor and Delivery

This chapter deals with those drugs that act upon the uterus and that are used during labor, delivery, and the postpartum period. The actions and uses of sex hormones for conception and throughout pregnancy are discussed in Chapter 27.

The process of labor is divided into three stages. Stage one begins with the onset of strong regular contractions of the fundus of the uterus and continues until the cervix is fully dilated. Stage two begins when the cervix is fully dilated and continues until the baby is completely delivered. Stage three begins after the baby is delivered and continues until the placenta has separated and is expelled. The time following the third stage of labor is referred to as the puerperium or postpartum, and is characterized by the involution of the uterus as it returns to its pregravid state, which takes about eight weeks.

OXYTOCIC DRUGS

Oxytocics are drugs that act on the smooth muscle of the uterus to increase its tone and motility. Uterine response to oxytocic drugs is related to the stage of pregnancy in which they are used. Large doses are needed in early pregnancy to achieve results similar to those achieved by smaller doses in late pregnancy, during labor, or during the puerperium. Uterine response to these drugs is dose-related, in that small doses may cause contractions and periods of relaxation similar to normal labor; larger doses may cause more powerful and longer-lasting contractions; and excessively high doses may cause sustained tetanic contractions of the uterus.

The two major types of oxytocic drugs employed in labor and delivery are oxytocin and the ergot alkaloids, such as ergonovine and methylergonovine. Oxytocin is one of the two hormones released by the posterior pituitary gland; it is normally responsible for causing uterine contractions. Oxytocic drugs used today, however, are synthetic (such as Pitocin) rather than natural hormones. Only oxytocin is administered to induce labor or to restart labor that has stalled (uterine inertia), because the ergot alkaloids can cause contractions that are too prolonged and too difficult to relax. In addition, oxytocin is considered safer in this situation, because it is more rapidly inactivated and would therefore wear off more quickly even if the uterine response were too strong.

Uses of Oxytocin

Induction of Labor. Early delivery is sometimes desirable for the safety of the mother and baby, as when the mother has diabetes or shows signs of pre-eclampsia, or when her membranes have ruptured prematurely and labor fails to begin spontaneously. Oxytocin is usually given by diluting ten units of the drug in 1000 cc. of an isotonic dextrose solution and administering the solution intravenously at a rate of not more than fourteen drops per minute. Patients receiving intravenous oxytocin should never be left unattended. Continuous observations of the frequency, strength, and duration of uterine contractions must be made, as well as frequent monitoring of fetal heart sounds. Care must be taken to avoid inducing contractions so strong that they force the fetus against the partially dilated cervix and tear cervical tissue, injure the fetus, or cause rupture of the uterine fundus. Sustained uterine spasm may also completely obstruct the blood flow from the mother's arteries into the placenta, causing fetal death or severe birth defects.

Oxytocin may also be given in the form of buccal tablets or by application of a solution to the nasal mucosa. A buccal tablet can be placed between the patient's cheek and gum; more tablets may be added every half hour until labor begins. If the contractions become too strong, the tablets may be removed or swallowed; they are destroyed in the gastrointestinal tract.

Other Uses of Oxytocin. Although not ordinarily injected during the first and second stages of labor, oxytocin may be used to stimulate labor that has stopped (uterine inertia) or labor that is proceeding so slowly that the mother is close to exhaustion.

This drug is occasionally used to expel a fetus that has died. Because the uterus is not very responsive to stimulation by oxytocin in the early months of pregnancy, a much larger dose must be used. This dosage can sometimes lead to water intoxication from the antidiuretic action of the drug, which is similar to that of the other posterior pituitary hormone, vasopressin (ADH).

Oxytocin is sometimes administered late in the second stage or during the third stage of labor to cause contraction of uterine muscle fibers and thus check postpartum bleeding. In such cases it is administered intramuscularly in a dose of three to ten units.

Oxytocin may also be used during the postpartum period to assist with lactation. Although this hormone is not responsible for the process by which the mammary glands make milk, it does make it easier for the baby to obtain the milk. When the mother uses a nasal spray of oxytocin, the alveoli of the breasts contract and force the milk into the larger ducts, where the baby can draw it more easily.

Cautions and Contraindications for Oxytocin

Oxytocin is contraindicated when there is cephalopelvic disproportion that would prevent a normal vaginal delivery. Abnormal position and abnormal presentation of the fetus are also contraindications. The cervix should be at least three cm. dilated and partially effaced, and the uterus should not be overdistended when oxytocin is to be used, to avoid injury to the mother and the fetus. Predisposition to uterine rupture also contraindicates use of oxytocin. Examples of this predisposition would be a primiparous patient over 35 years old; a multiparous patient (parity of four and over); previous cesarean section or other surgery of the cervix or the fundus of the uterus; a history of difficult delivery with trauma or sepsis of the uterus; and a previous hypertonic pattern of labor. Oxytocin should not be used when there is a predisposition to amniotic fluid embolism, as in the case of abruptio placentae or a dead fetus. Severe toxemia, fetal distress, and lack of adequate professional personnel for constant observation while the patient is receiving the drug are also considered contraindications for use of oxytocin.

Uses of the Ergot Alkaloids

Ergonovine maleate (Ergotrate) or methylergonovine maleate (Methergine) is usually administered intramuscularly in a dose of 0.2mg., during the third stage of labor or after spontaneous partial abortion. The drug acts in two to five minutes after administration, causing the uterus to contract and thus preventing excessive blood loss in the period of atony that ordinarily follows delivery of the placenta. Preferably, ergonovine is not given until after delivery of the placenta, although some physicians request that it be given after the delivery of the anterior shoulder. If ergonovine is given before delivery of the placenta and then the placenta does not spontaneously separate, the drug's action on the uterine muscle will cause the placenta to be trapped in the uterus. Manual removal will then be required. Too late an injection of ergonovine, on the other hand, can result in excessive maternal blood loss.

Ergot alkaloids are sometimes given during the puerperium to help hasten the involution of the uterus. The more rapid return of normal uterine tone is thought to lessen the likelihood of infection. Oral tablets are usually given three or four times a day during the first week postpartum. A mother who is breast feeding may receive a smaller dose of postpartum oxytocic drugs or may not receive any at all, because of the stimulation of natural oxytocin by the sucking infant.

Side Effects of the Ergot Alkaloids

Ergonovine maleate and methylergonovine maleate are relatively safe drugs when given in proper dosage, because their effects are largely limited to the myometrium of the uterus. Occasionally, they may have a stimulating effect on the blood vessels and cause a rise in blood pressure. The vasoconstriction can also lead to severe ischemia and even to gangrene in patients with obliterative type peripheral vascular disease.

Accidental ergotism is sometimes seen in women who take the drug for too long during the puerperium. Symptoms of ergotism include nausea, vomiting, abdominal cramping, headache, and confusion. Eventually, signs of circulatory impairment in the extremities appear, such as itching, tingling, numbness, and coldness.

During the early months of pregnancy, the uterus is not as responsive as the blood vessels to the effects of the ergot alkaloids. For this reason, overdose of these drugs, which may occur in an unskilled attempt to abort an unwanted baby, carries a great danger of gangrene.

PROSTAGLANDINS

The prostaglandins are a group of acidic lipids discovered forty years ago as being present in human semen. They have a stimulating effect on smooth muscle and a depressant effect on blood pressure. Only recently have they become the subject of much experimentation and medical literature. Prostaglandins are usually classified into general types (A, B, E, and F) according to their chemical structure. They have been found to influence the actions of the uterus, the fallopian tubes, the thyroid, and the nervous system, as well as affecting gastric secretions, fat metabolism, and blood pressure.

The pharmacological use of prostaglandins has not yet been fully established, but much of the experimentation with these factors (predominantly types E and F) has been in gynecology and obstetrics. Their uses in this field, discussed below, are still experimental.

The prostaglandins have been suggested for use in induction of labor, abortion, birth control, and treatment of infertility.

Use of Prostaglandins to Induce Labor

Intravenous infusion of prostaglandins to induce labor is useful, although the prostaglandins act much differently than oxytocin, the drug presently used for this purpose.

The onset of uterine activity is slower with prostaglandins than with oxytocin. It appears to be more difficult to provide an effective dose of prostaglandins without producing uterine hyperactivity from an excessive dose. Much more research is necessary before prostaglandins can be used routinely for this purpose, but initial studies suggest that they may be more useful than oxytocin for inducing preterm labor in such cases as diabetes and Rh incompatibility because of their cervical relaxation action.

Use in First Trimester Abortion

Because the prostaglandins have such side effects as nausea, vomiting, and diarrhea, and because of the low success rate, prostaglandins do not appear very useful for first trimester abortions; suction curettage remains the predominant method. However, since the prostaglandins cause dilation of the cervix, use of

these agents *before* suction curettage could theoretically decrease the need for forcible cervical dilation.

Use in Mid Trimester Abortion

At present, the majority of mid trimester abortions are performed with intrauterine instillation of saline. This type of abortion is about 85 percent effective, with about 48 hours elapsing between the saline instillation and the abortion.

Although intravenous infusion of prostaglandins has proved successful for mid trimester abortion, it is accompanied by the discomforting side effects of nausea, vomiting, and diarrhea. Intrauterine instillation of prostaglandins has also proved successful, *without* the discomforting side effects. This may become a useful alternative to saline-induced abortions, since the success rate is similar and abortion occurs in 20 to 36 hours. Presently there is a drug, dinoprost tromethamine (Prostin F2 alpha) available for intrauterine instillation.

Birth Control and the Treatment of Infertility

Hormones are presently the drugs of choice in these two areas; they are discussed fully in Chapter 27. It has been found that prostaglandins stimulate the pregnant uterus and make it sensitive to oxytocin as early as the first week of pregnancy. This suggests the possibility that vaginal administration of prostaglandins to a woman who has missed her menstrual period by 2 to 7 days might serve to induce menstruation.

It has also been found that in the nonpregnant female, the action of prostaglandins is to relax the uterus and constrict the portion of the fallopian tubes nearest the uterus, while relaxing the remaining portion of the tubes. This suggests that fertilization may be facilitated by retaining the ovum in the fallopian tubes. It is interesting to note that the husbands in some infertile couples have been found to have lower than average prostaglandin content in their semen. Prostaglandins, then, may be found useful in treating some types of infertility.

UTERINE RELAXANTS

Drugs capable of relaxing the smooth muscle of the uterus may be used to overcome premature labor and prevent threatened abortion, to relax tetanic contractions of the uterus during abnormal labor, or to reduce the severe uterine cramps of dysmenorrhea. The use of ovarian hormones in these situations is discussed in

Table 38-1. Drugs used in labor and delivery.

Generic Name	Trade Name	How Supplied	Routes	Usual Dose	Comments
methylergonovine maleate	Methergine	tablets 0.2 mg. ampuls 1 cc. 0.2 mg./cc.	P.O. I.V. I.M.	0.2 mg. P.O. t.i.d. or q.i.d. in puerperium for maximum 1 week. 0.2 mg. I.M. after delivery of placenta, after delivery of anterior shoulder, or during the puerperium.	Administration may be repeated at 2-4 hour intervals. Should not be administered I.V. routinely.
oxytocin	Pitocin	vial 10 cc. 10 U./cc. ampuls 1 cc. 10 U./cc. 0.5 cc. 5 U./0.5 cc.	I.V. I.M.	3-10 U. I.M. for postpartum bleeding. 10 U. added to 1000 cc. of 5% dextrose solution and infused I.V. at 10-14 gtt./ minute to induce labor.	Dosage determined by uterine response.
		nasal spray 40 U./cc.	intranasal	one spray 2-3 minutes prior to nursing.	
oxytocin citrate	Pitocin citrate	tablets 200 U.	buccal	200-3000 U.	

Chapter 27. The value of using two other nonsteroidal ovarian principles, lututrin (Lutrexin) and relaxin (Releasin), in these situations has not yet been established. The atropine type drugs (discussed in Chapter 16) have been used for treatment of dysmenorrhea, and a beta adrenergic stimulant, isoxsuprine hydrochloride (Vasodilan) has been used for dysmenorrhea as well as for relaxing uterine muscle in cases of premature labor.

REFERENCES

ARTHUR, H. R. "Active Management of Labor." *Nursing Times 69*:1654, December 1973.

BARR, WALLACE. "Prostaglandins." *Nursing Times 69*:1716, December 1973.

DiPALMA, JOSEPH R. "Prostaglandins, the Potential Wonder Drugs." *RN 35*:51, October 1972.

LAROS, RUSSELL K., Jr., et al. "Prostaglandins." *American Journal of Nursing 73*:1001, June 1973.

APPLICATION QUESTIONS

I. *True-False*

For each statement below, write **a** if the statement is true or **b** if it is false.

____ 1. Involution is the first normal menstrual period following delivery.

____ 2. Oxytocins are drugs that act on the smooth muscles of the uterus.

____ 3. The ergot alkaloids are not used before labor has begun.

____ 4. Oxytocin is responsible for the process by which the mammary glands make milk.

____ 5. Large doses of oxytocic drugs are needed in late pregnancy to produce the same effects that small doses produce in early pregnancy.

____ 6. Ergotamine is used when uterine inertia occurs.

____ 7. Patients receiving intravenous oxytocin should never be left unattended.

_____ 8. Large doses of oxytocin can cause excessive diuresis.

_____ 9. Oxytocins should not be used until the cervix is dilated at least 3 cm.

_____ 10. If ergotamine is given before delivery of the placenta, the placenta may be retained.

_____ 11. Breast-feeding mothers require higher doses of postpartum oxytocic drugs than nonbreast-feeding mothers.

II. *Multiple Choice*

For each of the following questions, indicate the letter providing the *best* answer.

_____ 1. If labor is being induced with buccal tablets of Pitocin, how can the strong contractions be relieved? (1) spit out the tablet (2) swallow the tablet (3) move the tablet under the tongue (4) neutralize the tablet with milk of magnesia (a) 1 (b) 1, 2 (c) 1, 2, 3 (d) 1, 2, 3, 4

_____ 2. When is the uterus least responsive to stimulation by oxytocin? (a) first trimester of pregnancy (b) second trimester of pregnancy (c) third trimester of pregnancy (d) during labor

_____ 3. Which of the following is an untoward symptom of large doses of oxytocin? (a) hypotension (b) liver failure (c) water intoxication (d) blurred vision

_____ 4. Which of the following best describes the function of oxytocin in the process of breast feeding? (a) it produces milk (b) it moves milk into large ducts (c) it dilutes milk by increasing vessel permeability (d) it stops milk flow when the baby is through nursing

_____ 5. How do ergot alkaloids prevent postpartum hemorrhage? (a) they act directly on the blood of the uterus, causing clotting (b) they act on the pituitary, causing a secondary contraction of the uterus (c) they stimulate systemic production of clotting factors in the blood (d) they act directly on smooth muscles of the uterus, causing them to clamp down on blood vessels

_____ 6. Which of the following oxytocic drugs is a natural glandular extract secreted by the pituitary gland? (a) ergonovine (b) oxytocin (c) lututrin (d) methylergonovine

_____ 7. Why is oxytocin safer than the ergot alkaloids for use in early labor? (a) it produces more forceful contractions (b) it is more rapidly inactivated (c) it does not cross the placental barrier (d) it is less likely to cause water intoxication

_____ 8. What are early signs of ergotism? (1) mental confusion (2) cold fingers and toes (3) vomiting (4) stiff neck (a) 1 (b) 3, 4 (c) 1, 2, 3 (d) 2, 3, 4

_____ 9. Possible adverse effects of all oxytocic drugs include which of the following? (1) tetanic uterine contractions (2) rupture of the uterus (3) damage to the baby's head (4) fetal anoxia (a) 2 (b) 1, 2, 4 (c) 1, 3, 4 (d) 1, 2, 3, 4

_____ 10. In which of the following patients would oxytocic drugs be contraindicated or used only with extreme caution? (1) a 20-year-old primipara in labor 12 hours with a fetus in transverse position (2) a 30-year-old gravida two in uterine inertia (3) a 37-year-old multiparous woman in hypertonic labor (4) a 35-year-old gravida two in early labor whose previous deliveries were done by cesarean section (a) 1, 2 (b) 2, 4 (c) 1, 3, 4 (d) 1, 2, 3, 4

39

Drugs Used in Cancer Chemotherapy

Cancer experts estimate that half the cases of cancer that develop each year could be cured by surgery or radiation if detected early. Cancer is best treated when it is still localized. After it has metastasized, surgery and radiation may not cure the condition. The major implication for nursing, then, is in the area of public education. Nurses should encourage people to have yearly physical examinations, including Papanicolaou smears for women. Women should be taught self breast examination; everyone should become aware of the major signs of cancer. Nurses should encourage those who discover a suspicious body change to seek medical attention immediately and not to delay because of fear.

USES AND TRENDS OF CANCER CHEMOTHERAPY

Anticancer drugs are used principally for treating advanced cases of disseminated cancer that can no longer be controlled by surgery or radiation, and for the treatment of leukemia, in which the cancer cells are spread throughout the body. Chemotherapy has played a part in "cures" in which patients with cancer have survived for longer periods than previously expected. For example, children with acute lymphocytic leukemia have survived for long periods following treatment with combinations of antileukemic drugs. Similarly, women with choriocarcinoma, a form of fetal membrane cancer, have now remained free of the disease for ten years or more after drug treatment. Chemotherapy has played a part in saving or prolonging the lives of patients with lymphatic tissue tumors, children with Wilms's tumor, men with

testicular tumors, and women with disseminated cancer of the breast and ovary.

Cancer chemotherapy is coming closer to its goal of destroying cancer cells without damaging normal body cells. For example, an enzyme called asparaginase (Elspar) is being used experimentally in the treatment of acute leukemia. This drug breaks down an amino acid called asparagine in body fluids. Leukemia cells require this substance for survival, whereas normal cells can make their own asparagine and are, therefore, unaffected by the drug. The early reports of remissions occurring with this drug, with relatively few toxic reactions, raise hopes that more chemicals will be found that take advantage of the differences between normal cells and cancer cells. Cancer cells are not ordinarily attacked by phagocytes and antibodies, as other foreign substances in the body are. However, recent evidence suggests that the immune systems do operate against some types of cancer. Immunotherapy is being used experimentally with some cases of inoperable malignant melanoma by inoculating the patient intradermally with tumor cells grown in tissue cultures, to produce antibodies against melanoma. Immunotherapy is another hopeful area on the horizon of cancer chemotherapy.

ANTICANCER DRUGS AVAILABLE TODAY

It is exciting to think about the possibilities of chemotherapy in the future. The reality of the anticancer drugs available today, however, is that their usefulness is limited by some serious drawbacks. The cytotoxic (cell poisoning) effects of anticancer drugs are unfortunately not limited to cancer cells. A major drawback of these agents, then, is the severe toxic reactions that occur from damage to normal tissues. The second major limitation of these drugs is that neoplastic cells develop new strains that are resistant to the anticancer drugs.

TOXICITY

Anticancer drugs interfere mainly with rapidly metabolizing tissues. This makes them useful for destroying cancer cells, of course, but they also destroy normal body tissues that metabolize rapidly, such as bone marrow, the epithelial lining of the gastrointestinal tract, and hair follicles.

Bone Marrow Depression

The two major dangers associated with bone marrow damage are the depression of white blood cells and the depression of platelets. Obviously, when a patient is taking an anticancer drug, frequent blood tests must be done.

If the white cell count is too low, the drug must be discontinued, because the patient will become very susceptible to infection. The patient and his family should be made aware of his decreased resistance, and people with any infection should postpone visiting him. The nurse caring for this patient should also consider his lowered resistance. The patient may be placed in reverse or protective isolation, but, even if he is not, the nurse may wish to cover her uniform with a clean gown before entering the room. Strict handwashing before coming in contact with the patient is also essential.

A reduction in platelets may lead to bleeding. The nurse must be observant for even small amounts of blood coming from any body orifice. She should also observe the patient for excessive bruising and for prolonged bleeding following an injection or a venipuncture. Patients taking anticancer drugs often receive transfusions of packed blood platelets.

Gastrointestinal Toxicity

Gastrointestinal side effects of anticancer drugs can be a great discomfort to the patient and may even make him request that the drug be discontinued. Antiemetics may be ordered to control the nausea and vomiting, and the patient should be encouraged and permitted to eat what he wants and when he wants. Ulcers in the mouth occur frequently, so a soft diet may be more tolerable. More dangerous gastrointestinal side effects include diarrhea, infection, and bleeding. Diarrhea can lead to dehydration and electrolyte imbalances; infection (especially if combined with a low white cell count) and bleeding (especially if combined with a decrease in platelets) can be very grave situations.

Baldness

Because of the damage to the hair follicles, patients taking anticancer drugs often lose some or all of their hair. Patients should be told of this possibility before treatment begins, since they may wish to purchase a wig to wear. Don't forget the selfconsciousness and self image of men as well as women. Many men do not appreciate being kidded about baldness, and they may be more comfortable with a wig as well.

In some cases, applying a head band during the administration of anticancer drugs may decrease hair loss by decreasing circulation to the scalp.

RESISTANCE

Administering combinations of several anticancer drugs simultaneously has been found to delay the emergence of drug-resistant cancer cell strains. Giving two drugs that act in different ways may kill a greater number of leukemic or lymphoma cells and thereby lengthen the remission of the disease. Stages III and IV of Hodgkin's disease are sometimes treated with a four-drug combination referred to as "MOPP" (mechlorethamine hydrochloride, vincristine sulfate [Oncovin], procarbazine, and prednisone).

CLASSIFICATION OF ANTICANCER DRUGS

There are six major classifications of anticancer drugs: (1) alkylating agents; (2) antimetabolites; (3) plant alkaloids and antibiotics; (4) steroid hormones; (5) radioactive isotopes; and (6) miscellaneous synthetic chemicals.

Alkylating Agents

These drugs interfere with the ability of cancer cells to reproduce and multiply, and thereby lead to their destruction. Mechlorethamine hydrochloride (Mustargen) was the first drug of this class used for treating cancer. This drug may be given intravenously or injected into body cavities to control fluid effusions, such as those resulting from local metastasis of breast and ovarian neoplasms. Care must be taken to avoid leaking this drug into subcutaneous tissues or splashing it on the skin or in the eyes. The local irritation occurring if the drug leaks into subcutaneous tissues can be counteracted by applying ice-cold compresses to the area or infiltrating the area with a sodium thiosulfate solution.

Cyclophosphamide (Cytoxan) can be given orally as well as parenterally, as it does not cause local tissue damage. It is converted to toxic metabolites in the liver and can cause severe bladder irritation when excreted in the urine. It is important to force fluids for a patient taking this drug, to keep him well hydrated to dilute the metabolites. If hematuria or painful urination occurs, the drug must be discontinued.

Mechlorethamine hydrochloride (Mustargen) and cyclophosphamide (Cytoxan) may be used in the treatment of lymphocytic cancers such as Hodgkin's disease. Mechlorethamine is very rapid acting and is also rapidly detoxified. Cyclophosphamide has a slower onset of action, but has a more prolonged effect.

Other drugs in this class include busulfan (Myleran), chlorambucil (Leukeran), and melphalan (Alkeran). Busulfan is used for treating chronic granulocytic leukemia. Chlorambucil is used for treating Hodgkin's disease, chronic lymphocytic leukemia, and choriocarcinoma. Melphalan is used for treating multiple myeloma and testicular and ovarian cancer.

Antimetabolites

These drugs have chemical structures resembling dietary substances needed by the cancer cells. They interfere with the biosynthesis of the cells' nucleic acids, including DNA and RNA, and thereby lead to the destruction of the cells.

Methotrexate was one of the first antimetabolites used in the treatment of leukemia. It interferes with the cell's utilization of folic acid. It is particularly effective when combined with other anticancer drugs for the treatment of acute lymphoblastic leukemia, the advanced stages of malignant lymphomas, and choriocarcinoma. This drug has also been used in the treatment of the nonmalignant skin disease psoriasis, because of its ability to slow the growth of rapidly reproducing skin cells. There is an antidote for this drug called folinic acid (Calcium Leucovorin), which can be used to counteract the drug's toxicity.

Mercaptopurine (Purinethol) is used mainly for providing prolonged periods of remission for children with acute leukemia. This drug, like some other anticancer drugs, increases the production of uric acid. The antigout drug allopurinol may be given to prevent uric acid crystals from causing kidney damage. However, allopurinol blocks the enzyme responsible for detoxifying mercaptopurine and can cause the drug to accumulate to toxic levels. It is important, therefore, to reduce the dosage of the anticancer drug if these drugs are given in combination.

Fluorouracil (5FU) has a narrow margin of safety and requires that patients be observed during administration. This drug, as well as floxuridine (FUDR), may be less toxic if injected directly into the arteries carrying blood to the affected area rather than by intravenous infusion.

Cytarabine (Cytosar), the most recent antimetabolite, is effective for advanced leukemia, especially if combined with thioguanine (6TG). Cytosar is best given by *rapid* intravenous infusion rather than by slow infusion. When signs of remission appear from this drug, treatment may be continued with subcutaneous injections.

Plant Alkaloids and Antibiotics

Vincristine sulfate (Oncovin) and vinblastine sulfate (Velban) are plant alkaloids useful for treating Hodgkin's disease; they are most often given in combination with other anticancer drugs. Toxic effects of these drugs are similar to those of other anticancer drugs, but Oncovin is less toxic to bone marrow. Both drugs can cause nervous tissue toxicity leading to severe psychomotor disturbances, including convulsions, mental depression, and psychotic reactions. Oncovin should be discontinued if the patient begins complaining of numbness and tingling in the fingers and toes.

The antibiotics used as anticancer drugs are too toxic for use against infection. Dactinomycin (Cosmegen) is useful for treating cancer in young children, including Wilms's tumor. Cosmegen, in combination with another antibiotic, mithramycin (Mithracin) is useful for treating metastatic testicular cancer.

Hormones

Corticosteroid hormones are useful for symptomatic relief of several kinds of cancer. They may also be used for reducing the high blood levels of calcium which can occur when breast cancer has spread to the bone.

Male or female sex hormones are useful for treating cancers dependent on the opposite hormone. Estrogen, for example, is used for treating metastatic cancer of the prostate, and androgens are used for treating metastatic cancer of the breast. The changes in secondary sex characteristics that can occur when these drugs are employed may be very upsetting to the patient, however.

Radioactive Isotopes

Radioactive isotopes such as sodium phosphate (P^{32}) and radiogold (Au^{198}) may be used in the treat-

Table 39–1. Drugs used in cancer chemotherapy.

Generic Name	Trade Name	How Supplied	Routes	Usual Dose	Comments
vincristine sulfate	Oncovin	ampuls 1 mg., 5 mg.	I.V.	adults: 1.4 mg./M.^{2} of body surface, administered at weekly intervals; children: 2 mg./M^2 of body surface, administered at weekly intervals.	Use extreme caution in administering the dose, since overdose may have a very serious or fatal outcome.
dactinomycin	Cosmegen	vials of powder 0.5 mg. supplied with mannitol	I.V.	dosage varies. adult: 0.01 mg./kg. body weight q.d. x5; children: 15 µg/kg. body weight q.d. x 5	Side effects are frequent and not dose dependent.
methotrexate	Methotrexate (formerly A-methopterin)	tablets 2.5 mg. vials 2 cc. 2.5 mg./cc., 25 mg./cc.	P.O. I.V. I.M. I.A. intrathecal	10–30 mg. q.d. x 5	Dosage may be repeated 3 to 5 times.
cytarabine	Cytosar	multiple dose vials 100 mg., 500 mg.	I.V. S.C.	initial: I.V. 2 mg./kg. q.d.x10 infusion: 0.5 mg.–1.0 mg./ k.g. q.d. maintenance: S.C. 1 mg./kg. weekly or semi-weekly	Obtain daily blood counts and monitor peripheral blood pressure daily. Increase dose as tolerated until therapeutic response achieved.
cyclophosphamide	Cytoxan	tablets 25 mg., 50 mg. vials: 100 mg., 200 mg., 500 mg.	P.O. I.M. I.V. intraperi-toneal and intrapleural	maintenance: 1–5 mg./kg. P.O. q.d.; 10–15 mg./kg. I.V. q. 7–10 days; 3–5 mg./kg. I.V. twice weekly	When mixing, allow solution to stand until clear before aspirating into a syringe.
mechlorethamine hydrochloride	Mustargen	20 cc. vials containing 10 mg. in dry form to be diluted with sodium chloride	I.V. (rapid) intracavity	200–600 microgram/ kg. per course of treatment	Dosage may be given all at once or spread out over several days. Avoid contaminating the eyes when handling the concentrated solution.

ment of chronic leukemia and polycythemia vera. The isotopes have more toxicity, especially to bone marrow, than other anticancer drugs; therefore, they are usually not the preferred choice for treatment.

Miscellaneous Synthetic Drugs

These are drugs that do not fall into any of the above classes, including procarbazine hydrochloride (Matulane), used for advanced Hodgkin's disease; and hydroxyurea (Hydrea), which is useful for treating melanoma and myelocytic leukemia. The mechanism of action of these two drugs is uncertain. Asparaginase (Elspar), the enzyme discussed at the beginning of this chapter, is also considered to be in this classification.

REFERENCES

HERBST, SUZANNE. "A New Approach to Parenteral Drug Administration." *American Journal of Nursing* 75:1345, August 1975.

HESS, CYNTHIA M. "Intra-Arterial Chemotherapy: Making It Safer and More Successful." *Nursing 74* 4:30 May 1974.

LIVINGSTON, B. M., and KRAKOFF, H. "L-Asparaginase." *American Journal of Nursing* 70:1910, September 1970.

LESSOF, M. H. "Immunosuppressive Drugs." *Nursing Times* 69:1648, December 1973.

McMULLEN, KATHLEEN. "When the Patient is on Bleomycin Therapy." *American Journal of Nursing* 75:964, June 1975.

RODMAN, MORTON J. "Anti-cancer Chemotherapy, Part 1: The Kinds of Drugs And What They Do." *RN* 35:45, February 1972.

RODMAN, MORTON J. "Anti-cancer Chemotherapy, Part 2: Against Solid Malignant Tumors." *RN* 35:61, March 1972.

RODMAN, MORTON J. "Anti-cancer Chemotherapy, Part 3: Against Leukemias and Lymphomas." *RN* 35:49, April 1972.

SCHUMANN, D., and PATTERSON, P. "The Adult with Acute Leukemia." *Nursing Clinics of North America* 7:743, December 1972.

TEITELBAUM, ANN C. "Intra-Arterial Drug Therapy." *American Journal of Nursing* 72:1634, September 1972.

APPLICATION QUESTIONS

I. *True-False*

For each statement below, write **a** if the statement is true or **b** if it is false.

_____ 1. Anticancer drugs are best used to counteract suspected malignancies before other therapy is begun.

_____ 2. Resistance may develop to anticancer drugs.

_____ 3. Mechlorethamine hydrochloride (Mustargen) may be taken orally.

_____ 4. Immunotherapy has been proven to be of no use in the treatment of cancer.

_____ 5. Cancer chemotherapy is aimed mainly at providing symptomatic relief, rather than at destroying cancer cells.

_____ 6. Cytarabine (Cytosar) is highly toxic and destructive to subcutaneous tissue.

_____ 7. The antibiotic anticancer drugs can be useful for treating very severe infections.

_____ 8. Corticosteroid hormones are sometimes used to increase blood calcium levels.

_____ 9. Female sex hormones are used for treating cancers dependent on male sex hormones.

_____ 10. Radioactive isotopes cause less toxicity than other anticancer agents.

_____ 11. Excessive bruising could indicate a decreased white blood cell count.

_____ 12. Gastrointestinal toxicity occurs only with orally administered anticancer drugs.

_____ 13. Administering several anticancer drugs simultaneously will delay the emergence of drug-resistant strains.

_____ 14. Cytarabine (Cytosar) is best administered by rapid intravenous injection.

II. *Multiple Choice*

For each of the following questions, indicate the letter providing the *best* answer.

_____ 1. Methotrexate may be used for treating which of the following conditions? (1) acute lymphoblastic leukemia (2) malignant lymphomas (3) choriocarcinoma (4) psoriasis
(a) 1, 2 (b) 1, 2, 3 (c) 3 (d) 1, 2, 3, 4

_____ 2. What is the major advantage of the experimental drug asparaginase (Elspar)? (a) it can be given orally once a day (b) it has a prolonged action that permits administration of medication only once a month (c) it interferes with cancer cells without interfering with normal cells (d) it is very inexpensive

_____ 3. Which of the following is an antidote for methotrexate? (a) thyroid extract (b) ascorbic acid (c) folinic acid (d) corticosteroids

3. Following administration of metyrapone (Metopirone), which of the following substances should be released in large quantities? (a) corticosteroid (b) epinephrine (c) ACTH (d) thyroxine

4. Before a patient is given sodium dehydrocholate (Decholin sodium) to determine circulation time, he should be told to be sure to indicate when he experiences which of the following? (a) bitter taste (b) warmth in his legs (c) feeling the need to void (d) nausea

5. Administration of ACTH stimulates the excretion of which of the following? (a) corticotropin (b) corticosteroids (c) epinephrine (d) vasopressin

6. When indocyanine green (Cardio-Green) is administered to determine cardiac output, which of the following specimens is needed for analysis? (a) urine (b) venous blood (c) arterial blood (d) capillary blood

7. Which of the following drugs would cause a decrease in blood pressure when used for the diagnosis of pheochromocytoma? (a) histamine (b) phentolamine mesylate (Regitine) (c) ACTH (d) atropine

8. Which of the following drugs could be used to determine whether gastric acid is being secreted in the stomach? (1) betazole hydrochloride (Histolog) (2) barium sulfate (3) iodine (4) histamine phosphate
(a) 2 (b) 4 (c) 1, 4 (d) 1, 3, 4

9. An overdose of histamine is marked by which of the following symptoms? (1) headache (2) shortness of breath (3) sleepiness (4) dryness of mucous membranes
(a) 1, 2 (b) 2, 3 (c) 3, 4 (d) 1, 2, 3, 4

10. What is the most common untoward side effect of injected phenolsulfonphthalein? (a) hypertension (b) allergic responses (c) hepatic failure (d) alopecia

11. Fluorescein may be used in diagnostic tests of which of the following organs? (1) gall bladder (2) eye (3) heart (4) pancreas
(a) 1, 3 (b) 1, 4 (c) 1, 2, 3 (d) 2, 3, 4

12. How might radiopaque media be administered? (1) orally (2) instilled into an organ (3) injected intravenously (4) injected intra-arterially
(a) 1 (b) 1, 2 (c) 1, 2, 3 (d) 1, 2, 3, 4

13. The common side effects of betazole hydrochloride (Histalog) are which of the following? (a) dry, hot skin; racing pulse; pinpoint pupils (b) cold, clammy skin; vertigo; anorexia (c) excessive hunger, thirst, and urination (d) sweating, flushed face, warmth

14. Which of the following specimen needed after azuresin (Diagnex Blue) diagnostic test for the flow of gastric urine (b) saliva (c) gastric contents (d) b

III. *Matching A*

Match each drug with the organ it evaluates.

1. radioactive sodium iodide

2. betazole hydrochloride (Histalog)

3. metyrapone

4. phentolamine mesylate (Regitine)

(a) pituitary gland

(b) stomach

(c) adrenal gland

(d) thyroid

IV. *Matching B*

Match each dye with the diagnostic test for which it is used.

1. phenolsulfonphthalein

2. sodium sulfobromophthalein (Bromsulphalein, BSP)

3. azuresin (Diagnex Blue)

4. Evans Blue

5. sodium dehydrocholate (Decholin Sodium)

(a) circulation time

(b) plasma volume

(c) kidney function

(d) liver function

(e) gastric acid secretion

V. *Discussion*

For each situation described below, write **a** if action by the nurse is required, or **b** if it is not. If action is required, describe what you would do.

1. You are helping a patient onto a stretcher to go to X-ray for a carotid angiogram. The patient says, "I sure hope they don't paint my skin with anything, because I'm allergic to iodine."

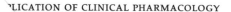

237

s would be
s given as a
acid? (a)
ood

s

possible to get some
ow, because she
ince she "swal-
ries two days

_____ 3. A patient is scheduled for a gastric analysis; and as you are collecting the histamine and naso-gastric tube for the doctor's use, the patient's daughter says to you: "Do you think Mom will be okay? You know she has asthma, but she won't tell anybody, and I'm just worried that her nervousness about this test might cause her to have an attack."

V. *Patient Situation*

1. b   2. a

CHAPTER 30

I. *True-False*

1. a	2. b	3. b
4. a	5. a	6. b
7. a	8. a	9. a
10. a		

II. *Multiple Choice*

1. d	2. c	3. c
4. b	5. b	6. a
7. c	8. a	

III. *Matching A*

1. b	2. c	3. a
4. b		

IV. *Matching B*

1. b	2. a	3. a
4. c		

CHAPTER 31

I. *True-False*

1. b	2. b	3. b
4. a	5. a	

II. *Multiple Choice*

1. a	2. c	3. b
4. d	5. c	

III. *Matching A*

1. a	2. b	3. c

IV. *Matching B*

1. d	2. a	3. c
4. b		

V. *Discussion*

1. a	2. b	3. a

CHAPTER 32

I. *True-False*

1. a	2. a	3. b
4. a	5. b	6. b
7. a	8. b	9. a
10. b	11. b	12. b

II. *Multiple Choice*

1. b	2. a	3.
4. a	5. a	6.
7. a	8. a	9. c

III. *Discussion*

1. b	2. a	3. a
4. a	5. a	6. a
7. a	8. a	9. b

V. *Calculation*

1. .4 cc.

CHAPTER 33

I. *True-False*

1. b	2. b	3. a
4. a	5. b	6. b
7. b	8. b	9. a
10. b	11. a	12. b
13. a	14. b	15. a
16. b	17. b	18. b
19. a	20. b	

II. *Multiple Choice*

1. c	2. c	3. a
4. c	5. b	6. a
7. a	8. c	9. c
10. b	11. b	12. c
13. a		

III. *Discussion*

1. a	2. b

CHAPTER 34

I. *True-False*

1. a	2. a	3. a
4. a	5. b	6. b
7. b	8. b	

II. *Multiple Choice*

1. a	2. c	3. d
4. b	5. a	

III. *Matching A*

1. b	2. a	3. b
4. b	5. a	

IV. *Matching B*

1. a	2. d	3. a
4. c	5. b	

3. c

CHAPTER 37

I. True-False

1.	b	2.	b	3.	a
4.	b	5.	b	6.	a
7.	a	8.	b		

II. Multiple Choice

1.	b	2.	d	3.	a
4.	b	5.	a	6.	b
7.	a	8.	d	9.	a
10.	d	11.	d		

III. Discussion

1.	b	2.	a	3.	a
4.	a				

3. b
6. a
9. a
12. a

a

1. b

e

2.	b	3.	b
5.	a	6.	b
8.	b	9.	a
11.	d	12.	a
13. b	14. a	15.	c
16. c	17. b	18.	c
19. c	20. c	21.	c

b

III. Discussion

1.	a	2.	a	3.	a
4.	a				

IV. Calculation

1.(a) 1200 mg.   (b) 300 mg.   (c) 12 cc.
2. 2.5 cc.

CHAPTER 38

I. True-False

1.	b	2.	a	3.	a
4.	b	5.	b	6.	b
7.	a	8.	b	9.	a
10.	a	11.	b		

II. Multiple Choice

1.	b	2.	a	3.	c
4.	b	5.	d	6.	b
7.	b	8.	c	9.	d
10.	c				

CHAPTER 36

I. True-False

1.	a	2.	a	3.	a
4.	a	5.	a	6.	b
7.	b	8.	a	9.	b
10.	b	11.	b	12.	a
13.	b	14.	a	15.	a
16.	b	17.	b	18.	b
19.	a	20.	b	21.	b
22.	b	23.	a		

II. Multiple Choice

1.	c	2.	a	3.	b
4.	c	5.	b	6.	a
7.	b	8.	a	9.	d
10.	b	11.	d	12.	b
13.	c	14.	b	15.	b
16.	c	17.	d	18.	b

III. Discussion

1.	a	2.	a	3.	a
4.	a	5.	a	6.	a

CHAPTER 39

I. True-False

1.	b	2.	a	3.	b
4.	b	5.	b	6.	b
7.	b	8.	b	9.	a
10.	b	11.	b	12.	b
13.	a	14.	a		

II. Multiple Choice

1.	d	2.	c	3.	c
4.	d	5.	b	6.	c
7.	a	8.	a	9.	b
10.	d				

III. Matching

1.	d	2.	c	3.	a
4.	b				

IV. Discussion

1.	a	2.	a	3.	a
4.	b	5.	a	6.	b

CHAPTER 40

I. *True False*

1. a   2. b   3. b

II. *Multiple Choice*

1. b	2. a	3. c
4. a	5. b	6. c
7. b	8. c	9. a
10. b	11. c	12. d
13. d	14. a	

III. *Matching A*

1. d   2. b   3. a
4. c

IV. *Matching B*

1. c   2. d   3. e
4. b   5. a

V. *Discussion*

1. a   2. a   3. a

Index

References to tabular material are given in *italics*

Abortion, 152, 225
Absorbable gelatin, 133
Acetaminophen, 65-66, *68*
Acetazolamide sodium, *8*, 112, *113*
Acetohexamide, 163
Acetylcysteine, *194*
Acetylsalicylic acid, *10*, *11*
   administration and dosage, *68*
   in arthritis, 175
   for pain, 65, 66
Achromycin, *201*
Acidifying salts, 114
Acidosis, 111-112, 164
Acidulin, 218
Acne, 187-188
Acne-dome, *190*
Acrisorcin, 190
ACTH, *see* Corticotropin
Activated charcoal, 17, 217
ADH, 144
Adrenalin, *see* Epinephrine
Adrenergic blocking agents, *see* Sympatholytics
Adrenergics, *see* Sympathomimetics
Adrenocorticosteroids, *see* Corticosteroids
Adrenocorticotropin, *see* Corticotropin
Akinetic seizures, 57
Akineton, *53*
Alcohol, *8*, *9*
   abuse
      organic effects, 26-27
      treatment, 25-26, 27, 43
   effects on body function, 25
   therapeutic uses, 27-28
Aldactazide, 112
Aldactone, *11*, 112, *113*
Aldomet, 116, *118*
Aldosterone, 169
Alevaire, *194*
Alkaloids
   ergot, 223, 224-225
   plant, 230
   rauwolfia, 37-38, 117
Alkalosis, 111
Alkeran, 230
Alkylating drugs, 229-230
Allergies, 180, 181
Allopurinol, *8*, *177*, 230

Alphaprodine hydrochloride, 64
Alpha receptors, 83-84
Aluminum acetate, 188
Aluminum hydroxide gel, 99
Aluminum nicotinate, 126
Aluminum salts, 217
Amantadine hydrochloride, *53*, 207
Amebiasis, 208-209
Amenorrhea, 152
Amethopterin, *10*, *231*
Amicar, *132*, 133
Aminocaproic acid, *132*, 133
Aminodur, *194*
Aminophylline, 193, *194*
Aminopyrine, 175
Aminosalicylic acid, *11*, 206-207, *210*
Amitriptyline hydrochloride, 38, *41*
Ammoniated mercury ointment, 188
Ammonium chloride, 114, *194*
Amobarbital, 31, *33*
Amodiaquin, 208
Amphetamines, *10*, 22, 43-44
Amphojel, 99
Amphotericin B, *8*, 190, 200
Ampicillin, 198, *201*
Amyl nitrite, 121
Amytal, 31, *33*
Anabolic agents, *12*, 150
Anabolin, 150
Analeptics, 25, 44-46
Analgesics, 21, 62-71, 137
   administration and dosage, 63-64, *67-68*
   in arthritis, 175-176
   pharmacological effects, 62-63
Androgen therapy, 148-150
Anectine, *9*, 73, *78*
Anemias, 139-141
Anesthetics, 31
   administration and dosage, 75-77
   classification and use, 72-74
Angina pectoris, 121-122
Anorexic drugs, 44
Antabuse, *8*, *9*, *12*, 27
Antacids, *11*, 99
Antepar, 209, *211*
Anthelmintics, 209
Anthralin, 188
Anthraquinone, 216
Antiamebics, 208-209

Antianemics, 139-141, *140*
Antianxiety drugs, 26, 31-35, 66
Antiarrhythmic drugs
    administration and dosage, *108*
    classification and use, 103, 107-109, 136
Antibiotics
    administration and dosage, *200-201*
    effects and use, 182, 194, 197-200
Anticholinergics, *see* Parasympatholytics
Anticholinesterases, 90, 91
Anticoagulants, *12*
    administration, 130
    uses, 129-131, *132*, 137
Anticonvulsants, 26, 56-57, *58*
Antidepressants, 38-39, *40-41*, 64
Antidiarrheals, 217, *219*
Antidiuretic hormone, 144
Antiemetics, 73, 217-219, *220*
Antihemophilic factors, *132*, 133
Antihistamines
    administration and dosage, *182*
    classification and use, 52, 180-183, 194, 218
Antihypertensives, 116-118
Anti-infectives, 10, 205-209, *210-211*
Anti-inflammatory drugs, *11*, 65, 175-178, *177*
Antilipemics, 126-128, *127*
Antilirium, 90, *92*
Antimalarials, 176, 208
Antimetabolites, 230
Antiparkinsonism drugs, 52-53
Antipyretics, 65, 175, 176
Antirheumatics, 175-176, *177*
Antithyroid drugs, 159
Antitussives, 62, 194
Antiviral drugs, 207-208
Anturane, 176
Anxiety, 31-32
A.P.C. tablets, 43
Apomorphine, 17, 27
Appetite
    stimulation, 150
    suppression, 44
Apresoline, 116, 118
Aqua Mephyton, 130, 132
Aquatag, 112, *113*
Aralen, 176, 208, 209, *211*
Aramine, *10*, 97, 136
Arfonad, 117
Aristocort, *see* Triamcinolone acetonide
Arlidin, *123*
Arrhythmias, 107-109, 136
Artane, 37, 52, *53*
Arthritis, 175-176
Ascariasis, 209
Ascorbic acid, 133
Asparaginase, 228, 232
Aspirin, *see* Acetylsalicylic acid
Asthma, 192-193
Atherosclerosis, 150-151
Atromid-S, *12*, 126, *127*
Atropine sulfate, 52, 73, 91, 96
    in arrhythmias, 103, 136
    as parasympatholytic, 97, *99*
Attapulgite, 217

Autacoids, 180
Autonomic nervous system
    classification and function, 82-84
    effects of drug administration, 84-85, 122-123
Azathioprine, *8*
Azo dye, 206
Azuresin, 235

Bacarate, 44, *45*
Bacitracin, 200
Baking soda, 17
BAL, 17
Baldness, 227
Banthine, *99*
Barbiturates, *12*
    administration and dosage, *33-34*
    uses, 26, 31-32, 73
Barium sulfate, 234, *236*
Benadryl, *53*, 181, *182*, 218
Benemid, *11*, 176, *177*
Benoxinate, 73
Benzalkonium chloride, 189, *190*
Benzathine penicillin G, 198, *200*
Benzedrine, 43
Benzocaine, 217
Benzophenone, 188
Benzthiazide, 112, *113*
Benztropine mesylate, 37, 52, *53*
Benzyl benzoate, 190
Bephenium hydroxynaphthoate, 209
Betaine hydrochloride, 218
Beta receptors, 83-84
Betazole hydrochloride, 234-235
Bethanechol chloride, 90, *92*
Bicarbonate, 27, 136
Bicillin, 198, *200*
Biguanides, 163
Bile salts, 218-219
Biliary disorders, 95-96
Biotransformation, 6
Biperiden, *53*
Birth control, 152-153, 225
Bisacodyl, 216, *219*
Bismuth salts, 217
Blood circulation, test for function, 235-236
Blood clotting, 129-133
Bone marrow depression, 229
Bonine, 218
Bradycardia, 103
Bromsulphalein, 235, *236*
Bronchodilators, 193
Bronchography, 234
BSP, 235, *236*
Burns, 188, 205
Busulfan, 230
Butabarbital, sodium, 31
Butazolidin, *see* Phenylbutazone
Butisol, 31
Butyrophenone derivatives, 37

Cadmium sulfide, 188
Caffeine, 43, *45*, 114
Caffeine sodium benzoate, 25

Calamine lotion, 187, 188
Calcium disodium edetate, 17
Calcium lactate, 146
Calcium phosphate, 99
Cancer, 228-232
    of breast, 149-150, 151
    of prostate, 151
Candicidin, 190
Cannabis derivatives, 22
Capreomycin, 207
Capsebon, 188
Carbachol, 90
Carbarsone, 208
Carbenicillin, 198
Carbon dioxide, 25
Carbonic anhydrase inhibitors, 112
Carboxymethylcellulose, sodium, 216
Cardiac disorders
    arrhythmias, 103, 107-109, 136
    coronary ischemia, 121-122
    myocardial infarction, 136-137
Cardiac function, test for, 235
Cardilate, 121
Cardio-Green, 235
Cardiotonic drugs, 103, *104*
Carisoprodol, 49, *50*
Cascara sagrada, 216
Castor oil, 216, *219*
Cathartics, 215-217
Caudal block, 74
CDC, 219
Cedilanid-D, 137
Central nervous system, effects of drug administration, 25, 96, 171-172
Central nervous system stimulants, 41-44, *43*
Cephalexin monohydrate, 199, *201*
Cephaloglycin dihydrate, 199
Cephaloridine, *8*, 199
Cephalothin, 199, *201*
Chelating agents, 17
Chemoprophylaxis, 206
Chenodeoxycholic acid, 219
Chloasma, 189
Chloral hydrate, 22, 26, 31, *33*
Chlorambucil, 230
Chloramphenicol, *12*, 200
Chlordiazepoxide hydrochloride
    administration and dosage, *34*
    effects and uses, 22, 26, 32, 135
Chlorguanide, 208
Chloroform, 72
Chloromycetin, *12*, 200
Chlorophenothane, 190
Chloroquine phosphate, 176, 208, 209, *211*
Chlorothiazide, 112
Chlorpheniramine maleate, 181, *182*
Chlorpromazine hydrochloride
    administration and dosage, 40
    effects and use, 26, 36, 37, 218
Chlorpropamide, 163
Chlorprothixene, 37
Chlorthalidone, *8*
Chlor-Trimeton, 181, *182*
Choleretics, 218-219

Cholesterol, 126-128
Cholestyramine, *12, 127*, 219
Cholinergic blocking agents, *see* Parasympatholytics
Cholinergics, *see* Parasympathomimetics
Cholinesterase inhibitors, 73
Choloxin, 127, 158
Chorionic gonadotropin, 148
Chrysotherapy, 176
Circulation of blood, test for function, 235-236
Citrated calcium carbimide, 27
Citrus juice, 17
Claysorb, 217
Climacteric, 149, 150
Clofazimine, 207
Clofibrate, *12*, 126, *127*
Clomid, 153, *154*
Clomiphene citrate, 153, *154*
Cloxacillin, 198
Coagulation, 129-133
Coal tar, 188
Coca Cola syrup, 218
Codeine, 62, 66, *67*
Cogentin, 52, *53*
Colace, 217, *219*
Colchicine, *177*, 178
Colds, 96, 181
Compazine, 36, 218
Comprehensive Drug Abuse Prevention and Control Act of 1970, 2-3
Conjugated estrogens, 150, *154*
Constipation, 63, 215-217
Contraceptives, 152-153
Convulsants, 46
Cordran, 188
Cortef, *172*
Cortef acetate, 170, *172*
Corticosteroids
    administration and dosage, 170-171, *172*
    adverse effects, 171-172
    as anti-inflammatory agents, 176, 207, 209
        dermatological uses, 186-187, 188
    classification, 169, 170
Corticotropin, 145
    mechanism, 169, 172-173
    uses, 178, 235
Cortisol, 169
Cortisone, 169
Cosmegen, 230, *231*
Cotazym, 218, *220*
Coumadin, 130, *132*, 137
Cretinism, 157
Cryptorchism, 149
Crystodigin, *104*
Crystoids, 209, *211*
Cuemid, *12, 127*, 219
Cyanocobalamin, *140*
Cyclandelate, 123-124
Cyclazocine, 21
Cyclizine, 218
Cyclogyl, 96, *99*
Cyclopentolate hydrochloride, *96, 99*
Cyclophosphamide, 229, *231*
Cyclopropane, 72, *76*
Cycloserine, 207

Cyclospasmol, 123-124
Cyproheptadine hydrochloride, 181
Cytarabine, 230, *231*
Cytomel, 158-159, *160*
Cytosar, 230, *231*
Cytoxan, 229, *231*

Dactinomycin, 230, *231*
Dalmane, 31
Dandruff, 188
Dapsone, 207
Darvon, 66
DBI, 163, *165*
DDT, 190
DEA, 3
Decadron, 170, *172*
Decholin sodium, *236*
Decongestants, 96, 181, *182*
Deferoxamine mesylate, 17, 139, *140*
Dehydroemetine, 208
Dehydrocholate, sodium, *236*
Delirium tremens, 26
Delivery (childbirth), 223-225
Demecarium bromide, 90
Demerol, *67*, 137
Depo-Testosterone cypionate, 149, *154*
Depressants, 21-22, 26, 32
Depression, 38-39, 44
Dermatological disorders, 186-190, 205-206
DES, 151-152
Desenex, 190
Desferal, 17, 139, *140*
Desipramine hydrochloride, 38
Deslanoside, 137
Desoxycorticosterone, 169
Dexamethasone sodium phosphate, 170, *172*
Dexedrine, 43, 44, *45*
Dextroamphetamine sulfate, 43, 44, *45*
Dextromethorphan, 62
Dextrothyroxine, sodium, 127, 158
Diabetes mellitus, 162-165
Diabinese, 163
Diagnex Blue, 235
Diagnostic tests, 152, 234-236
Diamox, *8*, 112, *113*
Diapid, 144
Diarrhea, 64, 217
Diazepam
    administration and dosage, *58*
    in alcoholic intoxication, 26
    in anxiety, 32, 64, 66, 73
    in status epilepticus, 57
    in tetanus, 49-50
Dibenzyline, 118-120
Dicloxacillin, sodium, 198
Dicyclomine hydrochloride, 99
Diethylpropion hydrochloride, 44
Diethylstilbestrol, 151-152
Digitalis, *8*, 103, *104*, 137
Digitoxin, *104*
Digoxin, *104*, 137
Dihydrotachysterol, *146*
Di-iodohydroxyquin, 208
Dilaudid, 62

Dilantin, *see* Diphenylhydantoin sodium
Dilation of pupil, 96
Dimenhydrinate, 218, *220*
Dimercaprol, 17
Dimethoxymethylamphetamine, 22
Dimethyl tubocurarine chloride, 73, *79*
Dioctyl sodium sulfosuccinate, 217, *219*
Diphenhydramine hydrochloride, 53, 181, *182*, 218
Diphenoxylate hydrochloride, 63
Diphenylhydantoin sodium, 9, *12*
    administration and dosage, *58*, 108
    in arrhythmias, 103, 107
    in seizures, 26, 56, 57
Diphylline, 193
Disodium carbenicillin, 198, 199
Disulfiram, *8*, *9*, *12*, 27
Diuretics
    administration and dosage, *113*
    classification and use, 26, 111-114, 116, 137
Diuril, 112
Dolophine, 21, 62
DOM, 22
Dopamine, 52
Doriden, 27
Double-blind study, 2
Doxapram hydrochloride, *45*
Doxepin hydrochloride, 38
Dramamine, 218, *220*
Droperidol, 37, 64
Drug Amendments of 1962, 2
Drug Enforcement Agency, 3
Drug abuse, 20-22
Drugs. *See also* classes of drugs and specific agents
    administration, 5-6, 7
        effects on nervous system, 25, 84-85, 96, 122-123, 171-172
    allergic reactions, 16, 198-199
    evaluation, 2
    excretion, 6
    idiosyncrasy, 16
    interactions, 6, *8-12*, 39
    legislation and standards, 2-3
    metabolism, 6, 171
    overdosage, 44, 64-65, 182
    poisoning, 16-17
"D.T.'s," 26
Dulcolax, 216, *219*
Durabolin, 150, *154*
Durham-Humphrey Amendment of 1951, 2
Dymelor, 163
Dynapen, 198
Dyrenium, *11*, 112
Dysentery, 208
Dysmenorrhea, 152
Dyspepsia, 218-219

Echothiophate iodide, *9*, 90, *92*
Eczema, 187
Edecrin, *8*, *9*, 112, *113*, 137
Edema, 103, 111, 112
Edrophonium chloride, 91, *92*
Efudex, 188
Elavil, 38, *41*
Eldoquin, 189, *190*

Eldoquin Forte, *190*
Elspar, 228, 232
Embolus, 130
Emetics, 17, 27
Emetine, 208, 209
Emetrol, 218
Emivan, 45-46
Emphysema, 45-46
Endocrine disorders, 144-146, 148-154
   adrenal cortex, 169-172
   pancreas, 162-165
   thyroid, 157-160
Enduron, 112
Enemas, 216, 234
Enterobiasis, 209
Ephedrine sulfate, *10*, 97, 193
Epilepsy, 56-58
Epinephrine, *9*
   administration and dosage, *99*
   uses, 74, 96, 97, 136
Epsom salts, 216
Equanil, 32, 49
Ergonovine maleate, 224
Ergot alkaloids, 224-225
Ergotamine tartrate, 66
Ergotism, 224
Ergotrate, 224
Erythrityl tetranitrate, 121
Erythrocytes, 139
Erythromycin, 199
Estrogens, 127, 150-152, 230
   administration and dosage, *154*
   gynecological uses, 152-153
Ethacrynate sodium, 137
Ethacrynic acid, *8, 9*, 112, *113*, 137
Ethambutol hydrochloride, 206, 207, *210*
Ethamivan, 45-46
Ethchlorvynol, 31
Ether, 72, *75*
Ethosuximide, 57, *58*
Ethyl alcohol, *see* Alcohol
Eunuchism, 148-149
Eunuchoidism, 148-149
Euthroid, 158, *160*
Eutonyl, 118
Evans Blue, 235, *236*
Expectorants, 194
Eyedrops, 90

FDA, 3
Fecal softeners, 216-217
Federal Food, Drug and Cosmetic Act of 1938, 2
Federal Trade Commission, 3
Fenfluramine, 44
Fentanyl, 64
Feosol, *140*
Ferrous sulfate, *140*
Fibrinolysin, 131
Fibrinolysis, 131
Field block, 74
Flagyl, 27, 209, *211*
Flaxedil, 73
Fleet enema, 216
Fluorescein, 235

Floxuridine, 230
Fluidextract of ipecac, 17
Fluorouracil, 188, 230
Fluothane, 72, *75*
Fluoxymesterone, 149
Flurandrenolide, 188
Flurazepam hydrochloride, 31
Flurothyl, 46
Folic acid, *140*, 141
Folinic acid, 230
Follicle stimulating hormone, 145, 148
Folvite, *140*, 141
Food and Drug Administration, 3
Formaldehyde, 187
FSH, 145, 147
5FU, 230
FUDR, 230
Fungal infections, 189-190, 200
Fungizone, *8*, 190, 200
Furosemide, *8*, 112, *113*, 137

Gallamine triethiodide, 73
Gamma benzene hexachloride, 190
Ganglionic blocking agents, 84, 117-118
Gantrisin, 205, *210*
Garamycin, 188, *202*
Gastric acid, 234-235
Gastrointestinal disorders, 27, 215-219, 229
   and parasympatholytics, 95-96, 97, 99
   and parasympathomimetics, 90
Gelusil, 99
Genitourinary disorders, 95-96
Gentamicin sulfate, 188, 200, *202*
Geocillin, 198
Geopen, 198, 199
Glaucoma, 90
Glucocorticoids, 169-170
Glutamic acid hydrochloride, 218
Glutethimide, 31
Goiter, 157
Goitrogens, 159
Gold salts, 176
Gonadotropic hormones, 145
   administration and dosage, *154*
   classification and use, 148-153
Gonadotropin, 148
Gout, 176-178
Grand mal seizures, 56
Griseofulvin, 190, 200
Guanethidine sulfate, *9*, 116, 117
Gynecological disorders, 149-150, 152-153
Gynergen, 66

Haldol, 37, *41*
Haldrone, 170
Hallucinogens, 22
Haloperidol, 37, *41*
Haloprogin, 190
Halotestin, 149
Halothane, 72, *75*
Hansen's disease, 207
Harrison Narcotic Act of 1914, 2
HCG, 148
Headache, *66-67*

Heart disease, *see* Cardiac disorders
Hematinics, 139-141, *140*
Hemofil, *132*, 133
Hemophilia, 133
Hemostatic agents, 131, 133
Heparin, 130, *132*, 137
Hexachlorophene, 189, *190*
Hexylresorcinol, 209, *211*
HGH, 145
Histalog, 234-235
Histamine, 180
Histamine phosphate, 234-235
Hodgkin's disease, 229, 230, 232
Homatropine hydrobromide, 96
Hookworm, 209
Hormones, *see* classes of hormones and specific agents
Humafac, *132*
Human growth hormone, 145
Hycodan, 62, 66
Hydralazine hydrochloride, 116, *118*
Hydrea, 232
Hydrochloric acid, 218
Hydrocodone, 62, 66
Hydrocortisone, 169-170, *172*, 187
Hydrocortisone acetate, 170, *172*
Hydrocortisone sodium succinate, 170
Hydromorphone, 62
Hydrophilic colloids, 216, *219*
Hydroquinone, 189, *190*
Hydroxyamphetamine hydrobromide, 97
Hydroxychloroquine, 176, 208
Hydroxyurea, 232
Hydroxyzine, 64
Hydroxyzine hydrochloride, 32, *34*
Hydroxyzine pamoate, *34*, 181
Hygroton, *8*
Hykinone, 133
Hyperglycemia, 164, *165*
Hyperkalemia, 111
Hyperkinesis, 44
Hyperlipidemia, 158
Hyperlipoproteinemia, 126-128
Hyperparathyroidism, 146
Hypertension, 116
Hyperthyroidism, 158-159
Hypocorticism, 169-170
Hypofibrinogenemia, 132
Hypoglycemia, 164, *165*
Hypoglycemics, 163-164
Hypogonadism, 151
Hypokalemia, 111
Hyponatremia, 112
Hypophysectomy, 145
Hyposensitization, 180-181
Hypotension, 95, 97
Hypothyroidism, 157
Hytakerol, 146

ICSH, 148
Idoxuridine, 207
Imferon, *140*
Imuran, *8*
Inapsine, 37, 64
Inderal, *11*, *108*, 109

Indigestion, 218-219
Indocin, 176, *177*, 178
Indomethacin, 176, *177*, 178
Infarction, myocardial, 136-137
Infertility, 153-154, 225
Inflammation, 170, 186-187
INH, *9*, 206, *210*
Innovar, 64, 72, 73
Insecticides, 90-91
Insomnia, 31
Insulin, 162-164, *165*
Insulin shock, 164
Interstitial cell stimulating hormone, 148
Intoxication, alcohol, 25-27, 43
Intrinsic factor, 141
Inversine, 117-118
Iodinated contrast media, 234
Iodine solutions, 159
Iodocyanine green, 235
Ipecac, 17, 194
Iron, 139, *140*
Irritants
    dermatological, 187
    intestinal, 216
Ischemia, 121-124
Ismelin, *9*, 116, 117
Isocarboxazid, 38
Isoflurophate, 90
Isoniazid, *9*, 206, *210*
Isopropamide, 181
Isoproterenol hydrochloride, 97, *98*, 103, 136
Isordil, 121
Isosorbide dinitrate, 121
Isoxsuprine hydrochloride, 123, 226
Isuprel, 97, *98*, 103, 136

Kafocin, 199
Kanamycin, 200
Kaolin, *9*, 217, *219*
Kaopectate, *9*, 217, *219*
Kefauver-Harris Act, 2, 3
Keflex, 199, *201*
Keflin, 199, *201*
Kenalog, 186, 187, *190*
Keratolytics, 187
Keratosis, 188
Ketamine hydrochloride, 72, *76*
Ketoacidosis, 164
Kidney, test for function, 235
Konakion, 133
Kynex, 205, *210*

Labor (childbirth), 223-226
Lactogenic hormone, 145
Lanoxin, *104*, 135
Larodopa, 52, *53*
Lasix, *8*, 112, *113*, 137
LATS, 158
Laxatives, 215-217
Leprosy, 207
Leucovorin, 230
Leukemia, 228, 230
Leukeran, 230
Levallorphan tartrate, 21, 64-65

Levarterenol bitartrate, *9*, *97*, *98*, 123, 136
Levodopa, *10*, 52, *53*
Levophed, *97*, *98*, 123, 136
Levoprome, 63, *67*
Levothyroxine, sodium, 158, *160*
LH, 145, 148
Librium, *see* Chlordiazepoxide hydrochloride
Lidocaine hydrochloride
    administration and dosage, 77, *108*
    uses, 103, 107, 136, 217
Lincomycin, 199
Liothyronine, sodium, 157, 159, *160*
Liotrix, 158, *160*
Lipids, 126-128, 225
Lithium salts, 39
Lithium carbonate, 39, *41*
Lithonate, 39, *41*
Liver
    effects of alcohol abuse, 26
    test for function, 235
Lixaminol, *194*
Lomotil, 63, *68*
Lorfan, 21, 64-65
Loridine, *8*, 199
"Low salt syndrome," 112
LSD, 22
LTH, 145
Lubricants (fecal), 216-217
Lugol's solution, 159
Luminal, 31, *33*, 56
Lung disease, 193-194
Luteinizing hormone, 145, 148
Luteotropin, 145
Lutrexin, 226
Lututrin, 226
Lypressin, 144

Maalox, 99
Mafenide acetate, 188, 205
Magnesium salts, 217
    hydroxide, 99
    sulfate, 216
Malaria, 208
Malathion, 91
Manic-depressive psychosis, 39
Mannitol, 26, 112, 114
MAO inhibitors, *10*, 38-39, 118
Marezine, 218
Marihuana, 22
Marplan, 38
Matulane, 232
MBD, 44
Mecamylamine hydrochloride, 117-118
Mechlorethamine hydrochloride, 229, 230, *231*
Mecholyl, 123
Meclizine hydrochloride, 218
Medroxyprogesterone acetate, *154*
Mefenamic acid, 176
Megaloblastic anemia, 140
Melanocyte-stimulating hormone, 145
Melasma, 189
Mellaril, 36, *40*
Meloxine, 189
Melphalan, 230

Menadione, 133
Menopause, 150
Menotropins, 153
Mental depression, 38-39, 44
Mental illness, 36-41
Meperidine hydrochloride, *67*, 137
Mephentermine sulfate, 97
Meprobamate, 32, 49
Mercaptomerin sodium, 113
Mercaptopurine, *8*, 230
Mercurials, 112
Mescaline, 22
Mesoridazine, 36
Mestinon, 91, *92*
Mestranol, 187
Metamucil, 216, *219*
Metandren, 149
Metaraminol bitartrate, *10*, 97, 136
Methacholine chloride, 123
Methadone hydrochloride, 21, 62
Methamphetamine hydrochloride, 43
Methantheline bromide, *99*
Methaqualone, 31
Methdilazine, 181
Methedrine, 43
Methenamine mandelate, *8*, 206
Methergine, 224, *226*
Methicillin, sodium, 198
Methimazole, 159, *160*
Methocarbamol, 49, 50
Methotrexate, *10*, 181, 230, *231*
Methotrimeprazine, 64, *67*
Methoxsalen, 189
Methoxyflurane, *11*
Methyclothiazide, 112
Methyl alcohol, 27
Methylandrostenediol dipropionate, 150
Methylcellulose, 216
Methyldopa, 116, 117, *118*
Methyldopate hydrochloride, *118*
Methylergonovine maleate, 224, *226*
Methylphenidate hydrochloride, 43, 44, *45*
Methylprednisolone sodium succinate, 170, *172*
Methyl salicylate, 65
Methyltestosterone, 149
Methyprylon, 31
Methysergide maleate, *67*, *68*
Metolazone, *8*
Metopirone, 235
Metrazol, 44, *45*, 46
Metronidazole, 27, 209, *211*
Metyrapone, 235
Mineralocorticoids, 169
Mineral oil, 216
Minimal brain dysfunction, 44
Miotics, 90
Mithracin, 230
Mithramycin, 230
Monoamine oxidase inhibitors, *10*, 38-39, 118
Monobenzone, 189
"MOPP," 229
"Morning after pill," 151-152
Morphine, *67*, 137
Morphine sulfate, 62, *67*

MSH, 145
Mucolytics, *194*
Mucomyst, *194*
Mucus, control, 193-194
Muscle relaxants, *11*, 49, *50*, 66
Musculoskeletal disorders, 49
Mustargen, 229, 230, *231*
Myambutol, 206, 207, *210*
Myasthenia gravis, 91
Mycostatin, 200, *202*
Mydriasis, 96
Mylanta, 219
Myleran, 230
Myocardial infarction, 136-137
Myoclonic seizures, 57
Mysoline, 56, 57, *58*
Myxedema, 157-158

Nafcillin, sodium, 198
Nalline, 21, 64
Nalorphine hydrochloride, 21, 64
Naloxone hydrochloride, 21, 63-64
Nandrolone phenpropionate, 150, *154*
Narcan, 21, 63-64
Narcolepsy, 43-44
Narcotic antagonists, 21, 64-65
Narcotics, 21, 62-65, *67*
Nardil, 38
National Formulary, 3
National Institutes of Health. Division of Biological
    Standards, 3
Nausea, 63, 217-218
Navane, 37
Nembutal, 31, *33*
Neomycin, 200
Neostigmine, 90, 91, *92*
Neo-Synephrine, *see* Phenylephrine hydrochloride
Neotep, 181, *182*
Neurolept analgesia, 64, 73
Neuroleptics, 64
Neurological disorders, 49
Neuromuscular blocking agents, 73
Neurospasmolytics, 49, *50*
N.F., 3
Nialamide, 38
Nicalex, 126
Nicotinic acid, 126
Nicotinyl alcohol, 123, 124
Nisentil, 64
Nitrates, 121-122, 137
Nitrites, 121-122
Nitro-Bid, *123*
Nitrofurantoin, 206
Nitroglycerin, 121-122, *123*
Nitrospan, *123*
Nitrous oxide, 72, 76
Noctec, 22, 26, 31, *33*
Noludar, 31
Nonsalicylates, 65-66
Nonsulfones, 207
Norethindrone, 152, *154*
Norflex, 49, *50*
Norinyl 28 Day, 152

Norlutin, 152, *154*
Norpramin, 38
Novocain, *77*, 217
Nydrazid, *210*
Nylidrin hydrochloride, *123*
Nystatin, 190, 200, *202*

Octyl nitrate, 121
Oleum ricini, *219*
Oligospermia, 149
Oncovin, 229, 231
Opiates, 21, 62-64, *68*
Opium camphorated tincture, 63, *68*
Orinase, 163, *165*
Ornade, 181
Orphenadrine citrate, 49, *50*
Ortho-Novum SQ, 152
Osmitrol, 26, 111, 114
Osmotics, 26, 111, 114
Osteoporosis, 150, 171
Oxacillin, sodium, 198
Oxethazaine, 217
Oxidized cellulose, 133
Oxtriphylline, 193
Oxybenzone, 188
Oxyphenbutazone, 175
Oxytetracycline, 208
Oxytocics, 223-224
Oxytocin, 144, 223, *226*

PABA, *10*, 188-189
Pain, 62-66
Pamisyl, 206-207, *210*
Pancrelipase, 218, *220*
Pancuronium bromide, 73
Panheprin, 130, *132*, 137
Papaverine hydrochloride, *123*, 124, 137
Para-aminobenzoic acid, *10*, 188-189
Para-aminosalicylic acid, *11*
Paral, 26, 31, *34*
Paraldehyde, 26, 31, *34*
Paramethasone acetate, 170
Parasitic infestations of skin, 190
Parasympathetic nervous system, 83, 84
Parasympatholytics, 84, 97, 99
    effects on body function, 95-96
    in parkinsonism, 52-53
    preoperative use, 73
Parasympathomimetics, 84
    administration and dosage, *92*
    effects and use, 89, 90-91
    as vasodilators, 123
Parathion, 90
Parathormone, 146
Paredrine, 96
Paregoric, 63, *68*
Pargyline hydrochloride, 118
Parkinsonism, 52-53
Parnate, 38, 41
PAS, *11*, 206-207, *210*
Pavabid, 124
Pavulon, 73
Pectin, *9*, 217, *219*

Penicillinase resistant drugs, 198
Penicillins
    administration and dosage, *200-201*
    classification and use, 182, 198
    side effects and alternatives, 198-199
Pentazocine, 64, 66, *67*
Penthrane, *11*
Pentobarbital, 22, 31, *33*
Pentothal, 31, 72, *76*
Pentylenetetrazol, 44, *45*, 46
Pepsin, 218
Peptic ulcers, 96, 97, 99, 171
Pergonal, 153
Periactin, 181
Perphenazine, 36, 37, *40*
Petit mal seizures, 57
Pharmacology, overview, 2
Phenacetin, *66*
Phenazopyridine hydrochloride, 206
Phendimetrazine tartrate, 44, *45*
Phenelzine sulfate, 38
Phenergan, 36, *39*, 135, 181
Phenformin hydrochloride, 163
Phenobarbital, 31, *33*
    in seizures, 56, 57, *58*
Phenolated calamine, 188
Phenolphthalein, 216, 235
Phenol red, 216, 235
Phenothiazines
    administration and dosage, *39-41*
    in alcoholic intoxication, 26
    in gastrointesinal disorders, 218
    as tranquilizers, 36-37, 73, *181*
Phenoxybenzamine hydrochloride, 118, 122
Phentolamine mesylate, 118, 123, 235
Phenylbutazone, *11*, 12
    administration and dosage, *177*
    uses, 66, 175, 178
Phenylephrine hydrochloride, *10*, 95, *98*
    as decongestant, 96, 181, *182*
Phenylpropanolamine hydrochloride, *10*, 181
Pheochromocytoma, 235
pHisoHex, *190*
Phospholine iodide, *9*, 90, 92
Phosphorylated carbohydrate solution, 218
Physostigmine salicylate, 90, *92*
Phytonadione, 130, 133
Picrotoxin, 44
Pigmentation disorders, 189
Pilocarpine hydrochloride, 90, *92*
Pima syrup, *194*
Pinworm, 209
Piperacetazine, 36
Piperazine, 36, 37, 209, *211*
Piperidyls, 36
Pitocin, 223, *226*
Pitressin, 144, *146*
Pituitary hormones, 144-146, 148-153, *154. See also*
    specific hormones
Pituitrin, 144
Placebos, 2
Placidyl, 31
Plantago seed, 216

Plant alkaloids, 230
Plasmin, 131
Plasminogen, 131
Polycarbophil, 217
Polycillin, *201*
Polymycin, 200
Polymyxin B, *11*
Pondimin, 44
Postencephalitic lethargy, 44
Postmenopause, 150
Potassium chloride, *11*
Potassium iodide, 159, *194*
Potassium penicillin G, 198, *200*
Potassium perchlorate, 159
Potassium phenoxymethyl penicillin, *200*
Pralidoxime chloride, 91
Prednisolone acetate, 170
Prednisone, 229
Premarin, 150, *154*
Premenstrual tension, 152
Primaquine, 208
Primidone, 56, 57, *58*
Priscoline, 122, *123*
Probenecid, *11*, 176, *177*
Procainamide hydrochloride, 107, *108*, 109, 135
Procaine hydrochloride, 77, 217
Procarbazine hydrochloride, 229, 232
Prochlorperazine maleate, 36, 218
Profibrinolysin, 131
Progesterone, 150, 152-153
Progestins, 152-153
Prolactin, 145
Promazine hydrochloride, 36
Promethazine hydrochloride, 36, *39*, 135, 181
Pronestyl, 107, *108*, 109, 136
Propacil, 159
Proparacaine, 73
Propoxyphene hydrochloride, 66
Propranolol hydrochloride, *11*, *108*, 109
Propylthiouracil, 159
Prostaglandins, 225
Prostaphlin, 198
Prostigmin, 90, 91, *92*
Protamine sulfate, 130
Protopam, 91
Protriptyline hydrochloride, 38
Provera, *154*
Pruritus, 127, 186-187
Pseudoparkinsonism, 37
Psoriasis, 188
Psychomotor seizures, 57
Psychomotor stimulants, 22, 43-44, *45*
Psychosis, 39
Psychotherapeutic drugs, 36-38, *39-41*
Psyllium hydrophilic mucilloid, 216, *219*
Pure Food and Drug Act of 1906, 2
Purinethol, 230
Purodigin, *104*
Pyrantel pamoate, *209*
Pyrazolon derivatives, *66*, 175
Pyribenzamine, 181
Pyridium, 206
Pyridostigmine bromide, 91, *92*

Pyrimethamine, 208
Pyrvinium pamoate, 209

Quaalude, 31
Questran, *12*, 127, 219
Quide, 36
Quinacrine, 208
Quinidex, 107, *108*, 136
Quinidine sulfate, *11*, 107, *108*, 136
Quinidine hydrochloride, *108*
Quinine, 208

Radioactive iodine, 159
Radioactive isotopes, 159, 230, 232
Radiogold, 230
Radiographic diagnosis, 234
Rauwolfia alkaloids, 37-38, 117
Red veterinary petrolatum, 188
Regitine, *118*, 123, 235
Relaxants
    muscle, *11*, 49, *50*, 66
    uterine, 225, 226
Relaxin, 226
Releasin, 226
Reserpine, 37-38, 117, *118*
Resorcinol, 187
Respiratory depression, 63
Respiratory disorders, 63, 96
Retin-A, 187
Rheumatoid disorders, 175-178
Rhinitis, 181
Rifadin, 206, 207, *210*
Rifampin, 206, 207, *210*
Riopan, 99
Ritalin, 43, 44, 45
Robaxin, 49, *50*
Romilar, 62
Roniacol, 123, 124
Roundworm, 209
Rubramin, *140*

Saddle block, 74
Salicylates, *10*, *11*
    administration and dosage, 68, *210*
    in acne, 187, *190*
    for pain, 65, 66, 175
    in tuberculosis, 206-207
Salicylic acid, 187, *190*
Saline solution, 225
Sansert, 67, *68*
Schizophrenia, 37
Scopolamine hydrobromide, 73, 97
Seborrhea, 188
Secobarbital, sodium, 31
Seconal, 31
Sedative-hypnotics
    administration and dosage, *33-34*
    classification and use, 22, 31-32, 66, 137
Seizures, 56-57
Selenium sulfide, 188, *190*
Selsun, 188, *190*
Serentil, 36
Serpasil, 37-38, 117, *118*

Sex hormones, *see* Gonadotropic hormones
Shock, *see* Hypotension
Silver nitrate, 187, 188
Simethicone, 219
Sinequan, 38
Skin disorders, 186-190, 205-206
Smallpox vaccination, *10*
Sodium bicarbonate, 27, 136
Sodium lactate, 27
Sodium phosphate, 216, 230
Sodium sulfate, 216
Solu-Cortef, 170
Solu-Medrol, 170, *172*
Soma, 49, *50*
Somatotropin, 145
Somophyllin, *194*
Sparine, 36
Spasms, 49
Spectinomycin, 200
Spironolactone, *11*, 112, *113*
SSKI, 159, *194*
Stanozolol, 150
Staphcillin, 198
Status epilepticus, 57
Stelazine, 36
Sterane, 170
Sterility, 149
Steroids, *see* Corticosteroids
Stevens-Johnson syndrome, 206
STH, 145
Stimulants, central nervous system, 22, 43-46
Stokes-Adams syndrome, 97
Stool softeners, 216-217
"STP," 22
Streptokinase, 131, *132*
Streptomycin sulfate, 206, 207, *210*
Strongyloides, 209
Sublimaze, 64
Succinylcholine chloride, *9*, 73, *78*
Succinylsulfathiazole, 205
Sulfamethoxypyridazine, 205, *210*
Sulfamylon, 188, 205
Sulfasuxidine, 205
Sulfinpyrazone, 176
Sulfisoxazole, 205, *210*
Sulfobromophthalein, sodium, 235, *236*
Sulfonamides, *10*
    classification and use, 112, 205-206, 208
Sulfones, 207
Sulfonylureas, 163
Sulfur, 187, *190*
Sulfurated lime solution, 187
Sulfurated potash, 187
Sulisobenzone, 188
Sunburn, 188-189
Surfak, 217
Symmetrel, *53*, 207
Sympathetic nervous system, 82, 83, 84
Sympatholytics
    administration and dosage, *92*
    classification, 90
    effects on body function, 84, 89
    in hypertension, 116-118, 122-123

Sympathomimetics
 administration and dosage, *98*
 in allergies, 180, 181, 193
 in cardiovascular disorders, 97, 123, 136
 in dysmenorrhea, 226
 effects on body function, 84, 95-96
Synkayvite, 133
Synthroid, 158, *160*
Syrup of ipecac, 17, 194

Tacaryl, 181
Tachyarrhythmias, 103
Talwin, 64, *66, 67*
Tandearil, 175
Tapazole, 159, *160*
Tapeworm, 209
Taractan, 37
Tegopen, 198
Temaril, 181, *182*
Temposil, 27
Tensilon, 90, *92*
Tenuate, 44
Teratogenicity, 16
Testosterone, 148-150, *154*
Tetanus, 49-50
Tetany, 146
Tetracyclines, *11*, 199, *201*, 208
6TG, 230
Thalidomide, 207
Theobromine, 114
Theophylline, 114, 193
Thiabendazole, 209
Thiazides, 112, 116
Thiethylperazine, *220*
Thiocarbamides, 159
Thioguanine, 230
Thiomerin, 113
Thiopental, 31, 72, *76*
Thioridazine hydrochloride, 36, *40*
Thiothixene, 37
Thioxanthene compounds, 37
Thorazine, *see* Chlorpromazine hydrochloride
Threadworm, 209
Thrombin, 131, 133
Thyroid hormones
 administration and dosage, *160*
 classification and use, 145, 157-159
Thyroid USP, *12, 160*
Thyrotoxicosis, 158-159
Thyrotropin, 145, 157
Thyroxine, 158
Thytropar, 145, 157
Tigan, 218, *220*
Titanium oxide, 188
Tolazamide, 163
Tolazoline hydrochloride, 122, *123*
Tolbutamide, 163, *165*
Tolinase, 163
Tolnaftate, 190
Torecan, *220*
Tranquilizers
 administration and dosage, *33-34, 39-41*
 in allergies, 181
 in anxiety, 26, 31-32, 65

Tranquilizers (*continued*)
 in gastrointestinal disorders, 218
 in mental illness, 36-38
Tranylcypromine, 38, *41*
Tretinoin, 187
Triamcinolone acetonide, 170, 182, 187, 188, *190*
Triameterene, *11*, 112
Trichinosis, 209
Trichloroacetic acid, 187
Trichloroethylene, 72
Trichuriasis, 209
Tricyclics, *9*, 38
Tridone, 57, *58*
Trifluoperazine hydrochloride, 36
Triflupromazine hydrochloride, 36
Triglycerides, 126-128
Trihexyphenidyl hydrochloride, 37, 52, *53*
Trilafon, 36, 37, *40*
Trimeprazine, 181, *182*
Trimethadione, 57, *58*
Trimethaphan camsylate, 117
Trimethobenzamide hydrochloride, 218, *220*
Trimethylene, 72, 76
Trioxsalen, 189, *190*
Tripelennamine, 181, 187
Trisoralen, 189, *190*
TSH, 145, 157
Tuberculosis, 206-207
Tylenol, 65-66, *68*
Tyloxapol, *194*
Tyrothricin, 200

Ulcers, peptic, 96, 97, 99, 170
Uncinariasis, 209
Unipen, 198
United States Pharmacopoeia, 3
Urea, 26, *113*, 114
Ureaphil, *113*
Urecholine, 90, *92*
Urevert, 114
Uricosuric drugs, 176-177
Urinary disorders, 90, 205-206
Urokinase, 131
Urotropin, *8*
Urticaria, 181
U.S.P., 3
Uterine bleeding, 152
Uterine relaxants, 225-226

Vaccines, *10*
Vaginitis, 151
Valium, *see* Diazepam
Varidase, 131, *132*
Vasal, *123*, 124, 137
Vascular disease, 121, 122-124, 150
Vasoconstrictors, 74
Vasodilan, 123, 226
Vasodilators
 administration and dosage, *123*
 classification and use, 121-124, 137
Vasopressin, 144, *146*
Vasopressors, 97
V-Cillin K, *200*
Velban, 230

Venereal disease, 198
Vesprin, 36
Vinblastine sulfate, 230
Vincristine sulfate, 229, 230, *231*
Vinegar, 17
Viomycin, 207
Viruses, 207-208
Vistaril, 32, 34, 181
Vitamins, *10*, 130, 133, *140*, 187
Vitiligo, 189
Vivactil, 38
Vleminckx's solution, 187
Volatile oils, 217
Volatile solvents, 22
Vomiting, 63, 217-218

Warfarin, sodium, *12*, 130, *132*, 137
Weight reduction, amphetamine-induced, 44

Winstrol, 150
Withdrawal
   from alcohol, 26
   from drugs, 21-22
Whipworm, 209
Worms, 209
Wyamine, 97

Xanthines, 114
Xylocaine, *see* Lidocaine hydrochloride

Zarotin, 57, *58*
Zaroxolyn, *8*
Zephiran, 189, *190*
Zinc oxide, 187, 188
Zinc sulfate, 187
Zincundecate, 190
Zyloprim, *8*, 177, 230